PROBLEM-BASED
Anatomy

PROBLEM-BASED
Anatomy

Craig A. Canby, Ph.D.

Associate Professor of Anatomy
Coordinator of University Accreditation
Des Moines University—Osteopathic Medical Center
Des Moines, Iowa

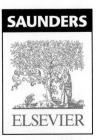

SAUNDERS

ELSEVIER

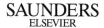

SAUNDERS
ELSEVIER

1600 John F. Kennedy Boulevard
Suite 1800
Philadelphia, PA 19103-2899

ISBN 13: 978-1-4160-2417-0
ISBN 10: 1-4160-2417-4

Problem-Based Anatomy

Library of Congress Cataloging-in-Publication Data

Canby, Craig A.
  Problem-based anatomy / Craig A. Canby
    p. ; cm.
  ISBN 1-4160-2417-4
  1. Human anatomy–Problem, exercises, etc. 2. Human anatomy–Case studies. 3. Physiology, Pathological–Problems, exercises, etc. 4. Physiology, Pathological–Case studies. I. Title.
  [DNLM: 1. Anatomy–Case Reports. 2. Anatomy–Problems and Exercises. QS 18.2 C214p 2006]
  QM32.C36 2006
  611'.0076–dc22

                                                                    2005042680

Acquisitions Editor: William Schmitt
Development Editor: Kevin Kochanski
Senior Project Manager: Mary Stermel
Marketing Manager: John Gore

Printed in China.

Last digit is the print number: 9 8 7 6 5 4 3 2 1

To my family for their blessings of love, support, and patience,

and to my students who have blessed my professional life.

PREFACE

Over the years, the curricula of health professions programs have evolved into a state of integration. From the first day of school, health professional students are immersed in a curriculum that exposes them to the basic sciences and the clinical sciences. This curricular shift has also impacted instruction in the discipline of anatomy. While anatomists remain passionate about the noble act of transferring the purity of anatomical knowledge onto future generations of students, they are also mindful that students in the health professions require a different fund of anatomical knowledge. These students must be able to apply their anatomical knowledge base to clinical situations. In response, anatomy educators are clearly emphasizing the clinical relevance of anatomy in their education of future generations of health professional students.

This text was written to further the clinical significance of anatomy. The text features 61 clinical cases divided into the traditional seven regions of the body: 1) back, 2) thorax, 3) abdomen, 4) pelvis and perineum, 5) lower limb, and 6) upper limb, and 7) head and neck. Each clinical case frames a set of study questions and accompanying answers. Another value-added attribute of this format is its integrated approach to the broad field of anatomy. Under the umbrella of anatomy are the subdisciplines of anatomic pathology, cell biology, embryology, gross anatomy, histology, neuroanatomy, and radiologic anatomy. The questions accompanying each clinical case are crafted, wherever possible, to include these anatomical subdisciplines. Additionally, 185 multiple choice questions are provided in Section VIII so that the student can assess his/her mastery of the material. Answers to the questions and references back to the text are also provided.

This text can be used by students as a clinically-oriented complement to standard anatomy-related texts in their courses. It should also be of educational utility for students preparing for national licensing examinations and to residents who are in the early years of their graduate medical training.

As with any intellectual pursuit, it is always proper to gratefully acknowledge the contributions that others have made to the outcome. To that end, I offer my profound gratitude to the authors of other textbooks who graciously granted permission to include their figures in this book. The textbooks are *Gray's Anatomy for Students* by Drake et al, *The Developing Human*, 7th edition by Moore and Persaud, *Sabiston Textbook of Surgery*, 17th edition by Townsend et al, *Robbins and Cotran Pathologic Basis of Disease*, 7th edition by Kumar et al, and *Color Textbook of Histology*, 2nd edition by Gartner and Hiatt. The student who desires a greater depth of knowledge in the topics covered in this book is encouraged to use these outstanding resources for additional information.

Anatomy is a wonderful, noble discipline filled with the awe and wonders of human form. It is a privilege and a blessing to be touched by the sanctity of its incredible beauty. I hope you are rewarded with the teachings of anatomy in your professional education and practice as I have been in my professional career. As learning colleagues of anatomy, please contact me directly with constructive criticisms about this text for incorporation into future editions.

CRAIG A. CANBY

ACKNOWLEDGMENTS

I am profoundly grateful to the many publication professionals who have played pivotal roles in shepherding this book through its preparation and production. Through their genuine diligence, creativity, and a keen eye to detail they have transformed a concept for a book and later a black and white manuscript into a vibrant and superbly edited publication. My special thanks go to William Schmitt for the opportunity to author this book and to Kevin Kochanski for his developmental acumen.

CONTENTS

Preface   vii

Acknowledgments   ix

SECTION I   BACK   1

CASE 1: Intervertebral disk herniation   3

CASE 2: Spina bifida   7

CASE 3: Spondylolisthesis   11

CASE 4: Vertebral compression fractures (osteoporosis)   13

SECTION II   THORAX   17

CASE 5: Achalasia   19

CASE 6: Atrial septal defect   23

CASE 7: Breast cancer   29

CASE 8: Cystic fibrosis (mucoviscidosis)   37

CASE 9: Emphysema   41

CASE 10: Lung hypoplasia   47

CASE 11: Mesothelioma   51

CASE 12: Myocardial infarction   55

CASE 13: Tetralogy of Fallot   67

SECTION III   ABDOMEN   69

CASE 14: Abdominal aortic aneurysm   71

CASE 15: Appendicitis   75

CASE 16: Cirrhosis   81

CASE 17: Congenital hypertrophic pyloric stenosis   87

CASE 18: Crohn's disease   89

CASE 19: Diabetes mellitus   93

CASE 20: Gallstones   97

CASE 21: Gastric esophageal reflux disease   101

CASE 22: Glomerulonephritis   105

CASE 23: Inguinal hernia   111

Case 24: Meckel's diverticulum   115

Case 25: Pancreatitis   119

Case 26: Peptic ulcer disease (gastric ulcer)   123

Case 27: Pheochromocytoma   129

SECTION IV   PELVIS AND PERINEUM   133

CASE 28: Bartholin cyst   135

CASE 29: Cryptorchidism   137

CASE 30: Hirschsprung's disease (congenital megacolon)   143

CASE 31: Leiomyoma (fibroids)   147

CASE 32: Ovarian tumor   153

CASE 33: Prostate cancer and prostatectomy   157

CASE 34: Testicular cancer   163

SECTION V   LOWER LIMB   167

CASE 35: Achilles tendon rupture   169

CASE 36: Dislocation of the hip   171

CASE 37: Duchenne's muscular dystrophy   177

CASE 38: Knee injury   181

CASE 39: Popliteal artery entrapment syndrome   189

CASE 40: Tibial fracture   193

SECTION VI   UPPER LIMB   197

CASE 41: Brachial plexus injury   199

CASE 42: Carpal tunnel syndrome   205

CASE 43: Dupuytren's contracture   209

CASE 44: Elbow dislocation   211

CASE **45:** Humeral shaft fracture   215

CASE **46:** Rotator cuff injury   219

CASE **47:** Shoulder dislocation   221

CASE **48:** Shoulder separation   225

CASE **49:** Ulnar nerve compression   227

SECTION **VII**   HEAD AND NECK   231

CASE **50:** Alzheimer's disease   233

CASE **51:** Basal cell carcinoma   237

CASE **52:** Bell's palsy   243

CASE **53:** Cleft palate   247

CASE **54:** Cushing's disease   251

CASE **55:** Glaucoma   257

CASE **56:** Grave's disease   263

CASE **57:** Parkinson's disease   267

CASE **58:** Primary hyperparathyroidism   271

CASE **59:** Torticollis   275

CASE **60:** Trigeminal neuralgia   277

CASE **61:** Watershed infarction   283

SECTION **VIII**   MULTIPLE CHOICE QUESTIONS AND ANSWERS   289

Bibliography   307

Index   309

SECTION I

Back

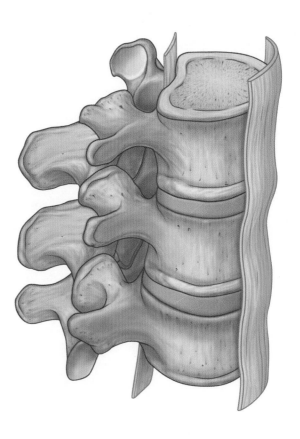

A 35-year-old man, a moving company employee for 15 years, complained of back pain and neurological symptoms after a full day of work moving a family to their new home. He went home and took some aspirin for the pain, but the symptoms persisted the next morning. Concerned, he visited his physician who conducted a neurological examination and ordered imaging studies. The MRI revealed a herniated intervertebral disc at L4/L5 (Fig. 1-1).

WHERE ARE INTERVERTEBRAL DISCS FOUND?

Intervertebral discs are found between the bodies of adjacent vertebrae from the axis to the sacrum (Fig. 1-2). A disc is not found between the atlas and the axis. The discs are thinnest between the cervical vertebrae and progressively thicken as they descend the vertebral column. In the secondary curvatures of the vertebral column (cervical and lumbar regions), the intervertebral discs are thicker anteriorly. This produces the anterior convexity of the cervical and lumbar segments of the vertebral column.

WHAT IS THE HISTOLOGY OF THE INTERVERTEBRAL DISC?

The intervertebral disc is composed of an outer ring, anulus fibrosus, and an inner core, nucleus pulposus (Fig. 1-2). The anulus fibrosus has an outer thin layer of dense collagenous tissue and an internal wider layer of fibrocartilage. The nucleus pulposus is derived from the notochord. It has a gelatinous consistency due to the presence of glycosaminoglycans (mucopolysaccharides) and proteins.

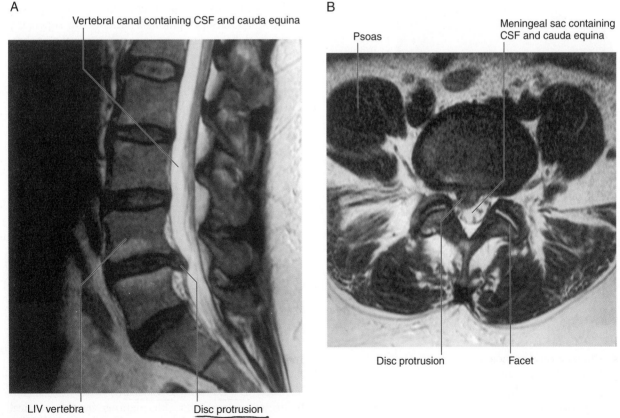

A

Vertebral canal containing CSF and cauda equina

B

Psoas

Meningeal sac containing CSF and cauda equina

LIV vertebra   Disc protrusion

Disc protrusion   Facet

FIGURE 1-1 MRI of a herniated disc between L4 and L5 vertebrae. **A**, Sagittal plane. **B**, Axial plane. (Drake R, Vogl W and Mitchell A: *Gray's Anatomy for Students*. Churchill Livingstone, 2004. Fig. 2-33.)

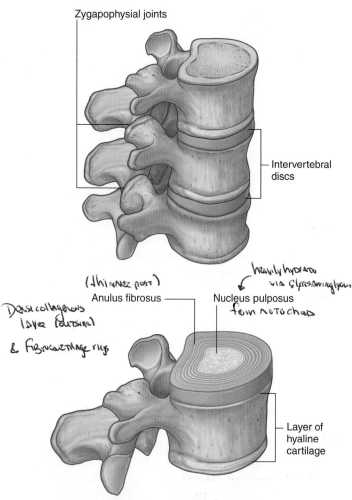

Zygapophysial joints

Intervertebral discs

(thinner post)

Anulus fibrosus

Nucleus pulposus

heavily hydrated via Glycosaminoglycans

from notochord

Dense collagenous layer (outside) & fibrocartilage rings

Layer of hyaline cartilage

FIGURE 1-2 Intervertebral joints. (Drake R, Vogl W and Mitchell A: *Gray's Anatomy for Students.* Churchill Livingstone, 2004. Fig. 2-31.)

WHAT OTHER LIGAMENTS ARE FOUND IN THE VERTEBRAL COLUMN?

Other ligaments of the vertebral column are the:

- Ligamenta flava
- Interspinous ligaments
- Supraspinous ligament
- Intertransverse ligaments
- Ligamentum nuchae
- Anterior longitudinal ligament
- Posterior longitudinal ligament

These ligaments, save for the anterior and posterior longitudinal ligaments, are described in the following paragraphs. The longitudinal ligaments are described later.

Ligamenta flava are comprised of yellow elastic tissue. Flavus is Latin for yellow so these ligaments are aptly named. The ligaments are attached to the laminae of adjacent vertebrae in the vertebral column. Specifically, their attachments are to the inferior anterior surface of the lamina above to the superior posterior surface of the lamina below. Regional differences exist in the basic appearance of the ligaments. In the cervical region the ligaments are thin and long, whereas in the lumbar region they are short and thick. The ligaments function to check flexion of the vertebral column and to assist in extending the column from a flexed position.

Interspinous ligaments are thin and weak as they attach to the spinous processes of adjacent vertebrae. The ligaments, which are poorly developed in the neck, are described by some authorities as being incorporated into the ligamentum nuchae. They are wider and thicker in the lumbar region.

The supraspinous ligament is a strong fibrous cord that attaches to the posterior tips of the spinous processes. The supraspinous ligament ends superiorly at the vertebra prominens (seventh cervical vertebra) where it becomes continuous with the ligamentum nuchae.

Intertransverse ligaments are weak fibers that attach to the transverse processes of adjacent vertebrae. They are poorly developed in the cervical region and are represented by cords in the thoracic region. In the lumbar region they are membranous.

The ligamentum nuchae is a fibroelastic membrane that attaches to the spinous process of the vertebra prominens, bifid spinous processes of the sixth to second cervical vertebrae, posterior tubercle of the atlas, and external occipital protuberance of the occipital bone.

WHERE DO HERNIATIONS OF THE INTERVERTEBRAL DISCS COMMONLY OCCUR?

Intervertebral disc herniations frequently involve the discs in the lumbar region. Most of these occur between L4/L5 and L5/sacrum, with L5/sacrum being more common. Herniations in the cervical region are more likely between C5/C6 and C6/C7, with C5/C6 occurring more frequently.

L5/sacrum & C5/C6

→ most common

[Handwritten: INVERT CANAL (NARROW)]

[Handwritten: Sup Layer / Central Bands / fan-like / expanses @ the IV / Discs / = Dentate]

[Handwritten: Deep Layer / Thinner central bands / w/ expanses dist / are just as wide / as the sup / layer]

[Handwritten: SACRUM → CC2 = Becomes Tectorial / membrane]

Posterior longitudinal ligament

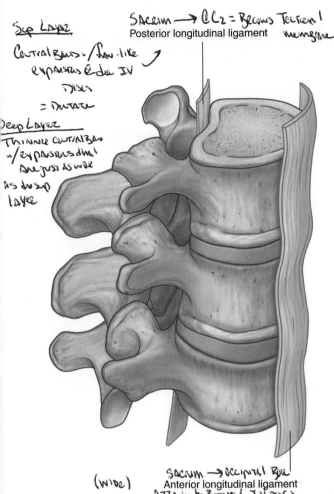

[Handwritten: (WIDE)]

[Handwritten: SACRUM → Occipital Bone / Attaches to Bodies & IV discs]

Anterior longitudinal ligament

FIGURE 1-3 Anterior and posterior longitudinal ligaments of vertebral column. (Drake R, Vogl W and Mitchell A: *Gray's Anatomy for Students*. Churchill Livingstone, 2004. Fig. 2-34.)

WHAT ARE THE STRUCTURES THAT SECURE THE INTERVERTEBRAL DISCS IN PLACE?

The anterior and posterior longitudinal ligaments maintain the intervertebral discs in position between the vertebral bodies (Fig. 1-3). The anterior longitudinal ligament extends along the anterior borders of the vertebral bodies and intervertebral discs from the sacrum to the occipital bone. Its function is to maintain the structural integrity of the intervertebral joints and to check hyperextension.

The posterior longitudinal ligament is the thinner, weaker cousin of the anterior longitudinal ligament. It extends along the posterior borders of the vertebral bodies and intervertebral discs from the sacrum to the axis. The superior continuation of the fibers is known

as the tectorial membrane. The posterior longitudinal ligament also maintains the structural stability of the intervertebral joints but limits hyperflexion of the vertebral column.

IN WHAT DIRECTION DO INTERVERTEBRAL DISCS HERNIATE?

A herniating intervertebral disc takes the path of least resistance, which is posterolateral. This path of least resistance is created by two structural features. The first is that the posterior part of the anulus fibrosus is weaker than it anterior margin. The other reason is that the posterior longitudinal ligament is narrower and weaker than the anterior longitudinal ligament.

[Handwritten: → weaker post lig / the post lig is weaker @ the spur & thinner anulus post. = post lat]

WHAT WOULD BE THE EXPECTED RESULTS OF THE NEUROLOGICAL EXAMINATION IN THE PATIENT WITH A HERNIATED DISC AT L4/L5 AND HOW COULD THIS BE DIFFERENTIATED FROM HERNIATIONS AT OTHER LUMBAR LEVELS?

A herniated intervertebral disc at the L4/L5 level will involve the extensor hallucis longus and will result in sensory deficits along the skin associated with the lateral leg and dorsum of the foot (Table 1-1). Herniations above or below the L4/L5 level can be differentiated on the basis of involved muscle, diminished reflex, and sensory deficit (Table 1-1).

HOW CAN YOU DIFFERENTIATE A HERNIATION OF THE INTERVERTEBRAL DISC BETWEEN C5/C6 AND C6/C7 BASED SOLELY ON NEUROLOGICAL SYMPTOMS AND PHYSICAL EXAMINATION?

Herniation of the intervertebral disc at the level of C5/C6 involves the nerve root of spinal nerve C6, whereas herniation between C6/C7 compresses the nerve root of spinal nerve C7. The levels of herniation can be differentiated by assessing muscle involvement, reflexes, and sensory deficits. These variables for cervical disc herniation are described in Table 1-2.

TABLE 1-1 Herniations of Lumbar Intervertebral Discs

Disc	Root	Muscles	Reflex	Sensation
L3/L4	L4	Tibialis anterior	Patellar tendon	Medial aspect of leg
L4/L5	L5	Extensor hallucis longus	None	Lateral aspect of leg, middle part of dorsum of foot, and digits 2–4
L5/S1	S1	Fibularis longus and fibularis brevis	Achilles tendon	Lateral aspect of foot

(Table adapted from p 66, Hoppenfeld, Orthopedic Neurology, 1997)

Table 1-2 Herniations of Cervical Intervertebral Discs

Disc	Root	Muscles	Reflex	Sensation
C4/C5	C5	Deltoid Biceps brachii	Biceps brachii	Lateral arm via axillary nerve
C5/C6	C6	Biceps brachii Wrist extensors	Brachioradialis	Lateral border of forearm via lateral antebrachial cutaneous nerve, digit one
C6/C7	C7	Triceps brachii Wrist flexors Finger extensors	Triceps brachii	Digits two, three, and four
C7/T1	C8	Intrinsic muscles of hand Flexors of fingers		Medial border of forearm via medial antebrachial cutaneous nerve and digit five
T1/T2	T1	Intrinsic muscles of hand		Medial border of arm via medial brachial cutaneous nerve

(Table adapted from p 38, Hoppenfeld, Orthopedic Neurology, 1997)

Compress the lower nerve @ level
  → Bledthe our @ upn Vert exits before the
    DISC
    & lue vert nerve crosses the
       DISC
★ L4/L5 → L4 is above disc & L5 crosses the disc

L4 = more medial / medial leg & sensay / Tib Ant. wrist medial Ant Comp Muscle / Patella Tendon medial

L5 = more Lat / ↓ sensay on middle of dorsum / By hallucis & Ext Digiterum ↓

S1 = even more LAT / ↓ LAT sensation of foot / Peronis muscles (Lateral) / Achilles reflex
  → Achilles one weakness = S1

C6 = Biceps / Lat. border of forearm
C7 = Triceps / Digits 2,3,4

To rule out chromosomal abnormalities and birth defects in the fetus of her 40-year-old gravid patient, the physician performs an amniocentesis and an ultrasound. The chromosomal analysis ruled out any chromosomal abnormalities; however, the amniocentesis showed that the alpha-fetoprotein (AFP) level was elevated. The ultrasound revealed that the fetus had spina bifida cystica.

WHAT FETAL STRUCTURES NORMALLY SYNTHESIZE AFP?

AFP, a glycoprotein, is synthesized by three fetal structures. These structures can be remembered by the acronym "GLY": gut, liver, and yolk sac. Although small amounts of AFP normally enter the amniotic fluid, elevated concentrations are markers for neural tube defects and defects of the ventral abdominal wall. Because these defects are not covered by skin, AFP freely enters the amniotic fluid from the fetal circulation. AFP is similar to adult albumin and is capable of binding to numerous ligands, such as fatty acids, steroids, bilirubin, and retinoids. Consequently, elevated AFP is a consequence of neural tube defects and not a cause.

HOW DO THE VERTEBRAE AND INTERVERTEBRAL DISCS FORM EMBRYOLOGICALLY?

The vertebrae and intervertebral discs develop from the mesenchyme of sclerotomes around the notochord (Fig. 1-4). Each sclerotome contains two layers of mesenchyme arranged cranially and caudally. The cranial layer of mesenchymal cells is loosely organized, whereas the caudal layer is dense in its arrangement. Between the sclerotomes are mesenchyme and intersegmental arteries. The intersegmental arteries ultimately become the intercostal and lumbar arteries in the thorax and lumbar regions, respectively.

Next, there is mesenchymal cell migration from one layer to the other. Within the same sclerotome, some mesenchymal cells migrate cranially from the inferior densely packed layer to the superior loosely organized layer. This movement results in the formation of the intervertebral disc. Other mesenchymal cells from the densely packed caudal layer of one sclerotome migrate inferiorly to the loosely organized cranial layer of the adjacent sclerotome. This cellular movement forms a mesenchymal centrum (body) of a primordial vertebra.

After the formation of a mesenchymal vertebral template, six chondrification centers appear during the sixth week of development (Fig. 1-5). Two chondrification centers develop in the centrum, two form where the vertebral arches join the centrum (these form transverse and articular processes), and two appear in the vertebral arches (these form the vertebral arches and spinous process). Waves of chondrification spread from these six centers, culminating in the formation of a cartilaginous vertebral template.

The last stage involves ossification (Fig. 1-5). Ossification is a lengthy process beginning during the last week (eighth) of the embryonic period and culminating by age 25. The first ossification centers appear in the centrum: one is ventral and one is dorsal. These centers fuse into one primary center of ossification. Two other primary ossification centers develop in right and left vertebral arches. Thus, three primary ossification centers develop by the end of the embryonic period. At birth, the three primary ossification centers have formed three bony elements: body and two vertebral arches. The arches are connected posteriorly by hyaline cartilage. Following puberty, five secondary ossification centers develop to complete the process:

- One appears in the spinous process.
- One appears in each transverse process (two transverse processes = two secondary centers of ossification).
- Two anular epiphyses. A superior anular epiphysis forms a peripheral ring around the superior surface of the vertebral body and an inferior anular epiphysis forms a ring on the inferior surface.

WHAT IS THE EMBRYOLOGICAL BASIS OF SPINA BIFIDA?

During normal development, the two halves of the vertebral (neural) arch join dorsally in the midline.

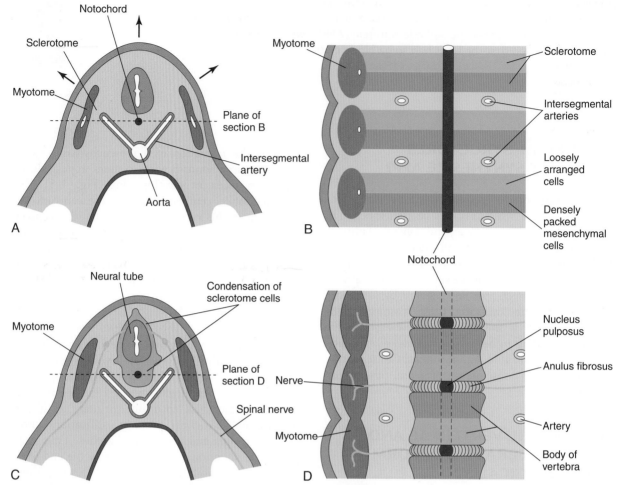

FIGURE 1-4 Development of vertebral column. **A,** Transverse section of a 4-week old embryo. **B,** Frontal section of embryo showing condensations of cells of the sclerotome. **C,** Transverse section of a 5-week old embryo showing development of a mesenchymal vertebra. **D,** Frontal section illustrating the development of the mesenchymal vertebral body and intervertebral disc. (Moore K and Persaud TVN: *The Developing Human,* 7e. WB Saunders, 2003. Fig. 15-7.)

Induction by the neural tube (ectoderm) causes adjacent mesoderm of the vertebral arches to form and to fuse. The induction is mediated by the homeobox gene, *Msx-2.* When the vertebral arches fail to develop and fuse, the vertebral arches remain open and the contents of the vertebral canal are exposed.

HOW IS SPINA BIFIDA CYSTICA DEFINED?

Spina bifida cystica is characterized by a cystlike sac that contains the meninges with or without the spinal cord (Fig. 1-6). If the sac contains meninges and cerebrospinal fluid, the cystic defect is called *spina bifida with meningocele.* When the sac contains meninges, cerebrospinal fluid, and the spinal cord, it is called *spina bifida with meningomyelocele.*

WHAT IS SPINA BIFIDA OCCULTA?

Spina bifida occulta (occult means hidden) is a minor form of a vertebral arch defect that is present in 5% to 10% of the population. The defect most frequently involves the fifth lumbar or the first sacral vertebrae and is typically asymptomatic. The only visible clue is a skin dimple with a tuft of hair overlying the defect. Visible confirmation of spina bifida occulta is usually an incidental radiological finding.

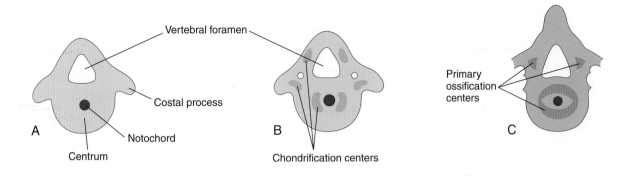

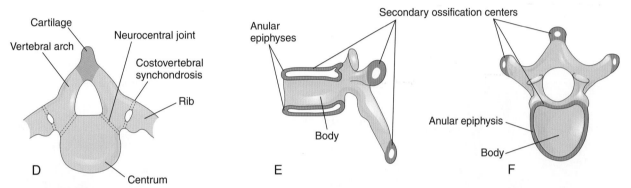

FIGURE 1-5 Chondrification and ossification of a vertebra. **A**, Mesenchymal vertebra. **B**, Appearance of chondrification centers at 6 weeks. **C**, Primary ossification centers at 7 weeks. **D**, Thoracic vertebra at birth demonstrating three osseous elements: centrum and two vertebral arches. **E** and **F**, Lateral and superior views of thoracic vertebra at puberty showing the secondary ossification centers. (Moore K and Persaud TVN: *The Developing Human,* 7e. WB Saunders, 2003. Fig. 15-8.)

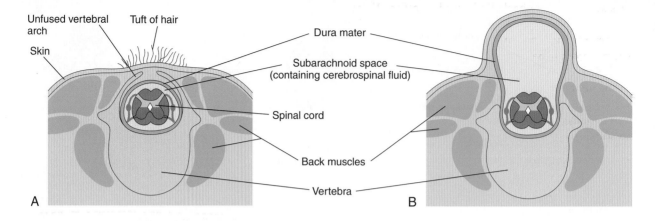

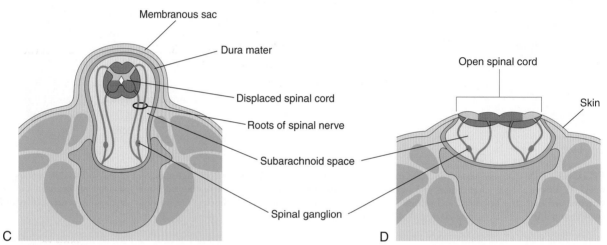

FIGURE 1-6 Illustrations of various types of spina bifida. **A,** Spina bifida occulta. **B,** Spina bifida with meningocele. **C,** Spina bifida with meningomyelocele. **D,** Spina bifida with myeloschisis. (Moore K and Persaud TVN: *The Developing Human,* 7e. WB Saunders, 2003. Fig. 18-12.)

As he was being tackled in a high school football game, the 17-year-old running back was speared in the back. As he walked off the field with difficulty, he complained of lower back pain and tightness of his hamstrings. He was transported by ambulance to the emergency department. The following observations were made during the physical examination: hyperlordosis of the lumbar region, unable to flex hips with knees extended, and a prominently palpable L5 spinous process. Obliquely-oriented x-rays of the lumbosacral region showed bilateral fractures of the pars interarticularis of vertebra L5 and a 35% anterior displacement (slippage) of its body. The diagnosis was spondylolisthesis with a high-grade slip, and spinal fusion surgery was performed to stabilize the segment of listhesis and to decompress the nerve roots.

WHAT IS THE DIFFERENCE BETWEEN SPONDYLOLYSIS AND SPONDYLOLISTHESIS?

The prefix *spondylo-* is derived from the Greek meaning vertebra. The suffixes *-lysis* and *-olisthesis* also are derived from Greek words meaning loosening and slipping, respectively. Therefore, spondylolysis occurs when there is degeneration or abated development of the vertebral arch, particularly the pars interarticularis. This can lead to slippage of the damaged vertebra upon the vertebra below. Slippage of the vertebra is spondylolisthesis.

WHAT IS THE PARS INTERARTICULARIS?

The pars articularis is the portion of the lamina between the superior and inferior articular processes of a lumbar vertebra.

AN OBLIQUE RADIOGRAPH OF A NORMAL LUMBAR SPINE SHOWS AN OUTLINE OF A "SCOTTIE DOG". WHAT STRUCTURES DEFINE THIS CANINE APPEARANCE?

The "Scottie dog" is a normal radiological feature of the lumbar spine in an oblique view and it is defined by the following vertebral structures (Fig. 1-7A):

- The pedicle represents the eye.
- The superior articular process represents the ears.
- The inferior articular processes form the legs.
- The superior articular process of the opposite side forms the tail.
- The lamina and spinous process form the body.

IN SPONDYLOLISTHESIS, THE "SCOTTIE DOG" IS WEARING A WIDE COLLAR. WHAT DOES THE WIDE COLLAR REPRESENT?

The wide collar of the Scottie dog represents the fracture (Fig. 1-7B) and separation of the vertebra from the pars interarticularis.

WHY WAS THE PATIENT UNABLE TO FLEX HIS THIGHS WITH HIS KNEES EXTENDED?

Spondylolisthesis of the fifth lumbar vertebra on the sacrum compresses the fifth lumbar and first sacral nerve roots. The ventral primary rami from L4 and L5 and S1–S3 form the sciatic nerve. Having the patient flex his thighs with knees extended stretches the sciatic nerves. Because the compressed L5 and S1 nerve roots contribute to the formation of the sciatic nerve, even slight tension on the nerve elicits enough pain to prevent the flexion.

WHAT ARE THE NEUROLOGICAL SYMPTOMS IF NERVE ROOT COMPRESSION ACCOMPANIES SPONDYLOLISTHESIS OF THE FIFTH LUMBAR VERTEBRA?

Spondylolisthesis of the fifth lumbar vertebra involves the roots of the fifth lumbar and first sacral nerves. Their muscular and sensory distribution and reflexes are described in Table 1-1. As an example, involvement of the first sacral nerve results in a diminished Achilles' tendon reflex, sensory disturbances over the lateral surface of the foot, and involvement of the fibularis longus and fibularis brevis muscles.

A

Superior articular process

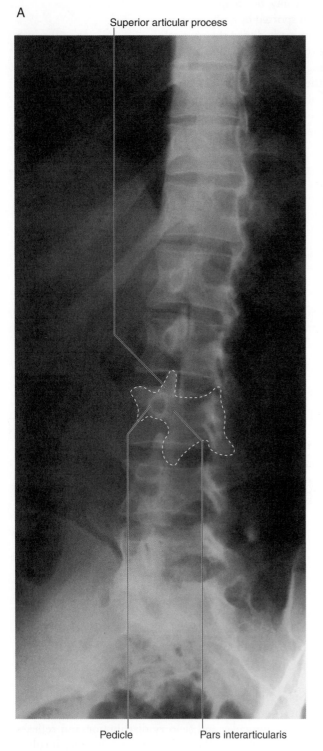

Pedicle   Pars interarticularis

B

Pars fracture

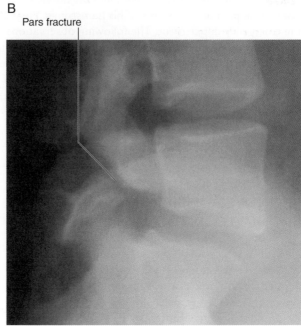

FIGURE 1-7 Radiograph of lumbar vertebra demonstrating the "Scottie dog" (oblique view). **A**, Normal lumbar vertebrae. **B**, Fracture of pars interarticularis with minimal slippage. (Drake R, Vogl W and Mitchell A: *Gray's Anatomy for Students*. Churchill Livingstone, 2004. Fig. 2-38.)

A 72-year-old woman presented to her geriatric physician with back pain that radiated laterally to the flanks. Upon examination, her physician noticed pronounced kyphosis of her vertebral column. Radiographs revealed vertebral compression fractures in the thoracic and upper lumbar regions. Bone densitometry showed significant loss of bone mineral density. The patient was diagnosed with senile osteoporosis (Fig. 1-8).

WHAT SKELETAL ELEMENTS ARE THE MOST SEVERELY DAMAGED BY THE OSTEOPOROTIC PROCESS?

In postmenopausal osteoporosis, the cancellous (spongy) regions of bones provide the greatest surface area for bone degradation by osteoclasts. Involvement of the cancellous bone in vertebral bodies may culminate in compression fractures.

In contrast, senile osteoporosis preferentially leads to pronounced bone resorption in cortical bone, which is composed of osteons (haversian systems). With excessive resorption, the cortical bone may resemble cancellous bone instead of compact bone with its haversian systems.

THE THORACIC REGION OF THE VERTEBRAL COLUMN EXHIBITS A NORMAL ANTERIOR CONCAVE CURVATURE (NORMAL KYPHOSIS). ANATOMICALLY, HOW IS THIS CURVATURE PRODUCED?

The primary curvatures (thoracic and sacral segments) of the vertebral column are formed from slight regional differences in the height of the thoracic vertebral bodies. Specifically, the anterior region of the body is shorter than its posterior aspect.

HOW WOULD YOU DESCRIBE A PRONOUNCED KYPHOSIS OF THE VERTEBRAL COLUMN?

Pronounced kyphosis is characterized by an exaggerated anterior curvature of the thoracic segment of the vertebral column. The exaggerated curvature produces a hunchback appearance.

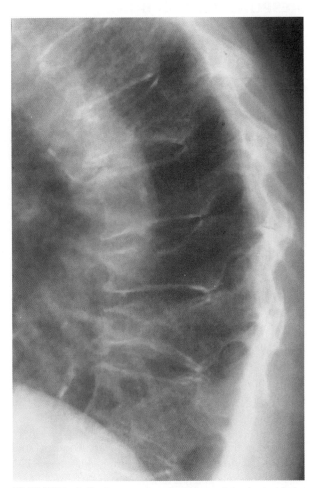

FIGURE 1-8 Compression fractures and kyphosis of the vertebral column in osteoporosis. (Goldman L and Ausiello D: *Cecil Textbook of Medicine, 22e*. WB Saunders, 2004. Fig. 258-4. From Cecil Textbook of Medicine, 22nd edition.)

FOSAMAX (ALENDRONATE SODIUM) WAS PRESCRIBED TO THIS PATIENT TO INHIBIT PROGRESSION OF OSTEOPOROSIS. ALENDRONATE, A BISPHOSPHONATE, INHIBITS THE ACTIVITY OF CELLS THAT RESORB BONE. WHAT CELL TYPE IS RESPONSIBLE FOR BONE RESORPTION? WHAT ARE THE SIGNATURE CHARACTERISTICS OF THIS CELL TYPE THAT WOULD ALLOW YOU TO IDENTIFY IT WITH LIGHT AND ELECTRON MICROSCOPY?

The osteoclast is the cell type responsible for bone resorption. At the light microscopic level with hematoxylin and eosin staining, the observed signature characteristics of the osteoclast are:

- Large cell (150 µm in diameter)
- Acidophilic cell
- Multinucleated (may have as many as 50 nuclei)
- Ruffled border.

The osteoclast exhibits the following characteristics at the ultrastructural level:

- Well-endowed with lysosomes, which are responsible for the cell's acidophilic cytoplasm
- Numerous enfoldings of the plasmalemma applied to the bone that is being resorbed. These enfoldings represent the ruffled border.
- Golgi apparatus is associated with each nucleus
- A pair of centrioles is associated with each nucleus
- Numerous mitochondria, which are concentrated in the region of the ruffled border
- Endoplasmic reticulum is scanty.

HOW DO OSTEOCLASTS RESORB BONE?

Active resorption of bone requires the osteoclast to acidify the microenvironment between the plasmalemma of its ruffled border and the surface of bone and the release of lysozymes from lysosomes. Osteoclasts that are actively resorbing bone are described as possessing four distinct morphological regions: (1) basal zone, (2) ruffled border, (3) clear zone, and (4) vesicular zone.

- Basal zone. This zone is well endowed with organelles and is the farthest zone from Howship's lacuna.
- Ruffled border. The ruffled border represents the site of active bone resorption within Howship's lacuna. The ruffled border is formed by finger-like extensions of the osteoclast's plasma membrane. The ruffled processes project toward the bone surface and serve to increase the surface area for resorption.
- Clear zone. This zone forms a belt around the ruffled border immediately deep to the plasma membrane. It is clear because of the absence of organelles, but it does contain abundant actin microfilaments. The actin microfilaments are anchored to integral proteins, called integrins, embedded in the plasma membrane of the clear zone. The integrin proteins attach the plasma membrane of the clear zone to the surface of bone around Howship's lacuna, thereby sealing off the ruffled border from the extracellular environment. The sealed-off space containing the ruffled border is known as the *subosteoclastic compartment*.
- Vesicular zone. This zone is located between the basal zone and ruffled border and is aptly named because of the abundant endocytotic and exocytotic vesicles found here.

Acidification of the subosteoclastic compartment involves the following steps:

- CO_2 is converted to H_2CO_3 (carbonic acid) in the cytoplasm of the osteoclast by the enzyme *carbonic anhydrase*.
- Being a weak acid, H_2CO_3 partially dissociates into H^+ and HCO_3^-.
- H^+ is then actively pumped out of the osteoclast and into the subosteoclastic compartment by transport proteins embedded in the plasma membrane of the ruffled border. Cl^- passively follows the movement of hydrogen ions.
- The acidification of the subosteoclastic compartment by the active transport of H^+ dissolves the inorganic elements of the bone matrix.
- The dissolved inorganic minerals are subsequently transported across the plasma membrane of the ruffled border and then transported out of the osteoclast to capillaries bordering the cell.

Lysosomes are membrane-limited organelles that contain degradative enzymes (lysozymes). Lysosomes represent the cell's digestive system as the organelles enzymatically digest endocytosed material or, as necessary, worn out organelles. Osteoclasts, however, use lysosomes and their lysozymes for another purpose—to degrade bone matrix. This is accomplished through the active secretion of lysozymes by the osteoclast where it abuts the surface of bone. This interface occurs between the osteoclast's ruffled border and Howship's lacuna.

HOW DOES ALENDRONATE AFFECT OSTEOCLASTS?

Alendronate does not affect recruitment and attachment of osteoclasts to the bone surface. Instead, it prevents the osteoclasts from developing their ruffled borders, which occurs when the cells are actively degrading bone.

Section II

Thorax

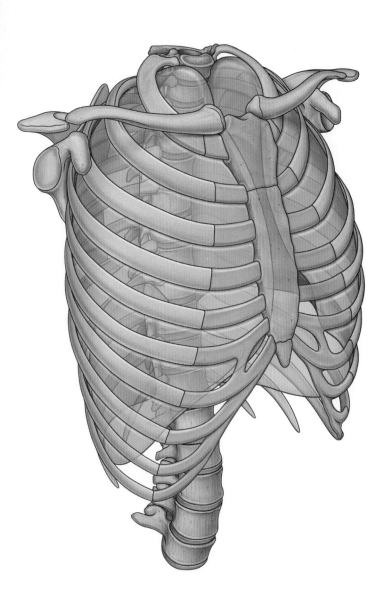

A 46-year-old woman presented to her physician complaining of dysphagia, regurgitation of undigested food and liquid and modest weight loss. The history revealed that the symptoms have lasted for 3 years and that she has a feeling of retrosternal fullness after meals. This feeling of fullness can be relieved at times by drinking a large glass of water and by standing with arms over her head. The radiographic imaging study (barium swallow and fluoroscopy) showed a dilated esophagus with a distinct air-fluid interface and a "bird's beak" silhouette (Fig. 2-1) in the region of the lower esophageal sphincter (LES) and no significant peristalsis in the esophagus. Save for an inflamed esophageal mucosa, the endoscopic examination was unremarkable. Esophageal manometry showed incomplete relaxation of the LES and aperistalsis of the esophagus. The patient was diagnosed with primary achalasia (unknown etiology), which was successfully treated with pneumatic dilation of the LES.

WHAT ARE THE VERTEBRAL RELATIONSHIPS OF THE ESOPHAGUS?

The esophagus begins at the level of the sixth cervical vertebra, which corresponds to the level of the cricoid cartilage of the larynx. The esophagus descends in the superior and posterior (division of the inferior mediastinum) mediastina and passes through the esophageal hiatus at the level of the tenth thoracic vertebra. The cardia of the stomach receives the abdominal esophagus at the level of the eleventh thoracic vertebra.

WHAT IS THE BLOOD SUPPLY TO THE ESOPHAGUS?

The esophagus is richly supplied by arteries. These arteries are:

- Esophageal branches of the inferior thyroid artery, a branch of the thyrocervical trunk
- Esophageal branches of the descending thoracic aorta
- Branches from the bronchial arteries. The right bronchial artery takes origin from the right third posterior intercostal artery, a branch of the descending thoracic aorta, whereas the left bronchial arteries issue directly from the descending thoracic aorta.
- Left gastric artery, a branch from the celiac trunk
- Left inferior phrenic artery, the first branch, along with its fellow, of the abdominal aorta

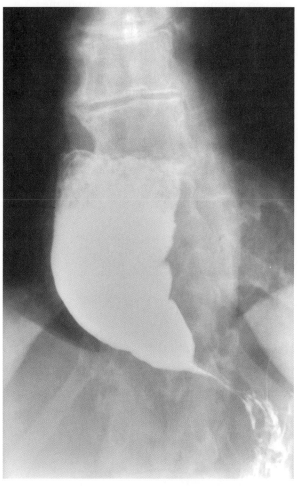

FIGURE 2-1 Esophagogram showing the characteristic "bird's beak" appearance of achalasia. (Towsend C et al.: *Sabiston Textbook of Surgery, 17e.* WB Saunders, 2004. Fig. 39-11. Courtesy of Ronella A. Dubrow, M.D., MD Anderson Cancer Center, Houston, TX.)

WHAT IS THE VENOUS DRAINAGE OF THE ESOPHAGUS?

The veins of the esophagus drain into the following:

● Inferior thyroid veins
● Azygos, hemiazygos, and accessory hemiazygos veins
● Left gastric vein

WHAT IS THE INNERVATION OF THE ESOPHAGUS?

The nerve supply to the esophagus is from the:

● Recurrent laryngeal nerves, branches of the vagi, provide motor innervation to the upper esophageal sphincter (cricopharyngeus muscle) and to the cervical segment of the esophagus. Injury to this nerve may result in dysfunction of the upper esophageal sphincter.
● Anterior and posterior vagal trunks
● Thoracic parts of the sympathetic trunk
● Greater and lesser splanchnic nerves. The greater splanchnic nerve originates from lateral gray horns from spinal cord segments T5–T9 and sometimes T10. The lesser splanchnic originates from T10–T11.
● Esophageal plexus. The esophageal plexus is an intermingling of nerve fibers from the vagus nerves and the sympathetic trunks.

HOW DO THE RIGHT AND LEFT VAGUS NERVES FORM THE VAGAL TRUNKS?

The anterior vagal trunk is a continuation of the left vagus nerve; conversely, the posterior vagal nerve is a continuation of the right vagus nerve. The reason this occurs is grounded in embryology. As the stomach develops, it undergoes 90 degrees of clockwise rotation about its longitudinal axis (Fig. 2-2). This rotation carries the left vagus nerve anteriorly and the right vagus nerve posteriorly. The acronym *LARP* is an excellent memory device to remember that the **l**eft vagus becomes **a**nterior and the **r**ight vagus becomes **p**osterior.

WHAT IS THE LYMPHATIC DRAINAGE OF THE ESOPHAGUS?

The mucosa and muscularis externa of the esophagus are well endowed with lymphatic plexuses. Lymphatic flow tends to flow cranially in the upper two-thirds of the esophagus and inferiorly in the lower one-third. Lymphatic flow from the plexuses drains into regional lymph nodes. The regional nodes are the:

● Internal jugular lymph nodes
● Paratracheal lymph nodes
● Subcarinal lymph nodes
● Paraesophageal lymph nodes

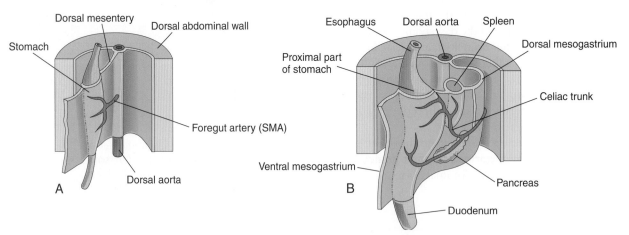

FIGURE 2-2 Rotation of the stomach. **A,** Starting point at 28 days. **B,** Clockwise rotation of the stomach at 35 days. (Moore K and Persaud TVN: *The Developing Human,* 7e. WB Saunders, 2003. Fig. 12-2.)

- Perigastric lymph nodes
- Left gastric artery lymph nodes
- Efferent lymphatic vessels from the perigastric and left gastric artery nodes convey lymph to celiac lymph nodes.

WHAT ARE THE ESOPHAGEAL CONSTRICTIONS THAT MUST BE NAVIGATED DURING INSTRUMENTATION OF THE ESOPHAGUS? HOW FAR ARE THESE CONSTRICTION SITES FROM THE INCISORS IN CENTIMETERS?

The esophagus has four points of constriction (Fig. 2-3), which are caused by the:

- Upper esophagus sphincter, which is formed by the cricopharyngeus muscle; 15 cm
- Arch of the aorta; 22.5 cm
- Left primary bronchus; 27.5 cm
- Esophageal hiatus in the diaphragm; 40 cm. This narrowed segment is clinically referred to as the *lower esophageal sphincter.*

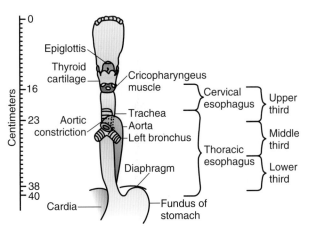

FIGURE 2-3 Segments and constrictions of the esophagus. (Towsend C et al.: *Sabiston Textbook of Surgery, 17e.* WB Saunders, 2004. Fig. 39-1.)

WHAT IS THE CLINICAL RELEVANCE OF THE TRANSITION IN FIBER ORIENTATION BETWEEN THE THYROPHARYNGEUS AND THE CRICOPHARYNGEUS MUSCLES?

The thyropharyngeus muscle represents the upper portion of the inferior constrictor muscle and the cricopharyngeus muscle is the lower part of the constrictor. Proceeding inferiorly from the thyropharyngeus muscle there is a change in fiber orientation. This transition between the upper and lower portions of the inferior constrictor is a point of weakness (Killian's triangle) that could be penetrated with instrumentation of the esophagus. The area of transition may form a pouch that protrudes externally. This is called a *pharyngoesophageal (Zenker's) diverticulum.*

WHAT DOES THE "BIRD'S BEAK" SILHOUETTE REPRESENT?

The "bird's beak" appearance is characteristic of achalasia (Fig. 2-1). It is seen by barium swallow, which shows a dilated esophagus with a narrowed distal segment. The stenotic segment is caused by failure of the lower esophageal sphincter to dilate. The dilated proximal segment of the esophagus represents the bird's head and the tapered segment is its beak.

WHY DO SOME PATIENTS WITH ACHALASIA SUFFER FROM DYSPNEA?

Extensive dilation of the esophagus causes compression of neighboring primary bronchi and this can compress the hilum of each lung.

WHAT ARE THE HISTOLOGIC CHARACTERISTICS OF THE ESOPHAGUS?

The wall of the esophageal tube is composed of four layers. From internal to external, these are the:

- Mucosa. The mucosal layer has three sublayers: epithelium and its supporting basal lamina, which are adlumenal, lamina propria, and muscularis mucosae (interna). The epithelium is stratified squamous, nonkeratinized to protect the esophagus against the abrasive nature of the food bolus. The only other place along the gastrointestinal tube where nonkeratinized, stratified epithelium is found is the distal one-third of the anal canal. The lamina propria contains loose connective tissue, blood vessels, lymphatics, and occasional glands. These glands are called *cardiac esophageal glands* to distinguish them from those in the submucosa and are limited to the proximal and distal segments of the esophagus.

- Submucosa. This layer is composed of moderately dense connective tissue, blood vessels, lymphatics, esophageal glands, and submucosal (Meissner's) plexus. The only segments of the gastrointestinal tube that contain glands in the submucosa are the esophagus and the duodenum.
- Muscularis externa (propria). The muscularis externa is arranged into two layers of muscle: inner circular and outer longitudinal. It is unique, however, in histologic composition. The proximal one-third is composed of skeletal muscle, the middle one-third is an admixture of skeletal and smooth muscle, and the distal one-third is smooth muscle. The myenteric (Auerbach's) plexus is located between the two layers of muscle.
- Adventitia/serosa. The thoracic segment of the esophagus is coated by a loose connective tissue layer, the adventitia. The intraabdominal segment does possess a serosa (visceral peritoneum).

WHAT MORPHOLOGIC CHANGES OF THE ESOPHAGUS ARE ASSOCIATED WITH PRIMARY ACHALASIA?

The esophagus in achalasia shows the following morphologic changes:

- The wall of the esophagus may be normal, thickened, or thinned. A thickened wall is caused by hypertrophy of the muscularis externa (propria), and dilation of the esophagus leads to it being thinner than normal.
- Myenteric (Auerbach's) ganglia are usually absent from the muscularis externa superior to the lower esophageal sphincter. The number of ganglia in the lower esophageal sphincter may be normal or decreased.
- The mucosa may be inflamed, fibrotic, ulcerated, or normal superior to the lower esophageal sphincter.

Achalasia may lead to the development of squamous cell carcinoma of the esophagus in up to 5% of affected patients. The cancer typically develops in the middle third of the esophagus.

A 2-year-old boy was brought to the physician's office by his mother who was concerned about the child's respiratory infection. During the physical examination, a heart murmur was detected. Antibiotics were prescribed for the infection and the child was referred to a pediatric cardiologist. The cardiologist ordered an EKG and echocardiography. The EKG showed atrial flutter accompanied by a rightward QRS axis. The echocardiogram revealed a dilated right atrium and ventricle consistent with an ostium secundum atrial septal defect. The defect was surgically closed.

WHAT ARE THE NORMAL EVENTS IN THE SEPTATION OF THE PRIMITIVE ATRIUM?

Complete division of the primitive atrium into right and left atria involves the following structures:

- Endocardial cushions
- Septum primum
- Septum secundum

The dorsal and ventral endocardial cushions are masses of tissue that develop toward the end of the fourth week (Fig. 2-4). Growth of the cushions by the invasion of mesenchymal cells during the fifth week ultimately results in their fusion. This event divides the common atrioventricular canal into right and left atrioventricular canals. Moreover, fusion of the endocardial cushions is required for complete septation of the primitive atrium. The fused endocardial cushions ultimately become dense collagenous connective tissue of the cardiac skeleton.

The formation of the endocardial cushions is orchestrated by an ensemble of molecules. The primitive myocardium induces the transformation of endothelial cells, which line the endocardium, into mesenchymal cells in the atrioventricular and outflow tract regions (Fig. 2-5). The inducible endothelial cells express the gene *Msx-1*. Endothelial cells that occupy other regions of the endocardium do not express *Msx-1*; therefore, they do not respond to the molecular inducer synthesized by the myocardium. The inducer, in part, is a molecular complex called *adheron*. Adherons, along with TGF-ß1 and TGF-ß3, are collectively responsible for the epithelial/mesenchymal transformation. In the absence of TGF-ß1 and TGF-ß3, the transformation of endothelial cells into mesenchymal cells fails to occur. The inducible endothelial cells also have to migrate from the endocardium into the cardiac jelly that occupies the space between the primitive myocardium and the endothelium. To migrate, the endothelial cells must decrease their synthesis of N-CAM, a protein that anchors the cells in place. The

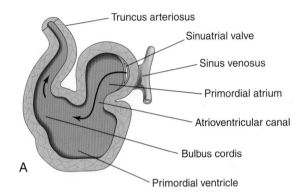

A

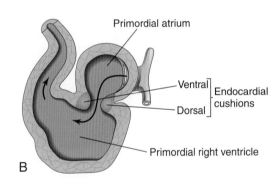

B

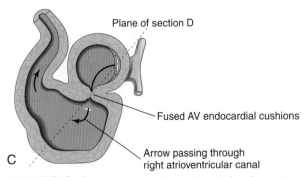

C

FIGURE 2-4 Development of the endocardial cushions. **A** to **C**, Sagittal sections of the heart during the fourth and fifth weeks. (Moore K and Persaud TVN: *The Developing Human*, 7e. WB Saunders, 2003. Fig. 14-11.)

23

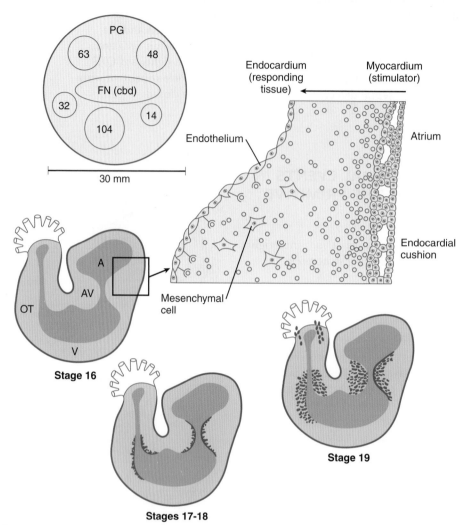

FIGURE 2-5 Molecular events in the development of the endocardial cushions. (Carlson B: *Human Embryology and Developmental Biology*, *3e*. Mosby, 2004. Fig. 17-18.)

down regulation of N-CAM ultimately allows these cells to become motile. Once these motile cells have morphed into mesenchymal cells, they inactivate adherons through the secretion of proteases. These molecular events are also required for normal development of the heart valves.

Septation of the primitive atrium begins at the end of the fourth week. The first structure to form is the septum primum (Fig. 2-6). The septum primum is a thin crescentic tissue membrane that grows from the cranial end of the primitive atrium toward the fused endocardial cushions. The opening between the rim of the membrane and the endocardial cushions is called the *foramen (ostium) primum*. The foramen primum is reduced in size by the continued growth of the septum primum. Before the foramen primum is obliterated by the fusion of the septum primum to the endocardial cushions, small openings are formed by apoptosis in the center of the septum. Coalescence of these openings occurs as the septum primum fuses with the endocardial cushions. This fusion produces a new foramen called the *foramen (ostium) secundum*. The foramen secundum permits shunting of blood from the right atrium to left atrium, thus bypassing the pulmonary circulation.

Next, a second crescentic membrane, called the *septum secundum*, grows from the ventro-cranial wall of the primitive atrium. The septum secundum grows on the right atrial side of the septum primum. Its growth culminates with fusion to the endocardial cushions. An oval opening in the septum secundum is called the *foramen (ostium) ovale*. The cranial margin of the

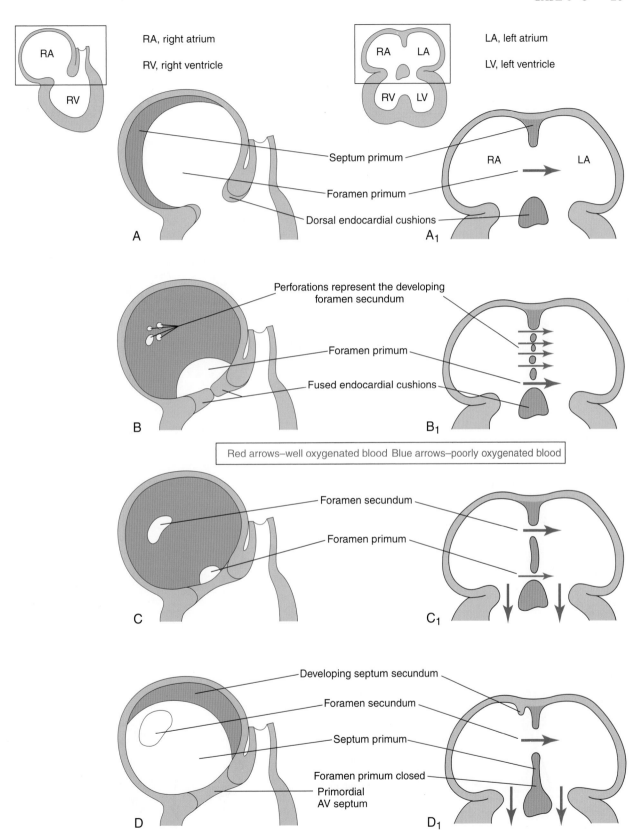

FIGURE 2-6 Septation of the primitive atrium. **A** to **H**, Sagittal view. **A1** to **H1**, Coronal view. (Moore K and Persaud TVN: *The Developing Human*, 7e. WB Saunders, 2003. Fig. 14-13.)

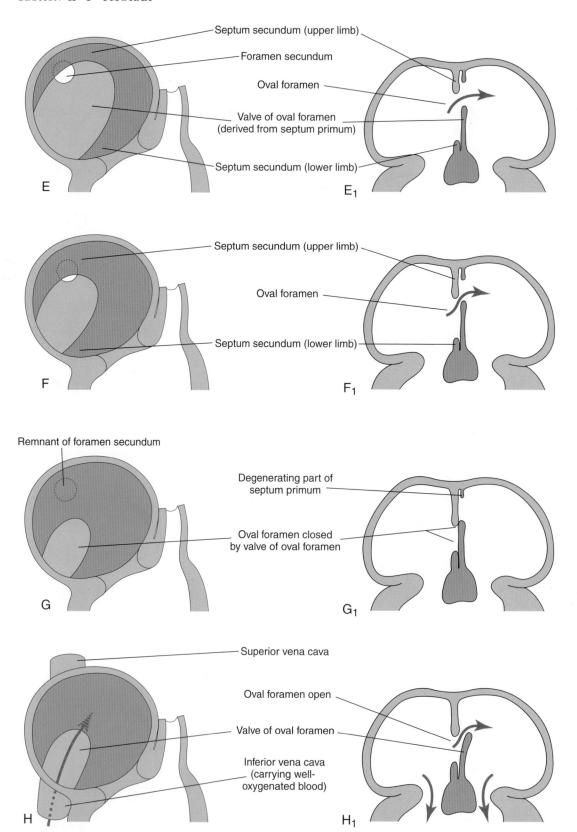

FIGURE 2-6, cont'd

septum primum undergoes apoptosis and disappears. This leaves the caudal end fused with the endocardial cushions. This free lip is long enough to cover the foramen ovale; hence, it is referred to as the *valve of the foramen ovale.*

In the fetal circulation, blood flows from the right atrium into the left by passing through the foramen ovale. After birth, left atrial pressure becomes greater than right atrial pressure, and this pressure gradient slaps the valve of the foramen ovale against the septum secundum. This action completely forms the inter-atrial septum, closing any communication between the two upper chambers.

WHAT STRUCTURES CONTRIBUTE TO THE FORMATION OF THE ATRIA?

The right atrium is formed by the primitive atrium and the right horn of the sinus venosus. The primitive atrium is responsible for the pectinate muscles that are found on the internal surface of the anterior wall of the right atrium. The smooth internal surface of its posterior wall is caused by the sinus venosus. This smooth portion is also known as the sinus venarum. The smooth part of the wall is separated from the rough part containing the pectinate muscles by the crista terminalis internally, and externally by the sulcus terminalis, a shallow groove.

In contrast to the right atrium, the primitive atrium does not contribute appreciably to the development of the left atrium. Instead, most of the left atrium is formed by the incorporation of the primitive pulmonary vein. As the pulmonary vein is incorporated into the expanding left atrium, its four distal branches (two on the right and two on the left) are brought to empty individually into the left atrium. The left auricle, which contains pectinate muscles, is derived from the primitive atrium.

WHAT IS THE EMBRYOLOGICAL BASIS OF ATRIAL SEPTAL DEFECTS?

Four types of atrial septal defects are of clinical importance. These are:

● Ostium primum defect
● Ostium secundum defect
● Sinus venosus defect
● Coronary sinus defect

An ostium primum atrial septal defect occurs when growth of the septum primum is insufficient to fuse with the endocardial cushions (Fig. 2-7E). As a result, the foramen primum remains patent and a cleft in the left atrioventricular (mitral) valve typically forms. Another type of this defect results with failure of the endocardial cushions to fuse. When this occurs, a large defect occurs in the atrioventricular septum and the atrioventricular valves are abnormal.

An ostium secundum atrial defect, the most common atrial septal defect, occurs in the vicinity of the foramen ovale. The defect can result from malformations of the septum primum, septum secundum, or both (Fig. 2-7A–D). Most commonly, the septum primum is involved. Apoptosis in abnormal areas of the septum primum produces fenestrations, or excessive regression of the septum primum produces a valve of the foramen ovale that is too short to cover the foramen ovale. When the septum secundum fails to develop properly, a large foramen ovale is formed. This prevents the normal valve from closing the large defect. When both septa are involved, the defect is excessively large.

Sinus venosus defects are uncommon. When they do occur, they are located in the cranial part of the interatrial septum adjacent to the ostium of the superior vena cava (Fig. 2-7F). This atrial septal defect occurs when reabsorption of the sinus venosus into the right atrium is incomplete or when there is a malformation of the septum secundum.

Coronary sinus atrial septal defects comprise less than 1% of all atrial septal defects. It is postulated that the defects result from the developmental failure of the wall between the coronary sinus and the left atrium to form properly.

The coronary sinus develops principally from the left common cardinal vein with an additional contribution from the left horn of the sinus venosus. The coronary sinus defect occurs in the inferior-anterior interatrial septum where the ostium of the coronary sinus is located. Consequently, the ostium of the coronary sinus communicates with the left atrium, and the defect in the interatrial wall allows the shunting of blood into the left atrium. This type of defect is often accompanied by a persistent left superior vena cava that empties into the coronary sinus.

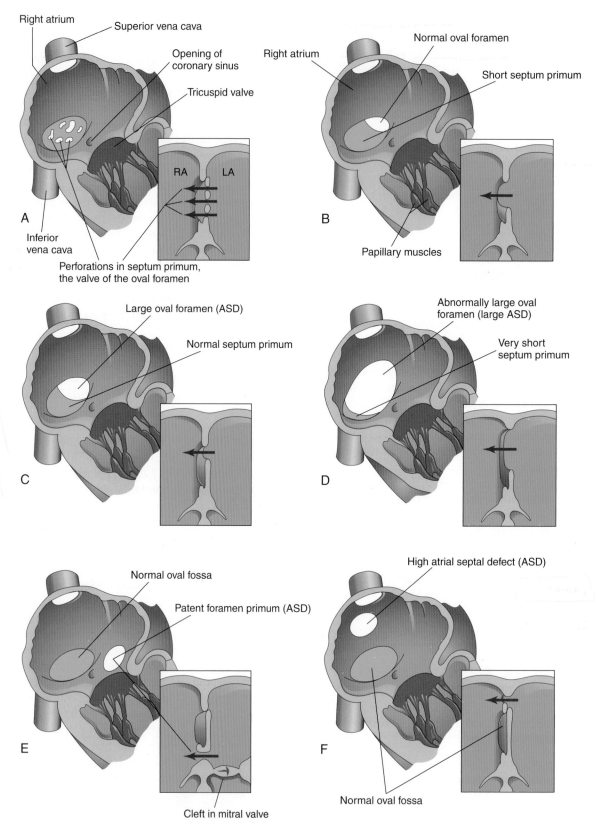

FIGURE 2-7 **A**, Patent foramen ovale caused by resorption in abnormal locations. **B**, Patent foramen ovale caused by a short septum primum. **C**, Patent foramen ovale resulting from a large foramen ovale. **D**, Patent foramen ovale caused by a short septum primum and a large foramen ovale. **E**, Endocardial cushion defect with primum-type atrial septal defect. **F**, Sinus venosus atrial septal defect. (Moore K and Persaud TVN: *The Developing Human*, 7e. WB Saunders, 2003. Fig. 14-26.)

A 62-year-old woman, concerned about a mass she detected during a breast self-examination, presented to the physician's office. The physician also detected the mass in the left breast and ordered a mammogram and ultrasound. The results of these studies revealed a solid mass (Fig. 2-8A). A core biopsy of the mass was obtained and sent to the pathologist. The pathologist's report provided a diagnosis of invasive carcinoma of no special type and confirmed the presence of estrogen and progesterone receptors on the tumor cells.

WHAT IS THE ARTERIAL SUPPLY TO THE FEMALE BREAST?

The breast is well equipped with an arterial blood supply (Fig. 2-9). The arteries that supply the breast are the:

- Internal thoracic (mammary) artery, a branch of the subclavian artery
- Intercostal arteries in the second to fourth intercostal spaces

- Superior thoracic artery, a branch of the first part of the axillary artery
- Pectoral branches of the thoracoacromial artery, which springs from the second part of the axillary artery
- Lateral thoracic artery, a branch of the second part of the axillary artery
- Subscapular artery, a branch of the third part of the axillary artery

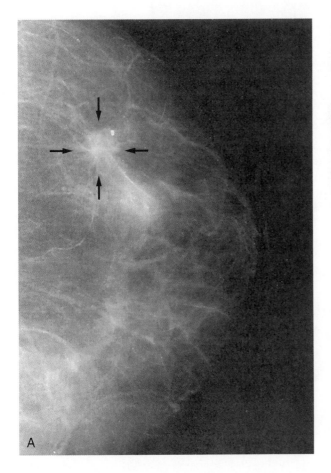

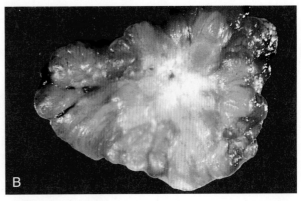

FIGURE 2-8 Invasive ductal carcinoma of the breast. **A,** Mammogram showing density at the arrows. **B,** Dense, white mass in yellow adipose tissue. (Kumar V, Abbas A and Fausto N: *Robbins & Cotran Pathologic Basis of Disease,* 7e. WB Saunders, 2004. Fig. 23-21. Part A Courtesy of Dr. Jack Meyer, Brigham and Women's Hospital, Boston, MA.)

WHAT IS THE VENOUS DRAINAGE OF THE FEMALE BREAST?

Venous drainage is principally to the axillary vein. Additional drainage is to the:

- Internal thoracic vein, which ends in the subclavian vein
- Lateral thoracic vein, which empties into the axillary vein
- Intercostal veins

WHAT IS THE LYMPHATIC DRAINAGE OF THE FEMALE BREAST?

An appreciation for lymph flow is important clinically because it is the primary route of metastasis of breast cancer and for performing and interpreting a sentinel node biopsy. Lymphatic drainage of the female breast is as follows (Fig. 2-9):

- 75% of the lymph drains to the axillary lymph nodes. The axillary nodes are clinically divided into

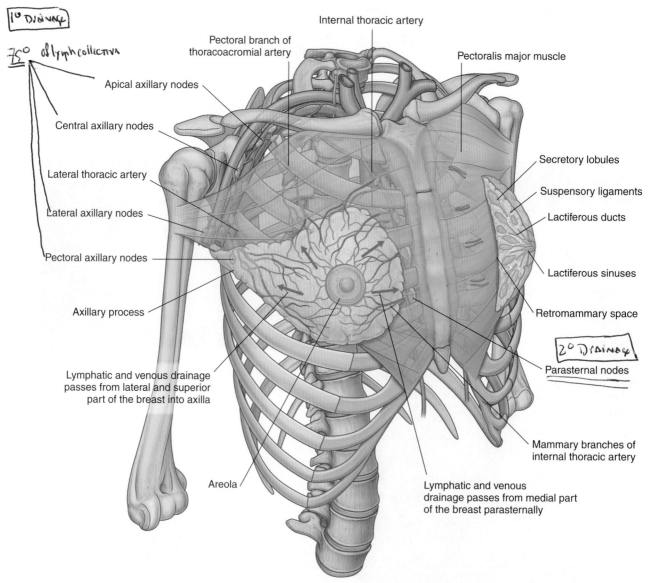

FIGURE 2-9 Arteries and lymphatics of the breasts. (Drake R, Vogl W and Mitchell A: *Gray's Anatomy for Students.* Churchill Livingstone, 2004. Fig. 3-16.)

three levels relative to the pectoralis minor muscle. Level I axillary lymph nodes are located lateral to the muscle, level II nodes are deep to it, and level III are located medial to the muscle.

- Lymph from the medial side of the breast flows into the parasternal (internal mammary) lymph nodes that accompany the internal thoracic artery and vein.
- Lymph from the deep surface of the breast empties into the apical group of axillary lymph nodes.
- Lymph from the skin covering the breast drains into abdominal lymph nodes and the opposite breast. Lymphatic channels deep to the nipple and areola form Sappey's plexus

A COMPLICATION OF DISSECTION OF THE AXILLARY LYMPH NODES IS LYMPHEDEMA OF THE UPPER EXTREMITY. WHAT IS THE ANATOMICAL EXPLANATION FOR THIS COMPLICATION?

Dissection (removal) of the axillary lymph nodes impedes lymphatic drainage of the involved upper extremity. This produces the lymphedema that usually accompanies dissection of the axillary lymph nodes.

WHAT IS A SENTINEL NODE BIOPSY?

Sentinel lymph nodes are the first nodes to receive lymph draining from a structure with a primary neoplasm. In breast cancer, the sentinel node is located in the ipsilateral axilla or parasternal (internal thoracic) lymph node chain and is the first to receive lymph from the tumor. Because the sentinel node is the first to receive the lymph, it is also more likely to contain metastatic tumor cells than other lymph nodes. The results of a sentinel lymph node biopsy determine whether a complete axillary dissection of lymph nodes is necessary.

A sentinel axillary lymph node can be located by the injection of a special blue dye. The axilla is then surgically dissected to locate and remove the sentinel node for histologic examination. If the examination is

negative, the patient is spared a complete axillary dissection.

WHAT IS THE NERVE SUPPLY OF THE FEMALE BREAST?

The breast is supplied by sensory and sympathetic nerve fibers that are conveyed in the lateral and anterior cutaneous branches of intercostal nerves that travel in the second to sixth intercostal spaces. The skin is supplied by the sensory fibers, and the sympathetic fibers innervate the glands and smooth muscle of blood vessels, areolae, and nipples.

WHERE DO MOST BREAST CANCERS DEVELOP?

The location and frequencies of cancerous lesions of the breast are:

- Most commonly (50%) located in the upper lateral quadrant.
- The upper medial and the lower lateral and medial quadrants each give rise to 10% of cancerous lesions.
- The remaining 20% of the lesions occur in the central (subareolar) area of the breast.
- The left breast develops cancer slightly more frequently than the right.

WHY DO LARGER INVASIVE CARCINOMAS OF THE BREAST PRODUCE A DISTINCTIVE PEAU D'ORANGE APPEARANCE?

Peau d'orange, which is French for *orange skin*, is caused when the expanding tumor compresses the lymphatic vessels draining the breast. Lymphedema results from the lymphatic obstruction producing elevations of the skin of the breast. The dimpling effect occurs where the suspensory ligaments (of Cooper) anchor the skin to the breast. The elevations and dimples mimic the appearance of an orange peel (Fig. 2-10).

WHAT NERVES ARE VULNERABLE TO INJURY DURING A MASTECTOMY?

As the breast tissue is surgically excised, caution is necessary in the axilla to avoid sacrificing nerves. Nerves in the axillary region that are vulnerable to injury are:

- Long thoracic nerve (external respiratory nerve of Bell) to supply the serratus anterior muscle
- Thoracodorsal nerve to innervate the latissimus dorsi muscle
- Medial pectoral nerve to supply the pectoralis major

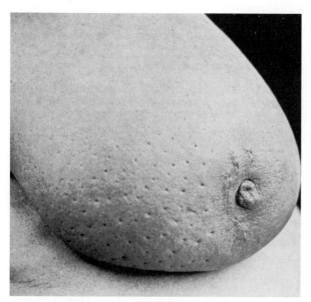

FIGURE 2-10 Peau d' orange of the skin of the breast. (Towsend C et al.: *Sabiston Textbook of Surgery, 17e*. WB Saunders, 2004. Fig. 32-6D.)

- Intercostal brachial nerve (T2) to supply the skin along the medial arm
- Medial brachial cutaneous nerve (C8 and T1) that also supplies the skin of the medial arm

These nerves are vulnerable to injury as the axillary tail (of Spence) of the breast is removed.

WHAT ARE THE HISTOLOGIC CHARACTERISTICS OF THE ADULT FEMALE BREAST?

The adult female breast is composed of variable amounts of glandular tissue, fibrous connective tissue, and fat (Fig. 2-11). Fibrous suspensory ligaments of the breast (Cooper's ligaments) attach to the dermis of the skin of the breast and to the deep fascia associated with the pectoralis major. Fat is an important element with respect to mammography as it provides better contrast to differentiate changes in the breast.

The glands of the breast are classified as compound tubuloalveolar arranged into 15 to 20 lobes. The lobes are separated from one another by fat and collagenous tissue. The basal domains of the glandular cells are separated from the basal lamina by myoepithelial cells. The myoepithelial cells also embrace the cells lining the duct system. The basal lamina is a clinical landmark in differentiating a noninvasive carcinoma from one that is invasive. Breast cancers that have not penetrated through the basal lamina are noninvasive (carcinoma in situ) and those that have penetrated through the basal lamina into the stroma are invasive.

The breast contains an elaborate system of ducts. Small ducts leaving each secretory unit within a lobe are lined by simple columnar epithelium. These small ducts

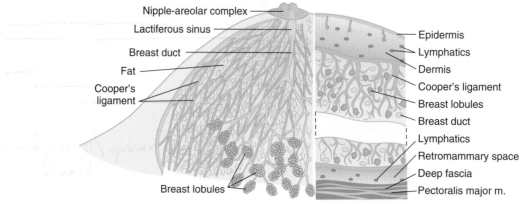

FIGURE 2-11 Illustration of the internal structure of the breast. (Towsend C et al.: *Sabiston Textbook of Surgery, 17e*. WB Saunders, 2004. Fig. 32-1.)

converge to form a large lactiferous duct. This means that the breast contains 15 to 20 lactiferous ducts, one from each of the 15 to 20 lobes. The lactiferous duct is lined by stratified cuboidal epithelium as it extends towards the nipple. Near the nipple, the duct dilates to form the lactiferous sinus, which also is lined by stratified cuboidal epithelium. The short segment of the duct between its sinus and opening at the nipple is lined by stratified squamous epithelium. Bilateral discharge or discharge from several ducts does occur in normal breasts; however, if the discharge is from just one duct, this may indicate underlying disease in the involved duct.

WHAT IS THE MORPHOLOGY OF INVASIVE CARCINOMA OF NO SPECIAL TYPE? *= INVASIVE DUCTAL CARCINOMA*

Invasive carcinoma of no special type has the following morphologic characteristics:

- Most are hard to firm and are described as possessing an irregular border
- The central region of the carcinoma contains small foci of streaks of chalky white degenerating collagen fibers having the appearance of elastic tissue. Small calcification centers may be present.

- Some tumors are well differentiated (Fig. 2-12A) and usually express estrogen and progesterone receptors and do not overexpress human epidermal growth factor receptor 2, HER2.
- Other tumors are not well differentiated. Instead they consist of connecting sheets of pleomorphic (different sizes and shapes) cells (Fig. 2-12B). These pleomorphic cells less frequently express estrogen and progesterone receptors and more likely overexpress HER2.
- Most tumors result in an increase in dense fibrous tissue (Fig. 2-8B) which replaces the adipose tissue. The accumulation of fibrous tissue imparts a hard consistency to the breast that can be detected upon palpation and mammography.

WHAT IS THE MORPHOLOGY OF LYMPH NODES?

Lymph nodes are oval to kidney-shaped structures that are 0.1 to 2.5 cm long. A slight indentation, the hilum, is found on their side. The hilum is the doorway through which blood vessels enter and leave and efferent lymphatic vessels, which are equipped with valves, exit. The lymph node is surrounded by a fibrous connective capsule.

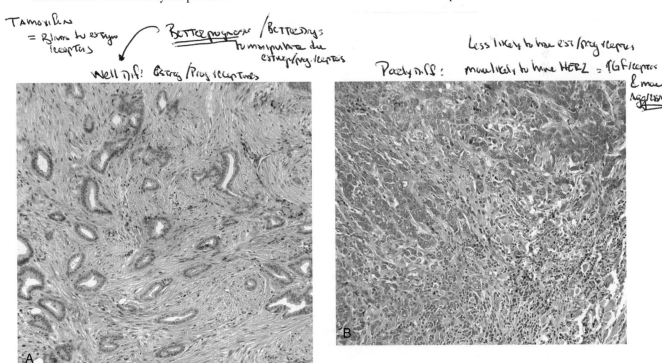

FIGURE 2-12 **A,** Well-differentiated invasive carcinoma of no special type. **B,** Poorly differentiated invasive carcinoma of no special type. (Kumar V, Abbas A and Fausto N: *Robbins & Cotran Pathologic Basis of Disease,* 7e. WB Saunders, 2004. Fig. 23-22.)

Histologically, three distinct zones are observed: cortex, paracortex, and medulla. The zones are described below.

● Cortex. The cortex is the outermost zone of the lymph node. It is incompletely subdivided into compartments by extensions of the fibrous capsules called *trabeculae*. The compartments of the cortex are distinguished by the presence of lymphoid nodules. Because these lymphoid nodules frequently contain pale central regions (germinal centers), they are called *secondary lymphoid nodules (follicles)*. Secondary lymphoid nodules only form in response to an antigenic challenge. Lymphoid nodules are heavily populated by B lymphocytes, and germinal centers, when present, are the site of plasma cell production. Because of the intense mitotic proliferation of small B lymphocytes, the periphery of the secondary lymphoid nodule is darkly stained. Dendritic follicular cells also are found in the nodules. These cells are a type of antigen-presenting cell and they participate in stimulating the formation of plasma cells.
● Paracortex. T lymphocytes are the primary cellular residents of the paracortex. When challenged by antigens from antigen-presenting cells, T-helper cells become activated. After activation, T-helper cells proliferate and migrate into the medullary sinus where they ultimately exit the lymph node. After leaving the node, the T cells travel to the front of antigenic invasion. High endothelial venules are found in this region. These are unique blood vessels because they are lined by simple cuboidal epithelium rather than simple squamous epithelium.
● Medulla. The hallmark feature of this region is the presence of medullary cords. The medullary cords consist of lymphocytes, plasma cells, macrophages, reticular cells, and reticular fibers. Lymphocytes from this region leave the lymph node through efferent lymphatic vessels.

HOW ARE BREAST CANCERS CLINICALLY STAGED?

Breast carcinomas are clinically staged based on the following characteristics:

● Invasive nature of the cancer
● Size of the neoplasm
● Nodal involvement
● Distant metastases

These factors led to the development of five clinical stages, which are described in Table 2-1.

Another classification paradigm for staging breast cancer is the TNM system. The TNM system stages breast cancers on the basis of tumor size (T), nodal status or involvement (N), and metastases (M). The system is defined in Table 2-2.

TABLE 2–1	Clinical Stages of Breast Cancer and Their Morphologies	
Clinical Stage	**Morphology**	**5-Year Survival Rate**
Stage 0	Carcinoma in situ—the cancer is confined to the ductal system of the breast.	92%
Stage 1	Cancer has invaded stroma of breast.	87%
	Is less than or equal to 2 cm in diameter.	
	Lymph nodes are uninvolved.	
Stage 2	Cancer has invaded stroma of breast.	75%.
	Cancer is less than or equal to 5 cm in diameter.	
	One to three axillary nodes are involved.	
	It is also at stage 2 if the cancer is greater than 5 cm in diameter and nodes are uninvolved.	
Stage 3	Cancer has invaded stroma of breast.	46%
	Cancer is less than or equal to 5 cm in diameter.	
	Four or more axillary lymph nodes are involved.	
	It is also stage 3 if:	
	Cancer is greater than 5 cm in diameter with involvement of axillary lymph nodes, or	
	Cancer is invasive and 10 or more axillary lymph nodes are involved, or	
	Cancer is invasive and ipsilateral parasternal (internal thoracic) lymph nodes are involved, or	
	Cancer is invasive and involves skin, fixation of chest wall, or inflammatory cancer	
Stage 4	Distant metastases are present	13%

TABLE 2-2 TNM System of Breast Cancer Classification

Primary Tumor Size

TX	Primary tumor cannot be evaluated.
T0	No evidence of primary tumor.
Tis	Carcinoma in situ: intraductal carcinoma, lobular carcinoma in situ, or Paget's disease of the nipple with no tumor.
T1	Tumor < 2 cm in greatest dimension.
T2	Tumor > 2 cm and ≤ 5 cm in greatest dimension.
T3	Tumor > 5 cm in greatest dimension.
T4	Tumor of any size with direct involvement to the chest wall or skin (includes inflammatory carcinoma).

Nodal Involvement-N (Nodal Status)

NX	Regional lymph nodes cannot be assessed.
N0	No regional lymph node metastases.
N1	Metastasis to movable (nonfixed) ipsilateral axillary lymph nodes.
N2	Metastases to ipsilateral axillary lymph nodes fixed to one another or to other structures.
N3	Metastases to ipsilateral parasternal (internal thoracic) lymph nodes.

Metastases

M0	No evidence of distant metastasis.
M1	Distant metastases; including metastases to ipsilateral supraclavicular lymph nodes.

(Table adapted from page 1234, Goldman and Ausiello, Cecil Textbook of Medicine, 22nd edition, 2004.)

SOME TUMOR CELLS HAVE DEVISED MECHANISMS TO RESIST THE EFFECTS OF CHEMOTHERAPEUTIC AGENTS. ONE MECHANISM IS THE IMPLEMENTATION OF MDR-1. WHAT IS MDR-1 AND HOW DOES IT CONFER RESISTANCE?

MDR-1 (P-glycoprotein) is a member of a multidrug-resistant protein family. Some types of tumor cells contain a gene that encodes MDR-1 and its over-expression has enabled the tumor cells to resist the action of antimitotic agents. The mechanism is nefariously ingenious. Once the MDR-1 proteins are synthesized, they are transported to and inserted into the plasma membranes of tumor cells. As chemo-therapeutic agents gain entry into the tumor cells, they are immediately pumped out of the cell by the action of the MDR-1, thus protecting the cell from the cytotoxic effects of the pharmacologic agent.

To restore efficacy to chemotherapy, the expression of MDR-1 must be blocked. Investigators are

⌐ not abnormal / just over-expressed

experimenting with RNA interference as a means to inhibit the cancer cell's ability to render itself immune to the action of chemotherapeutic agents. In RNA interference, small interfering RNA fragments (siRNA) are introduced to the tumor cell's genetic machinery for protein synthesis. For example, double-stranded RNA that matches the gene for MDR-1 is introduced into the cell. The introduced double-stranded RNA is subsequently cut into fragments of 21 to 25 nucleotides called *small interfering RNAs*. The enzyme responsible for enzymatically creating the small interfering RNA is the ribonuclease Dicer. Dicer is localized at the endoplasmic reticulum and its ribonuclease activity occurs at the interface of the endoplasmic reticulum and cytoplasm. The small interfering RNAs then instruct another nuclease complex, called the *RNA-induced silencer complex*, to enzymatically destroy the messenger RNA for the MDR-1. This action effectively silences the gene encoding MDR-1 by eliminating its transcript product (mRNA) for translation into the protein. The RNA-induced silencer complexes have been shown to be associated with ribosomes.

While MDR-1 was first discovered in tumor cells, it is also expressed by normal cells. For example, MDR-1 is found in the gastrointestinal tract, kidney, and liver. Its presence in these tissues allows it to limit drug absorption in the gastrointestinal tract and to eliminate what is absorbed into the bile and urine.

SOME TUMOR CELLS HAVE ALSO DEVISED MECHANISMS TO RESIST THE EFFECTS OF RADIATION TREATMENT. HOW DO CANCER CELLS ENDOW THEMSELVES WITH THE ABILITY TO RESIST RADIATION THERAPY?

Cancer cells become desensitized to radiation treatment by overexpressing peroxiredoxins. Peroxiredoxins are a family of peroxidases that protects normal cells against reactive oxygen species. Radiation treatment generates reactive oxygen species that ultimately lead to death of cancer cells. By upregulating perox-iredoxins, cancer cells increase their ability to eliminate generated reactive oxygen intermediates. This desensitizes them to the damaging effects of radiation. This again illustrates just how formidable a foe are cancer cells.

WHAT ARE THE CHECKPOINTS IN THE CELL CYCLE THAT PREVENT A MUTATED CELL FROM ENTERING MITOSIS?

Cells rolling through the cell cycle have evolved quality control mechanisms to maintain the fidelity of the genetic apparatus. The two principal checkpoints in the cell cycle occur at the G_1/S and G_2/M transitions. Cells in the G_1 phase must check the quality of their DNA before entering the S phase, the point of no return. If DNA damage is detected in the G_1 phase, then this phase is braked to a stop to allow time for repair of the DNA. If the damaged DNA is beyond repair, then the apoptotic pathway is triggered to eliminate the cell.

The second checkpoint, G_2/M, serves to assess the fidelity of DNA replication and whether the environment is suitable for the cell to continue into mitosis. Cells with abnormal DNA from the S phase would be prevented from continuing in the cell cycle.

The checkpoints are molecularly regulated. The best characterized molecular police of the cell cycle is p53. The p53 molecule induces p21, a cell-cycle inhibitor, to arrest a cell in the G_1 phase. This molecule also participates in monitoring the G_2/M checkpoint. Defects in these cell-cycle checkpoint molecules are a major cause of allowing genetically unstable cancer cells to run unabated through the cell cycle.

Women with mutations in their BRCA-1 and BRCA-2 genes are at an increased risk of developing breast cancer. Normal BRCA genes play an active role in tumor suppression, regulation of transcription, and repair of DNA.

The mother of a 5-year-old boy, concerned about his inability to gain weight and his coughing and wheezing, appeared in the pediatrician's office. The history revealed that the boy's coughing and wheezing were worse at night and upon wakening and that his stools were foul smelling. The laboratory evaluation showed that sputum culture was positive for *Pseudomonas aeruginosa* and that the chloride sweat test was positive. Chest radiographs revealed hyperinflation, peribronchial cuffing, and mild bronchiectasis. A head x-ray showed opaque paranasal sinuses. The boy was diagnosed with cystic fibrosis. He was treated with gentamicin and piperacillin to eradicate the *Pseudomonas aeruginosa*, pancrelipase, and fat-soluble vitamins A, D, E, and K.

WHAT ARE THE PARANASAL SINUSES AND WHERE DO THEY DRAIN?

The paired, paranasal sinuses reside in the bones of the skull that surround the nasal cavity (Fig. 2-13). The sinuses are lined by ciliated, pseudostratified columnar epithelium containing goblet cells. The thickened mucus produced and secreted by the goblet cells contributes to their opaqueness in cystic fibrosis. The paranasal sinuses and their drainage are (Fig. 2-14):

- Frontal sinuses. Each drains into the frontonasal duct that empties into the anterior portion of the middle meatus.
- Ethmoidal air cells. These are divided into three groups: anterior, middle, and posterior. The anterior and middle air cells drain into the middle meatus and the posterior air cells empty into the superior meatus, however, one or more may open into the adjacent sphenoidal sinus.
- Sphenoidal sinuses. These open into the sphenoethmoidal recesses.
- Maxillary sinuses. These sinuses empty into the middle meatus.

WHICH LOBE OF THE LUNGS IS MOST OFTEN AFFECTED FIRST?

For reasons that have yet to be elucidated, the superior lobe of the right lung is most often the first lobe to show cystic fibrosis-related changes. Figure 2-15 shows pathologic changes in the lung with advanced cystic fibrosis.

WHAT IS THE ETIOLOGY OF CYSTIC FIBROSIS?

Cystic fibrosis is caused by a mutation in the gene that encodes for a chloride ion membrane channel protein. This chloride channel protein is called cystic fibrosis transmembrane conductance regulator (CFTR). When CFTR is expressed normally in epithelial cells lining the respiratory passageways (Fig. 2-16) and the pancreatic ducts, chloride ions are transported out of the cell and into the lumen. CFTR also inhibits the action of the epithelial sodium channel (ENaC). Inhibition of ENaC reduces the reabsorption of sodium ions from the lumina of the respiratory passageways. This action also reduces water reabsorption. The upshot of this is that the mucus is fluid and does not clog the lumina. With defective CFTRs, chloride ions are not secreted and there is increased sodium ion and water reabsorption by the epithelial cells. This enhanced reabsorption leads to the development of thick mucus. Consequently, the lumina of the respiratory passageways become plugged.

Pancreatic insufficiency is usually associated with cystic fibrosis. The insufficiency of pancreatic secretions is also due to a mutation in the CFTR gene. The defective CFTR, however, fails to move bicarbonate ions, rather than chloride, into the lumina of the pancreatic ducts. Failure to add bicarbonate results in a pancreatic juice that is acidic. The acidic juice causes mucins to precipitate and the ducts plug as a result (Fig. 2-17).

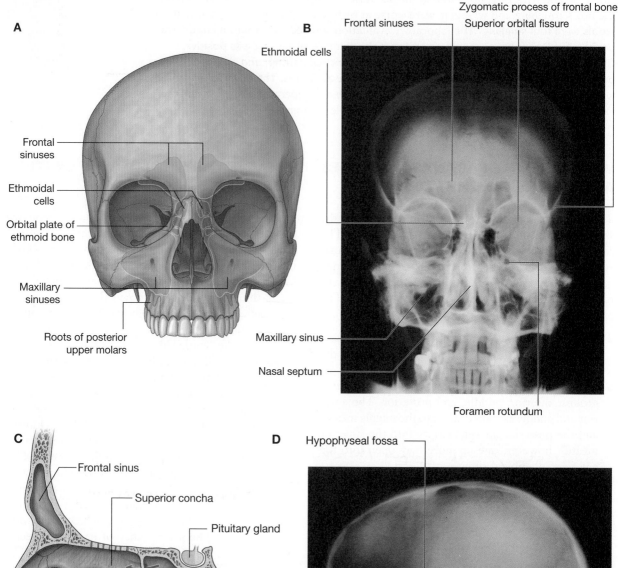

FIGURE 2-13 Paranasal sinuses. **A,** Anterior view. **B,** Posteroanterior skull radiograph. **C,** Parasagittal view of right nasal cavity. **D,** Lateral skull radiograph. (Drake R, Vogl W and Mitchell A: *Gray's Anatomy for Students*. Churchill Livingstone, 2004. Fig. 8-222.)

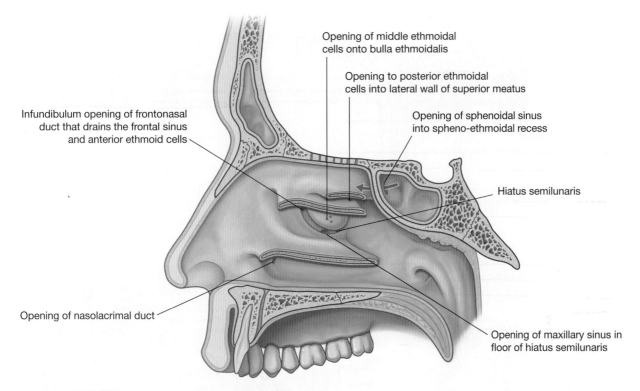

Opening of middle ethmoidal cells onto bulla ethmoidalis

Opening to posterior ethmoidal cells into lateral wall of superior meatus

Opening of sphenoidal sinus into spheno-ethmoidal recess

Infundibulum opening of frontonasal duct that drains the frontal sinus and anterior ethmoid cells

Hiatus semilunaris

Opening of nasolacrimal duct

Opening of maxillary sinus in floor of hiatus semilunaris

FIGURE 2-14 Lateral wall of nasal cavity showing drainage of the paranasal sinuses. (Drake R, Vogl W and Mitchell A: *Gray's Anatomy for Students*. Churchill Livingstone, 2004. Fig. 8-226.)

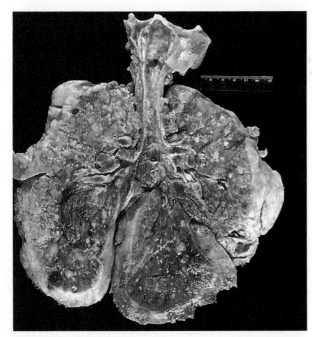

FIGURE 2-15 Lungs with cystic fibrotic changes. Note the extensive nature of mucus plugging and dilation of respiratory passageways. There is also consolidation of the lung tissue. (Kumar V, Abbas A and Fausto N: *Robbins & Cotran Pathologic Basis of Disease*, 7e. WB Saunders, 2004. Fig. 10-23. Courtesy of Dr. Eduardo Yunis, Children's Hospital of Pittsburgh, Pittsburgh, PA.)

IF CYSTIC FIBROSIS CAUSES DECREASED CHLORIDE ION SECRETION, WHY IS THERE CHLORIDE IN SWEAT?

The CFTR in epithelial cells lining sweat gland ducts plays by a different set of rules. Sweat gland ductal cells are specialized to reabsorb chloride and sodium ions. Therefore, CFTR causes movement of chloride ions into the ductal cell and activation of ENaC transport of sodium ions into the cell (Fig. 2-16). When CFTR is defective, the ENaC is inactivated. This results in increased sodium and chloride ion secretion in sweat and a positive chloride sweat test.

WHAT ARE THE PRINCIPLE PANCREATIC DUCTS AND WHERE DO THEY EMPTY?

The pancreas possesses two pancreatic ducts that empty into the second (descending) part of the duodenum. The main pancreatic duct (of Wirsung) joins the

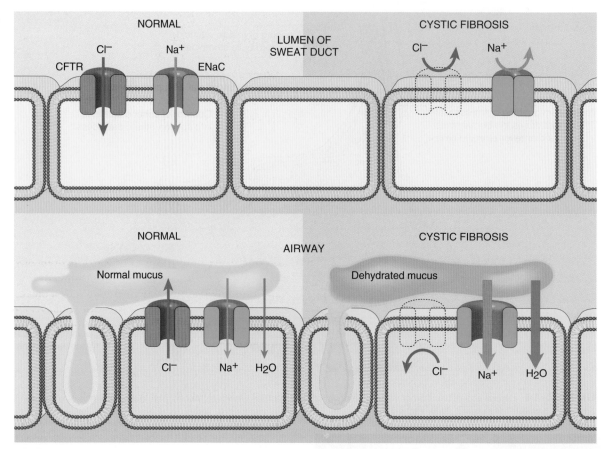

FIGURE 2-16 *Upper figure.* Chloride channel defect in duct of sweat gland increases sodium and chloride concentration is sweat. *Lower figure.* Defective chloride channels in respiratory passageways causes a decrease in chloride secretion and an increase in sodium ion and water reabsorption. This leads to the formation of thick mucus. (Kumar V, Abbas A and Fausto N: *Robbins & Cotran Pathologic Basis of Disease*, 7e. WB Saunders, 2004. Fig. 10-21.)

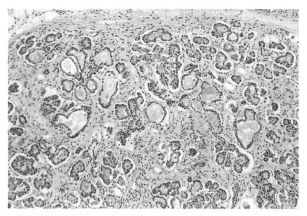

FIGURE 2-17 Changes in the pancreas due to cystic fibrosis. Ducts are dilated and plugged with acidophilic mucus. Glands are shrunken (atrophic) and replaced by collagenous connective tissue. (Kumar V, Abbas A and Fausto N: *Robbins & Cotran Pathologic Basis of Disease*, 7e. WB Saunders, 2004. Fig. 10-24.)

common bile duct at the hepatopancreatic ampulla (of Vater). A thickened circular band of smooth muscle, hepatopancreatic sphincter (of Oddi), regulates the flow of pancreatic juice and bile into the duodenum at the major duodenal papilla. The other duct is called the accessory duct (of Santorini). This duct empties into the duodenum at the minor duodenal papilla, which is located 2 cm proximal to the major duodenal papilla.

A 64-year-old man, presented to his physician complaining of dyspnea. The patient, a smoker (2 packs a day for 45 years), stated that several months ago he noticed that his breathing was labored when he walked up the stairs of his home and that it has progressively worsened. The physical exam results were: height = 70 inches, weight = 150 lb, blood pressure = 135/85, and respiratory rate = 28. Additionally, peripheral cyanosis was noted, breath sounds were markedly diminished, lungs were hyperresonant upon percussion, expirations were prolonged and the patient exhaled through pursed lips, had a barrel chest (anterior-posterior chest dimension was increased), and accessory muscles of respiration were being used for breathing. Lab results for arterial blood gases were: PO_2 = 70 (normal: 75–100), PCO_2 = 52 (normal: 35–45), and pH = 7.30 (normal: 7.35–7.45). Pulmonary function tests indicated the following: increased residual volume, increased total lung capacity, decreased forced expiratory volume, and decreased vital capacity. The patient was diagnosed with emphysema.

WHAT ARE THE ACCESSORY MUSCLES OF RESPIRATION?

There are several accessory muscles of respiration. The muscles for inspiration and expiration are listed in Table 2-3.

DECREASED ARTERIAL OXYGEN SATURATION STIMULATES RESPIRATORY DRIVE. WHERE ARE THE PERIPHERAL CHEMORECEPTORS FOR ARTERIAL OXYGEN LOCATED AND HOW IS THIS SENSORY INFORMATION TRANSMITTED TO THE CENTRAL NERVOUS SYSTEM?

The arterial chemoreceptors are the carotid and aortic bodies. The left and right carotid bodies are reddish-brown and are located in the fork of the bifurcation of the common carotid (Greek for *deep sleep*) artery or posterior to its bifurcation. The carotid branches of the glossopharyngeal nerve (CN IX) innervate each body. This innervation is complemented by a plexus of nerve fibers from the vagus (Latin for *wanderer*) and sympathetics. The glossopharyngeal nerves convey impulses regarding the oxygen saturation to the dorsal respiratory area of the medulla oblongata.

Other small bodies of chemoreceptors are principally located near the aortic arch. These structures are called the *aortic bodies*. Some other bodies are found in the vicinity of the right subclavian vein. The vagus nerves (CN X) transmit impulses regarding the oxygen status to the dorsal respiratory area of the medulla oblongata. In addition to monitoring oxygen, the peripheral chemoreceptors also are specialized to detect changes in carbon dioxide and hydrogen ion concentrations.

WHAT ARE THE HISTOLOGIC CHARACTERISTICS OF THE PERIPHERAL CHEMORECEPTORS?

The carotid and aortic bodies are enveloped by a fibrous capsule, which sends septa into the body that divide it into lobules. Each lobule contains a collection of two cell types: glomus cells (type I cells) and sustentacular cells (type II cells).

Glomus cells are more numerous than the sustentacular cells. They are described as moderately large cells with large nuclei. A few dendritic processes are seen and they contain the usual array of organelles. Secretory granules contain dopamine and the protein glomin.

Sustentacular cells have a role similar to that of glial cells. The long processes of the sustentacular cells wrap almost completely around the glomus cells and the

TABLE 2-3 Accessory Muscle of Respiration	
Inspiration	**Expiration**
Pectoralis major	Quadratus lumborum
Pectoralis minor	Serratus posterior inferior
Serratus anterior	External abdominal oblique
Sternocleidomastoid	Internal abdominal oblique
Scalenus anterior	Transversus abdominis
Scalenus medius	Rectus abdominis
Scalenus posterior	
Serratus posterior superior	
Levatores costarum (longi and breves)	

sustentacular cells support nerve cell processes that lost their Schwann cells when they penetrated the substance of the body

WHAT ARE THE GROSS ANATOMICAL CHARACTERISTICS OF THE RIGHT AND LEFT LUNGS?

The gross anatomical characteristics of the right and left lungs are summarized in Table 2-4.

WHAT IS THE ARTERIAL SUPPLY TO THE LUNGS?

The lungs receive a dual arterial supply. The principal arterial supply is from the right and left pulmonary arteries. These arteries transport deoxygenated blood to the lungs to unload carbon dioxide and to load oxygen. Consequently, these arteries are not responsible for oxygen and nutrient delivery to the lung tissue. Instead, bronchial arteries are responsible for this task. The paired left bronchial arteries supply the left lung and originate directly from the thoracic aorta. The single right bronchial artery usually springs from the right third posterior intercostal artery. The right and left bronchial arteries course along the posterior borders of the bronchi as they penetrate the lung tissue. The bronchial arteries end at the respiratory bronchioles.

WHAT IS THE VENOUS DRAINAGE OF THE LUNGS?

The lung also has a dual system of veins that drain it of venous blood. The right superior and inferior and left superior and inferior pulmonary veins deliver oxygen-enriched blood to the left atrium.

Bronchial veins drain venous blood from the larger branches of the bronchial tree. The two bronchial veins from the right lung empty into the azygos vein, whereas the two left bronchial veins drain into the accessory hemiazygos vein or the left superior intercostal vein. The bronchial veins do not drain all of the blood that is delivered to the lungs by the bronchial arteries. Blood not drained by the bronchial veins is returned to the left atrium by the pulmonary veins.

WHAT IS THE LYMPHATIC DRAINAGE OF THE LUNGS?

Maintaining our dual theme, lymph from the lungs is drained by two lymphatic plexuses. These two lymphatic systems communicate with one another and are called the *superficial (subpleural)* and *deep plexuses*.

The superficial (subpleural) lymphatic plexus, which drains lymph from the visceral pleura and lung, resides internal to the visceral pleura. Lymph from this plexus drains into bronchopulmonary lymph nodes located in the hilum. Lymph then proceeds to superior and inferior tracheobronchial lymph nodes located above and below the tracheal bifurcation.

The deep lymphatic plexus resides in the middle layer of the bronchi, the submucosa, and the adventitia of the bronchi. Lymph then drains into the pulmonary lymph nodes that run along the large branches of the primary bronchi. From the pulmonary lymph nodes, lymph proceeds to the bronchopulmonary lymph nodes in the hilum of each lung. Next, lymph flows into the tracheobronchial lymph nodes (see above).

The tracheobronchial nodes, which receive lymph from the superficial and deep lymphatic plexuses, drain into the right and left bronchomediastinal trunks (Fig. 2-18). The trunks are formed by the efferent lymphatic vessels of parasternal, tracheobronchial, and anterior mediastinal lymph nodes. Both bronchomediastinal trunks empty into the junction of the internal jugular and subclavian veins of its respective side. Alternatively, the trunks may drain into the right lymphatic trunk or thoracic duct.

TABLE 2-4 Features of the Right and Left Lungs		
Feature	**Right Lung**	**Left Lung**
Shape	Short and stout	Tall and narrow
Fissures	Oblique and horizontal	Oblique
Lobes	Three: superior, middle, and inferior	Two: superior and inferior
Bronchopulmonary segments	Ten	Ten
Weight	625 g in average adult	565 g in average lung

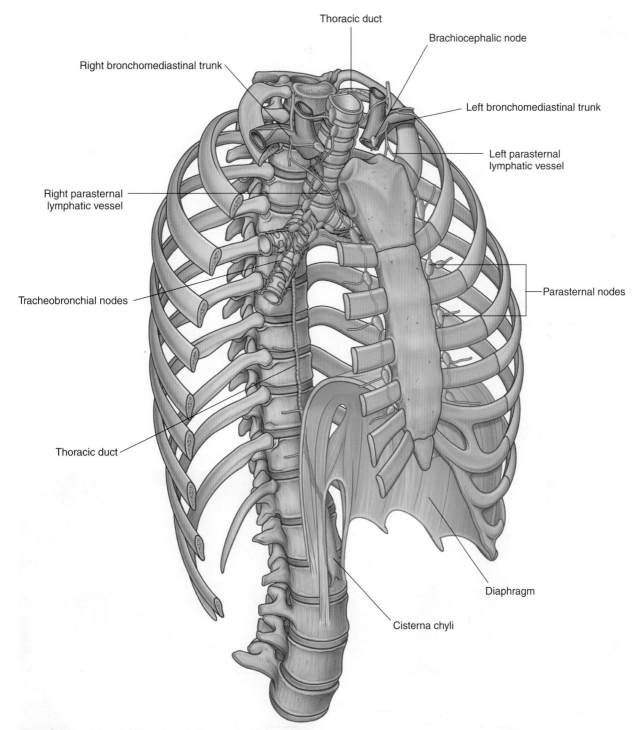

FIGURE 2-18 Lymphatic drainage of lungs. (Drake R, Vogl W and Mitchell A: *Gray's Anatomy for Students*. Churchill Livingstone, 2004. Fig. 3-47.)

WHAT STRUCTURAL ELEMENTS FORM THE BLOOD-AIR BARRIER?

The lungs contain approximately 300 million alveoli with an estimated surface area exceeding 140 square meters. To further the function of gas exchange, the lung is endowed with the highest capillary density of any organ in the body. The number of capillaries ensures that the alveoli are literally bathed with blood. Specifically, the structural components that form the thin blood-air barrier are the (Fig. 2-19):

● Attenuated epithelium of the type I pneumocyte
● Basal laminae of the type I pneumocytes and the endothelial cells
● Endothelial cells of the continuous capillaries

WHAT ARE THE ANATOMICAL RELATIONSHIPS OF THE TRACHEA?

The trachea begins at the level of the sixth cervical vertebra inferior to the cricoid cartilage of the larynx. It descends into the superior mediastinum, where it divides into the right and left primary bronchi. The bifurcation of the trachea, carina (Fig. 2-20), is at the level of the intervertebral disc between the fourth and fifth thoracic vertebrae.

WHAT ARE THE MORPHOLOGIC CHANGES OF THE LUNG THAT ACCOMPANY EMPHYSEMA?

There are four major types of emphysema:

● Centriacinar (Figs. 2-21 and 2-22)
● Panacinar (Figs. 2-21 and 2-22)
● Distal acinar
● Irregular

The four types and their characteristics are described in Table 2-5.

Of these four types, the centriacinar and panacinar forms cause clinically significant airway obstruction. Of these two, centriacinar occurs more frequently.

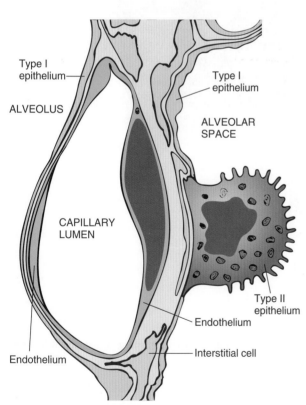

FIGURE 2-19 Microscopic structure of the blood-air barrier. (Kumar V, Abbas A and Fausto N: *Robbins & Cotran Pathologic Basis of Disease*, 7e. WB Saunders, 2004. Fig. 15-1.)

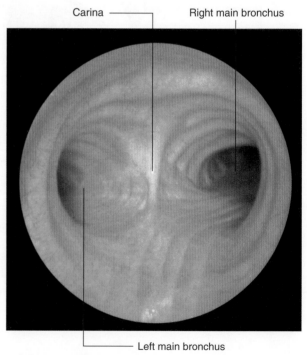

FIGURE 2-20 Bronchoscopic view of the tracheal carina. (Drake R, Vogl W and Mitchell A: *Gray's Anatomy for Students*. Churchill Livingstone, 2004. Fig. 3-48.)

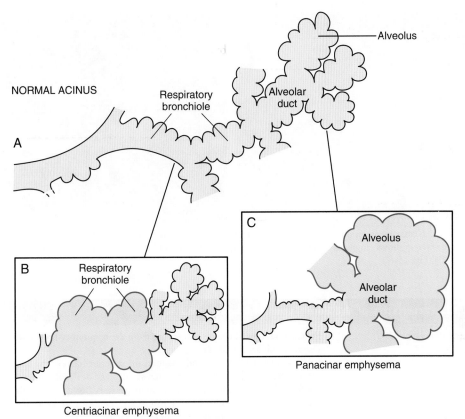

FIGURE 2-21 **A**, Illustration of the normal structure of the acinus. **B**, Centriacinar emphysema showing initial dilation of the respiratory bronchioles. **C**, Panacinar emphysema showing initial involvement of the alveolus and alveolar duct. (Kumar V, Abbas A and Fausto N: *Robbins & Cotran Pathologic Basis of Disease*, 7e. WB Saunders, 2004. Fig. 15-5.)

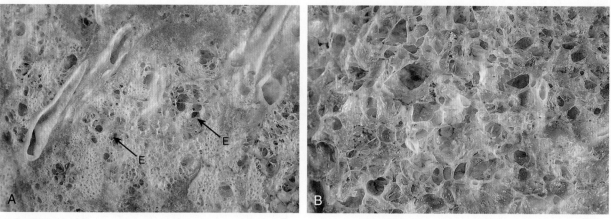

FIGURE 2-22 A, Centriacinar emphysema. Central areas of emphysematous damage are indicated by the arrows. **B**, Panacinar emphysema. The entire tissue shows emphysematous damage. (Kumar V, Abbas A and Fausto N: *Robbins & Cotran Pathologic Basis of Disease, 7e.* WB Saunders, 2004. Fig. 15-6.)

TABLE 2-5 Characteristics of the Four Types of Emphysema

Centriacinar (centrilobular)	Proximal regions of alveoli that spring from the respiratory bronchioles are diseased. Distal alveoli are not affected. Lesions are more frequent and severe in the superior lobes of the lungs. More severe forms result in more extensive damage of the alveoli.
Panacinar (panlobular)	Uniform damage to the alveoli from the respiratory bronchioles to the distal alveoli. Occurs frequently in the inferior portions and anterior margins of the lungs. Tends to be more severe at the bases of the lungs. Associated with alpha$_1$-antitrypsin deficiency.
Distal acinar (paraseptal)	Distal part of alveolus is chiefly damaged. Proximal segments are normal. More severe in superior half of lungs. Enlarged air spaces may form cystlike structures.
Irregular	Air space enlargement is accompanied by fibrosis. Alveoli are irregularly involved.

A full-term, newborn infant was suffering from respiratory distress and cyanosis after his birth. Imaging studies demonstrated lung hypoplasia owing to a decreased thoracic volume.

HOW DO THE LUNGS DEVELOP?

The lungs and their bronchi develop from the lung bud (Fig. 2-23). The lung bud is an outgrowth of the caudal end of the laryngotracheal tube during the fourth week of development. The next event is division of the single lung bud into two bronchial buds (right and left) of endoderm. Each bronchial bud expands to form the primordium of its respective primary bronchus. As in the adult, the embryonic right primary bronchus is larger and more vertically oriented than the left. Each primary bronchus subsequently divides into two secondary or lobar bronchi. The superior secondary bronchus supplies the superior lobe of its respective lung. The right inferior secondary bronchus divides into middle and inferior secondary bronchi that supply the middle and inferior lobes of the right lung. The left inferior secondary bronchus supplies the inferior lobe of the left lung.

Lungs undergo four periods of maturation (Fig. 2-24) beginning at 5 weeks of development and ending in childhood. The four periods of lung maturation are described in Table 2-6.

WHAT IS THE EMBRYONIC BASIS OF LUNG HYPOPLASIA?

The most common cause of lung hypoplasia (reduced lung size) is congenital diaphragmatic hernia (CDH),

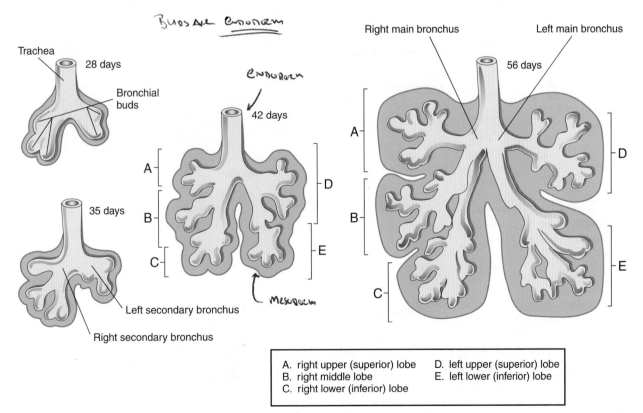

A. right upper (superior) lobe D. left upper (superior) lobe
B. right middle lobe E. left lower (inferior) lobe
C. right lower (inferior) lobe

FIGURE 2-23 Developmental stages of bronchial buds, bronchi, and lungs. (Moore K and Persaud TVN: *The Developing Human,* 7e. WB Saunders, 2003. Fig. 11-8.)

4 stages

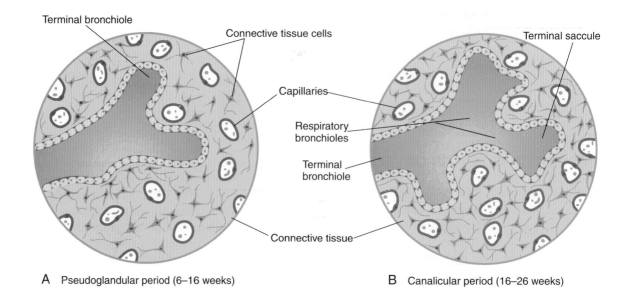

A   Pseudoglandular period (6–16 weeks)

B   Canalicular period (16–26 weeks)

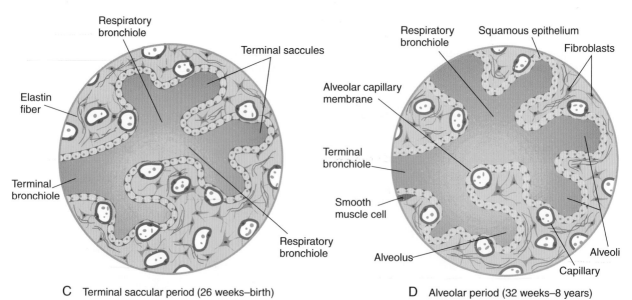

C   Terminal saccular period (26 weeks–birth)

D   Alveolar period (32 weeks–8 years)

FIGURE 2-24 Illustrations of the four periods of lung development. (Moore K and Persaud TVN: *The Developing Human*, 7e. WB Saunders, 2003. Fig. 11-9.)

specifically a Bochdalek hernia. A Bochdalek hernia is located in the left posterolateral region of the diaphragm and is responsible in 85% to 90% of the CDH cases. The embryologic basis of a Bochdalek hernia is failure of the left pleuroperitoneal membrane to form and/or fuse with the other parts of the diaphragm (Fig. 2-25). As a consequence of the defect in the diaphragm, abdominal viscera herniate into the thoracic cavity. Occupancy of the thoracic cavity by

abdominal organs reduces the volume for lung growth and expansion. This leads to lung hypoplasia.

Another cause of lung hypoplasia is a reduction in lung fluid. Fetal lung development is dependent on an adequate volume of fluid in the lungs. Lung fluid, which comprises over 90% of the weight of the lungs in the last trimester, is produced by the lung's epithelial cells. The epithelial cells express chloride ion transporters that move chloride ions into the lumina of the

TABLE 2-6 Periods of Lung Maturation

Period of Maturation	Time Band	Characteristics
① Pseudoglandular	5–17 weeks	Lung has appearance of exocrine. At end of this period all lung structures have developed except the respiratory exchange units.
② Canalicular	16–25 weeks	Cranial segments of lung develop faster than caudal segments. Luminal diameter of bronchi and terminal bronchioles become larger. Lung tissue becomes more vascular. Respiratory bronchioles branch from the terminal bronchioles at end of this period. Alveolar ducts begin to develop from the respiratory bronchioles. Primordial alveoli (terminal sacs) are present.
③ Terminal sac	24 weeks–birth	Rapid development of terminal sacs. Epithelium of terminal sacs becomes greatly attenuated. Capillaries become intimate with the primordial alveoli: blood-air barrier is formed. Type II pneumocytes (alveolar cells) are the first to develop in the alveoli. Type I pneumocytes differentiate from type II pneumocytes and from a population of endodermal cells lining the alveoli. Type II pneumocytes ramp up synthesis of surfactant during the last 2 weeks prior to birth.
④ Alveolar	Late fetal period to childhood	Proliferation of alveoli is rapid the last 4 weeks of the fetal period. 95% of alveoli develop postnatally. Lungs of the newborn contain only 50 million alveoli; the full adult complement of 300 million alveoli is achieved at 8 years of age.

(Handwritten annotations:) = Terminal bronchus develop.
= 1) Dev. of resp. passageways 2. ↑ Vasc 3. Terminal sacs develop
= Develop Blood–Air Barrier

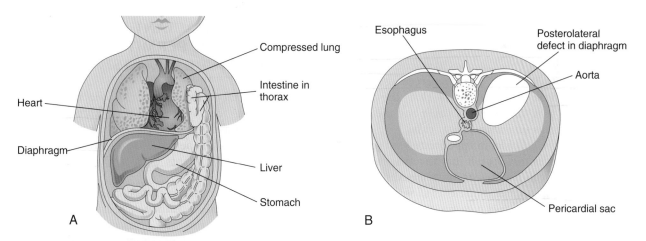

FIGURE 2-25 A, B, Herniation of the intestines through a posterolateral defect in the left side of the diaphragm. (Moore K and Persaud TVN: *The Developing Human,* 7e. WB Saunders, 2003. Fig. 9-10.)

(Handwritten: Amniotic fluid ↑ inhibits by this / heavy = ↓ lung growth)

respiratory passageways. The efflux of chloride ions is accompanied by water. The expanding fluid volume stimulates epithelial cell proliferation and lung growth through mechanical stretching. Any reduction in pulmonary fluid volume removes the stimulus of stretch causing lung hypoplasia.

Lung hypoplasia is associated with the following conditions:

(Handwritten: ↓ amniotic fluid)

- Oligohydramnios (little amniotic fluid)
- Prune-belly syndrome (abdominal wall muscles are poorly developed)

- Dextrocardia
- Abnormal pulmonary vein that empties directly into the inferior vena cava
- Genitourinary malformations

AT WHAT VERTEBRAL LEVEL WOULD THE STOMACH HERNIATE THROUGH THE DIAPHRAGM?

The stomach would herniate into the thoracic cavity through the esophageal hiatus of the diaphragm. The esophageal hiatus is located at the level of the tenth thoracic vertebra.

WHAT ARE THE CYTOLOGIC CHARACTERISTICS OF TYPE II PNEUMOCYTES?

Type II pneumocytes are also known as type II alveolar cells, great alveolar cells, and septal cells. The type II pneumocyte possesses the following cytologic attributes:

- The type II pneumocyte is more abundant than the type I pneumocyte. In spite of its abundance in the alveolar wall, it only comprises 5% of its surface. This quantitative conflict is reconciled by the extremely attenuated morphology of the type I pneumocyte. This means that one type I pneumocyte occupies a large percentage of the alveolar wall. An analogy is that the type I pneumocyte is like a sheet of paper and the type II pneumocyte is similar to a sugar cube.
- The cells are cuboidal in appearance with rounded apical surfaces that project into the alveolar space. Short microvilli are present on its apical surface.
- The centrally located nucleus is slightly irregular and clumps of heterochromatin are found adjacent to the inner nuclear envelope.
- A large volume of rough endoplasmic reticulum and a well-developed Golgi apparatus are appreciated at the level of the electron microscope.
- Mitochondria are present.

- Type II pneumocytes are connected to type I pneumocytes by occluding (tight) junctions.
- The signature feature is the presence of lamellar bodies. Lamellar bodies contain pulmonary surfactant which is synthesized by the rough endoplasmic reticulum and packaged by the Golgi apparatus into composite bodies. Composite bodies then form the lamellar bodies. Pulmonary surfactant is an admixture of phospholipids and surfactant proteins A, B, C, and D. The principle phospholipids are dipalmitoyl phosphatidylcholine and phosphatidylglycerol.
- Lamellar bodies confer a foamy appearance to the cytoplasm.

Pulmonary surfactant functions to prevent alveolar collapse and decreases the work of lung inflation by reducing the surface tension of water molecules along the adlumenal surface of the alveolar cells. To prevent excessive accumulation of surfactant in the alveoli, it is phagocytosed by type II pneumocytes and alveolar macrophages.

Another function of type II pneumocytes is to regenerate the alveolar epithelium. Not only do type II pneumocytes undergo mitosis to replenish themselves, they also regenerate type I pneumocytes.

WHEN IS SURFACTANT PRODUCTION SUFFICIENT TO PERMIT SURVIVAL OF PREMATURE INFANTS?

During the fetal period, surfactant production is most robust during the last two weeks before birth (38 weeks' total gestation). Though surfactant synthesis is reduced prior to this period, it is usually sufficient to permit survival of infants born at 26 to 28 weeks' gestation.

Two hormones play a pivotal role in regulating surfactant production. Although there are probably many more, thyroxine and corticosteroids increase surfactant synthesis. Consequently, corticosteroid therapy was routinely used to treat premature infants. This therapy is being supplanted by the administration of exogenous surfactant.

A 65-year-old retired plasterer presented to his physician with complaints of chest pain and difficulty breathing. He also complained of weakness. The physical examination was unremarkable. Chest radiographs indicated a large diffuse mass in the right pleural cavity. A thoracotomy was performed to obtain a biopsy. The pathologist's report concluded that the patient had malignant mesothelioma.

WHAT ARE THE SURFACE MARKINGS OF THE INFERIOR LIMITS OF THE PARIETAL PLEURA, VISCERAL PLEURA, AND LUNGS AFTER EXPIRATION?

The inferior surface markings of these structures are based on three vertical lines. These are midclavicular, midaxillary, and vertebral. The structures that define the inferior limits are the ribs. Moving from the midclavicular to vertebral lines, the inferior limits of the parietal pleura are represented by ribs 8, 10, and 12 (Fig. 2-26). Because the visceral pleura is adhered to the surface of the lung, both these structures share the same limits. Again, proceeding from the midclavicular to the vertebral lines, the inferior limits are ribs 6, 8, and 10 (Fig. 2-27).

WHAT ARE THE HISTOLOGIC CHARACTERISTICS OF THE PARIETAL AND VISCERAL PLEURAE?

The parietal and visceral pleurae comprise a layer of mesothelial cells supported by a basal lamina. Deep to the basal lamina are elastic and collagen fibers, ground substance, macrophages, fibroblasts, lymphatics, and neurovascular structures. The mesothelial cells have microvilli and cilia on their luminal surfaces, and the cells contain numerous micropinocytotic vesicles. Mesothelial cells are specialized for the secretion of proteoglycans rich in hyaluronic acid, a glycosaminoglycan. The proteoglycans are responsible for reducing the friction between the visceral and parietal layers of the pleura.

WHAT IS THE ARTERIAL SUPPLY OF THE PARIETAL AND VISCERAL PLEURAE?

The parietal pleura receives its arterial supply from vessels that supply the body wall. These vessels are the:

- Anterior and posterior intercostal arteries
- Internal thoracic artery
- Musculophrenic artery

The visceral pleura receives its blood supply from the right and left bronchial arteries. Two left bronchial arteries arise from the aorta. The single right bronchial artery springs from the third right posterior intercostal artery, which is the first posterior intercostal artery that issues from the aorta.

WHAT IS THE LYMPHATIC DRAINAGE OF THE PARIETAL AND VISCERAL PLEURAE?

The lymph from the parietal pleura flows to the body wall. From the body wall, lymph drains to the:

- Intercostal lymph nodes
- Parasternal lymph nodes
- Posterior mediastinal lymph nodes
- Diaphragmatic lymph nodes

The visceral pleura is drained by the superficial (subpleural) lymphatic plexus. This lymphatic network is visible as fine black lines on the external surfaces of lungs of older people owing to the accumulation of small particulate material that has

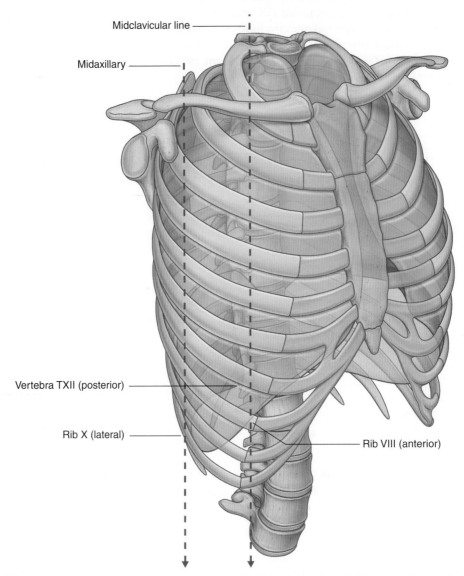

Midclavicular line

Midaxillary

Vertebra TXII (posterior)

Rib X (lateral)

Rib VIII (anterior)

FIGURE 2-26   Topography of the parietal pleura to the ribs. (Drake R, Vogl W and Mitchell A: *Gray's Anatomy for Students*. Churchill Livingstone, 2004. Fig. 3-37.)

been inspired over their lifetime. Lymph is conveyed from this superficial plexus to the bronchopulmonary lymph nodes located in the hilum of each lung.

WHAT IS THE INNERVATION OF THE PARIETAL AND VISCERAL PLEURAE?

The parietal pleurae receive their nerve supply from the intercostal and phrenic (C3-C5) nerves. The visceral pleurae are supplied by sympathetic and parasympathetic fibers that originate from lateral gray horns of spinal cord segments T2-T4 and the vagus

nerves, respectively. The autonomic fibers commingle in the anterior and posterior pulmonary plexuses and their fibers accompany the respiratory passageways and vessels into the lung.

WHAT ARE THE MORPHOLOGIC CHARACTERISTICS OF A MALIGNANT MESOTHELIOMA?

A malignant mesothelioma is an aggressive tumor that proliferates diffusely in the pleural cavity. Grossly, it appears as a grayish-pink layer of gel-like tissue that

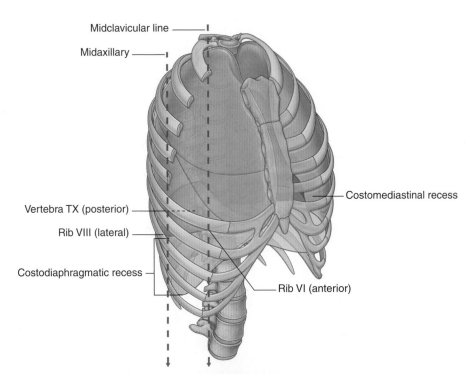

Midclavicular line

Midaxillary

Vertebra TX (posterior)

Rib VIII (lateral)

Costodiaphragmatic recess

Costomediastinal recess

Rib VI (anterior)

FIGURE 2-27 Topography of the visceral pleura and lungs to the ribs. (Drake R, Vogl W and Mitchell A: *Gray's Anatomy for Students.* Churchill Livingstone, 2004. Fig. 3-38.)

envelops the lung (Fig. 2-28). Microscopically, two types of cells can be identified: epithelium-like lining cells and mesenchymal stromal cells.

The epithelioid cells have the following characteristics:

- Appear as flattened, cuboidal, or columnar cells. The cells may be arranged so that they resemble an adenocarcinoma.
- Exhibit pronounced staining for the intermediate filament keratin. Keratin staining shows a greater accumulation of keratin around the nucleus (perinuclear) than at the cell's periphery.
- Carcinoembryonic antigen (CEA) is not expressed; therefore, staining for this marker is negative. Staining for CEA is positive in pulmonary adenocarcinoma.
- Long, slender microvilli and abundant tonofilaments are observed with electron microscopy. In contrast, cells of pulmonary adenocarcinoma possess microvilli that are short and stout. Electron microscopy is considered the gold standard in differentiating mesothelioma from pulmonary adenocarcinoma.

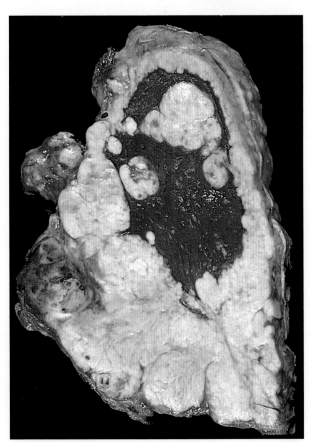

FIGURE 2-28 Malignant mesothelioma. The mesothelioma is the thick, white growth that envelops the lung. (Kumar V, Abbas A and Fausto N: *Robbins & Cotran Pathologic Basis of Disease,* 7e. WB Saunders, 2004. Fig. 15-48.)

A 62-year-old man complaining of crushing chest pain was rushed to the emergency room by ambulance. The physical examination showed that his pulse was 105 beats per minute (sinus tachycardia) and regular, arterial pressure was 130/92, and his respiratory rate was 26 breaths per minute (normal is 12–22). His EKG showed ST segment elevation and the patient was prophylactically administered aspirin and atenolol, a beta$_1$-selective adrenergic antagonist. A blood sample from the patient revealed that the serum cardiac marker, cardiac-derived troponin I (c-TnI), was elevated. An angiogram was performed and the results showed that the proximal one-third of the left anterior descending artery was 95% occluded, the proximal one-third of the circumflex artery was 80% occluded, and the proximal one-third of the right coronary artery was 75% occluded. Because of the multiple stenotic lesions, a triple coronary bypass was performed. The bypass procedure was successful, but the patient's ejection fraction was below normal. Digoxin was prescribed to improve contractile activity.

WHAT IS THE ARTERIAL SUPPLY TO THE HEART?

The heart is supplied by the right and left coronary arteries (Fig. 2-29). The ostia of these vessels are located in the aortic sinuses (of Valsalva) superior to the right and left coronary cusps of the aortic semilunar valve.

The right coronary artery travels in the atrioventricular (coronary) sulcus around the right margin of the heart and continues in the posterior interventricular sulcus as the posterior interventricular artery. The posterior interventricular artery issues septal branches that penetrate and supply the posterior one-third of the interventricular septum. Along its course it gives rise to the sinuatrial (sinoatrial) nodal artery, the right marginal artery, and the atrioventricular nodal artery.

The left coronary artery is a short vessel (average length of 2 cm) that promptly divides into the larger anterior interventricular artery (known clinically as the left anterior descending artery) and the circumflex artery. The anterior interventricular artery runs in the anterior interventricular sulcus giving rise to one or more diagonal branches. Diagonal arteries course obliquely across the anterior surface of the left ventricle toward its left border. Septal branches issue from the anterior interventricular artery and penetrate the interventricular septum. The anterior and posterior interventricular arteries anastomose in the vicinity of the apex. The circumflex artery travels in the coronary sulcus and wraps around the left border of the heart. At the left border it issues a marginal artery. Posteriorly, the circumflex artery normally anastomoses with the right coronary artery.

WHAT ARE SOME OF THE VARIATIONS IN THE CORONARY ARTERIES?

Variations in the coronary arteries are common. Some of these variations are:

- Coronary circulation is left dominant. In this arterial pattern, the left coronary artery, rather than the right, continues as the posterior interventricular artery. This occurs in about 15% of the population.
- The coronary arterial circulation is balanced; neither coronary is dominant.
- Only one coronary artery is present.
- Three coronary arteries are present.

WHAT IS THE FUNCTION OF THE AORTIC AND PULMONIC SINUSES?

The aortic and pulmonic sinuses are dilatations of the aorta and pulmonary trunk just superior to each of the semilunar cusps. When blood is ejected from each ventricle, its flow creates eddy currents between the open valve cusps and the sinuses. This prevents the valves from being slapped against the outflow arteries. This allows the cusps to close quickly during diastole. If the sinuses were absent, the cusps would be forced against the vascular wall during systole. This would ultimately delay their closing during ventricular relaxation.

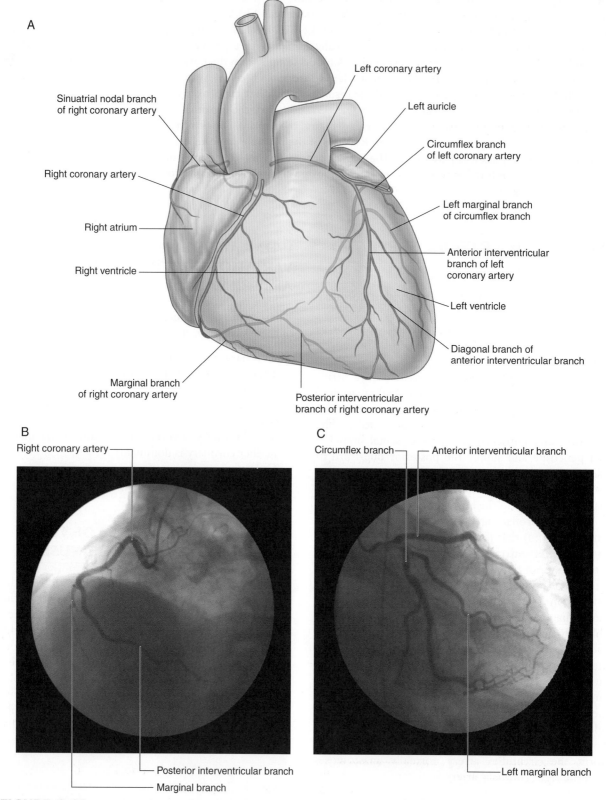

FIGURE 2-29 **A**, Anterior view of the coronary arteries. **B**, Left anterior oblique arteriogram of right coronary artery. **C**, Right anterior oblique arteriogram of left coronary artery. (Drake R, Vogl W and Mitchell A: *Gray's Anatomy for Students.* Churchill Livingstone, 2004. Fig. 3-72.)

WHAT IS THE VENOUS DRAINAGE OF THE HEART?

There are three systems of veins that drain the heart: (1) coronary sinus and its tributaries, (2) anterior cardiac veins, and (3) venae cordis minimae.

- Coronary sinus. Most of the cardiac veins empty into the coronary sinus. The coronary sinus is nestled in the posterior aspect of the atrioventricular (coronary) sulcus between the left atrium and left ventricle. The coronary sinus empties into the right atrium. The semilunar valve of the coronary sinus prevents retrograde blood flow into the coronary sinus during right atrial contraction.
- Great cardiac vein. This vein begins at the apex of the heart and accompanies the anterior interventricular artery. It reaches the coronary sulcus and courses to the left to terminate in the coronary sinus.
- Middle cardiac vein. This vein begins at the apex and accompanies the posterior interventricular artery. It ends in the coronary sinus just before it empties into the right atrium.
- Posterior vein of the left ventricle. This vein travels on the diaphragmatic surface of the left ventricle to the left of the middle cardiac vein to end in the coronary sinus.
- Oblique vein of the left atrium. This small vein courses obliquely along the posterior surface of the left atrium to empty into the coronary sinus before it ends in the right atrium. The oblique vein of the left atrium is a remnant of the left common cardinal vein.
- Anterior cardiac veins. These veins (usually two to three) drain the anterior part of the right ventricle. After crossing the coronary sulcus they empty directly into the right atrium.
- Venae cordis minimae (Thebesian veins). These minute veins empty into all four cardiac chambers, being more numerous in the atria.

WHAT IS THE INNERVATION OF THE HEART?

The heart is innervated by the parasympathetic and sympathetic nervous systems, which form a cardiac plexus. Parasympathetic innervation is provided by the vagus nerves as follows:

- Cardiac branches from the vagus nerves convey preganglionic fibers.
- Preganglionic parasympathetic fibers synapse in ganglia located in the cardiac plexus or in the wall of the atria.
- Postganglionic fibers leave the ganglia to innervate the atrial muscle.

Sympathetic innervation to the heart is provided as follows:

- Preganglionic sympathetic fibers originate from the lateral gray horns of thoracic spinal cord segments T1-T5.
- Preganglionic fibers synapse with ganglia located in the cervical and superior thoracic segments of the sympathetic trunk.
- Postganglionic fibers leave cervical and upper thoracic ganglia and proceed to the heart by passing through the cardiac plexus.

WHAT CORONARY ARTERY IS MOST FREQUENTLY NARROWED OR THROMBOSED?

The frequencies at which the coronary arteries are lesioned or thrombosed are:

- Anterior interventricular artery (left anterior descending): 40% to 50%
- Right coronary artery: 30% to 40%
- Circumflex artery: 15% to 30%

WHAT BLOOD VESSELS CAN BE USED FOR CORONARY ARTERY BYPASS GRAFTS?

Several vessels (veins and arteries) may be used as coronary artery bypass grafts. Most commonly, the great saphenous vein is used as a graft. The small saphenous vein may be used if the great saphenous vein is unsuitable or unavailable (e.g., harvested for a previous bypass procedure).

The preferred vascular conduits, however, are the right and/or left internal thoracic arteries. Arteries are preferred because they are more likely to remain patent over a 10-year period than venous conduits. The left internal thoracic artery is typically used to bypass the anterior interventricular artery, whereas the right internal thoracic artery is used to bypass the right coronary artery. If the right internal thoracic artery is sufficiently long, it can be grafted to the posterior interventricular artery or branches of the left coronary artery. The radial and gastro-omental arteries can also be used as bypass grafts.

The great saphenous vein begins anterior to the medial malleolus of the tibia as a continuation of the medial marginal vein. It then ascends subcutaneously along the medial leg and thigh. At the height of its ascension, it passes through the fossa ovalis, an opening in the fascia lata, to terminate in the femoral vein. Harvesting the great saphenous vein requires ligation of its tributaries. To prevent injury to the valves in the saphenous graft, the inferior end of the vein graft is anastomosed to the proximal end of the coronary artery and the superior end of the vein is sutured to the distal end of the coronary artery. This maintains anterograde blood flow through the venous graft.

The small saphenous vein begins posterior to the lateral malleolus of the fibula as a continuation of the lateral marginal vein and ends in the popliteal vein.

The internal thoracic artery takes origin from the first part of the subclavian artery. It courses inferiorly along the lateral margins of the sternum until it terminates at the level of the sixth intercostal space by dividing into the superior epigastric and musculophrenic arteries. The main branches springing from the internal thoracic artery are the anterior intercostal arteries to the first six intercostal spaces and the pericardiacophrenic artery. The anterior intercostal arteries to intercostal spaces seven to nine issue from the musculophrenic artery. The branches of the internal thoracic artery must be ligated before the vessel can be used for a coronary bypass. The artery is mobilized and an end-to-end anastomosis connects its divided end to the coronary artery. Thus, blood flows from the subclavian artery to the internal thoracic to reach the coronary circulation.

HOW IS ARTERIAL FLOW TO THE INTERCOSTAL SPACES MAINTAINED IF THE INTERNAL THORACIC ARTERY IS USED AS A CONDUIT FOR CORONARY BYPASS?

The intercostal spaces also are supplied by posterior intercostal arteries, which anastomose with the anterior intercostal arteries springing from the internal thoracic and musculophrenic arteries. There are 11 pairs of posterior intercostal arteries in contrast to the 9 pairs of anterior intercostal arteries. The last two intercostal spaces do not extend far enough anteriorly to require anterior intercostal arteries. The posterior intercostal arteries spring from two sources:

- Superior intercostal artery. This artery divides into the posterior intercostal arteries that supply the first two intercostal spaces. It branches from the costocervical trunk, which springs from the second part of the subclavian artery.
- Aorta. The aorta issues the posterior intercostal arteries that supply the inferior nine intercostal spaces. The third posterior intercostal artery, the first posterior intercostal artery that originates from the aorta, forms an anastomosis with the superior intercostal artery.

SOME PATIENTS EXPERIENCE SENSORY DEFICITS IN THEIR LOWER EXTREMITY AFTER HARVESTING OF THE GREAT SAPHENOUS VEIN. WHAT IS THE ANATOMICAL BASIS OF THIS SENSORY DEFICIT?

The saphenous nerve (L3-L4) accompanies the great saphenous vein in the leg and may be injured during the harvesting of the vein. The nerve, a branch of the femoral nerve (L2-L4), is purely sensory in its distribution. The saphenous nerve branches from the femoral nerve in the femoral triangle and accompanies the femoral artery and vein into the adductor canal. It exits the adductor canal, proximal to the adductor hiatus, by passing between the sartorius and gracilis muscles, emerging subcutaneously into the leg. The saphenous nerve innervates the skin on the medial side of the knee, leg, and foot (Fig. 2-30).

WHAT ARE THE HISTOLOGIC CHARACTERISTICS OF THE ARTERIAL AND VENOUS SEGMENTS OF THE CIRCULATORY SYSTEM?

The histologic characteristics of arteries and veins are described in Table 2-7.

WHAT ARE THE TYPES OF CAPILLARIES, THEIR CHARACTERISTICS, AND LOCATION?

The three types of capillaries, their characteristics, and their location are described in Table 2-8.

As shown in Table 2-8, cardiac muscle tissue is endowed with continuous capillaries. Because the

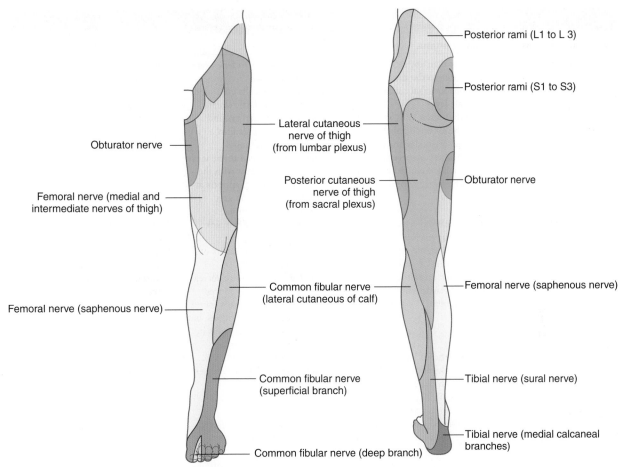

FIGURE 2-30 Areas of skin innervated by the saphenous and other peripheral nerves. (Drake R, Vogl W and Mitchell A: *Gray's Anatomy for Students*. Churchill Livingstone, 2004. Fig. 6-19.)

heart is dependent on aerobic metabolism to generate adenosine triphosphate (ATP), the active organ is supplied by 2,000 to 5,000 capillaries per mm² of tissue.

BY WHAT PROCESS IS LOW-DENSITY LIPOPROTEIN (LDL) TAKEN UP BY CELLS, THEREBY LOWERING ITS CONCENTRATION IN THE BLOOD?

Most cells use receptor-mediated endocytosis to selectively take up cholesterol. Cholesterol is transported in the blood by LDL. To take up cholesterol for the synthesis of membranes, cells synthesize LDL receptors and insert them into their plasma membrane. The LDL receptors aggregate within clathrin-coated pits. The aggregation is accomplished by cytosolic proteins, called *adaptins*, that link LDL receptors to the clathrin of the coated vesicle. The receptors are now positioned to bind with their ligand.

The binding of LDL to its receptor results in the internalization of the LDL through the formation of coated vesicles. The coated vesicles then shed their clathrin coat. The contents of the naked vesicles are delivered to early endosomes. In the harsh acid environment of the endosomes, the LDL dissociates from its receptor and is ultimately transported to lysosomes. The action of lysozymes forms free cholesterol, which is used by the cell for membrane synthesis.

Cholesterol uptake is tightly regulated by the cell. If free cholesterol becomes too abundant intracellularly, the cell responds by:

● Stopping synthesis of cholesterol
● Shutting down synthesis of LDL receptors

Both of these mechanisms lead to an intracellular decrease in free cholesterol.

Conversely, if intracellular free cholesterol is too low, the cell quickly responds by ramping up synthesis

TABLE 2-7 Histologic Characteristics of the Vascular Segments

Vascular Structure	Tunica Intima	Tunica Media	Tunica Adventitia
Elastic artery	Thicker than any arterial vessel. Thick due to the thick subendothelial connective tissue layer. Smooth muscle cells are found in the subendothelial layer. Internal elastic lamina is difficult to observe since it is readily confused with the elastic lamellae of the media.	Concentric sheets of fenestrated elastic lamellae. Smooth muscle cells are found between the elastic sheets. Reticular fibers and ground substance (chondroitin sulfate) is also found. External elastic membrane is not always evident with the light microscope; appears at high magnification as a discontinuous lamina.	Thin. Elastic and collagen fibers. Vasa vasorum—may penetrate as far as into the outer half of the media.
Muscular artery	Subendothelial layer is thicker than an arteriole but thinner than an elastic artery. Smooth muscle cells are found at branching sites. Internal elastic lamina is prominent.	Smooth muscle is the major tissue. Up to 40 concentric layers of smooth muscle. Elastic lamellae steadily decrease as the diameter is reduced. External elastic lamina is found in large muscular arteries, but is thin and discontinuous in small muscular arteries.	Thick: inner dense region; outer loose layer. Elastic and collagen fibers. Vasa vasorum—may penetrate into the outer media in larger vessels.
Arteriole	Subendothelial layer is thin. Internal elastic lamina is only found in larger arterioles (>50 µm).	1–2 layers of smooth muscle. External elastic lamina is absent.	Thin. Vasa vasorum are absent.
Venule	Endothelium and basal lamina. Thin subendothelial layer. Internal elastic lamina is absent.	Thin. 0–2 layers of smooth muscle. Media may be absent in small venules where pericytes would relate to its relative position. External elastic lamina is absent.	Thin in small venules. Thickest layer in large venules.
Small and medium veins	Thin. Subendothelial layer is thin or absent. Poorly defined internal elastic lamina. May form valves.	2–4 layers of smooth muscle. Collagen, elastic, and reticular fibers. Thin. External elastic lamina is absent.	Well-developed. In medium veins, it's the thickest layer. Collagen fibers and some smooth muscle cells. Vasa vasorum.
Large vein (i.e., IVC)	Well developed. Internal elastic lamina is present.	Poorly developed. Few smooth muscle cells. Abundant connective tissue. External elastic lamina is poorly defined or absent.	Thickest of the three tunics. Collagen and smooth muscle fibers (longitudinally arranged). Vasa vasorum. Cardiac muscle fibers near the heart.

of cholesterol and LDL receptors. The additional LDL receptors increase uptake of LDL by the cell.

Some individuals have a corrupt regulatory pathway for cholesterol uptake. In familial hypercholesterolemia, individuals possess mutations in the gene encoding LDL receptors. This derangement in LDL receptor synthesis reduces LDL uptake by the cells, causing elevated LDL levels in the blood. In a rare form of hypercholesterolemia, the defect is not with the receptor but with the cytosolic protein adaptin. In this case, LDL binds to its receptor, but the receptor and its ligand are unable to link to the clathrin vis-à-vis adaptin. Therefore, LDL is not endocytosed. Plasma cholesterol levels are typically 300 to 500 mg/dL, but in rare cases, 800 to 1,000 mg/dL have been measured.

TABLE 2-8 Characteristics and Location of Capillaries

Type of Capillary	Characteristics	Location
Continuous	10 µm in diameter. Tight junctions (complete belts or incomplete) between endothelial cells. Endothelial cells lack pores or fenestrae. Endothelial cells contain numerous pinocytotic vesicles. Well-developed basal lamina. Pericytes are enclosed by the basal lamina and processes make physical contact with the endothelial cell.	Brain (tight junctions are continuous). Muscle. Connective tissue. Exocrine glands.
Fenestrated	10 µm in diameter. Fenestrae (pores) are present in the walls of endothelial cells. Pores are usually closed by a thin diaphragm. Basal lamina is continuous. Pericytes are enclosed by the basal lamina and processes make physical contact with the endothelial cell.	Kidney, nonglomerular. Kidney, glomerulus—diaphragms are absent. Endocrine glands. Intestines.
Sinusoidal	30–40 µm in diameter. Discontinuous endothelial lining: large opening between endothelial cells. Discontinuous or absent basal lamina. Macrophages are associated with these vessels.	Red bone marrow. Liver. Spleen. Adrenal cortex.

WHAT ARE THE CYTOLOGIC EVENTS IN THE DEVELOPMENT OF ATHEROSCLEROSIS?

It is hypothesized that the pathogenesis of atherosclerosis is caused by chronic endothelial cell injury. Chronic cell injury leads to inflammation and an activation of repair processes that, when unchecked, cause intimal thickening, which obstructs the vascular lumen. This theory, which is illustrated in Figure 2-31, proposes that the following cytologic interactions occur:

- Endothelial cells become damaged because of chronic injurious stimuli (e.g., hyperlipidemia, hypertension, elevated homocysteine, and smoking).
- The endothelium becomes dysfunctional. There is increased permeability, with leukocyte adhesion and migration of monocytes into the subendothelial layer.
- Lipoproteins accumulate and are oxidized in the tunica intima.
- Platelets adhere to denuded endothelium. Irreversibly damaged endothelial cells die off, exposing the underlying subendothelial layer. These areas represent denuded endothelium.
- Endothelial cells, macrophages, and platelets release an ensemble of cytokines and growth factors that cause smooth muscle cells to migrate from the tunica media to the subendothelium, morph into a synthetic phenotype, and proliferate. The synthetic phenotype is responsible for the elaboration of extracellular matrix elements (i.e., proteoglycans and collagen fibers and elastin).
- Macrophages and smooth muscle cells imbibe oxidized lipoproteins. Because of their voracious appetite for oxidized lipoproteins, macrophages and smooth muscle cells appear foamy with microscopic observation. Macrophages and smooth muscle cells that have acquired this appearance are appropriately called *foam cells*. Most of the foam cells are macrophages.
- The accumulation of lipoproteins, deposition of extracellular matrix material, proliferation of smooth muscle cells, and the continued emigration of monocytes into the intima all contribute to intimal thickening and the development of atherosclerotic plaque.

TABLE 2-9 Characteristics of Infarcted Cardiac Tissue Over Time

Time	Gross Features	Light Microscopic Features	Electron Microscopic Features
Reversible Injury			
0–1/2 hr	None	None	Relaxation of myofibrils; loss of glycogen, swelling of organelles (e.g., mitochondria)
Irreversible Injury			
1/2–4 hr	None	Usually none to muscle fibers exhibit variable waviness at borders	Disruption of sarcolemma; amorphous densities form in mitochondria.
4–12 hr	Occasional dark spotting (mottling)	Beginning of coagulation necrosis; edema; hemorrhage.	
12–24 hr	Dark spotting	Ongoing coagulation necrosis; pyknotic nuclei; myocyte hypereosinophilia; marginal contraction band necrosis; neutrophils begin to infiltrate.	
1–3 days	Spotting with yellow-tan infarct center	Coagulation necrosis with loss of nuclei and striations; neutrophils have infiltrated interstitium.	
3–7 days	Hyperemic (increased blood flow) border; softening of yellow-tan infarct center.	Dead cardiomyocytes begin to disintegrate; dying neutrophils; dead cells are phagocytosed by macrophages at infarct margin.	
7–10 days	Infarct center is maximally yellow-tan and soft; infarct margins are depressed and red-tan in color.	Prolific phagocytosis of dead cells; early formation of fibrovascular granulation tissue at margins.	
10–14 days	Depressed infarct borders are red-gray	Granulation tissue is well-developed; new blood vessel formation; collagen deposition.	
2–8 weeks	Gray-white scar, progressive from border toward core of infarct	Increased collagen deposition; decreased cellularity	
> 2 months	Scarring process is complete	Dense collagenous scar	

(Table adapted from 579, Kumar et al., Robbins and Cotram Pathologic Basis of Disease, 7th edition, 2005)

WHAT IS THE CELLULAR MECHANISM BY WHICH MONOCYTES ADHERE TO THE ENDOTHELIUM?

Endothelial cells contain genes that encode various adhesion molecules. Vascular cell adhesion-1 (VCAM-1) plays a pivotal role in attracting monocytes. Expression of VCAM-1 on the plasmalemma of endothelial cells causes monocytes to adhere to its surface. Once adhered, monocytes emigrate into the subendothelium.

A LIFE-THREATENING COMPLICATION THAT MAY FOLLOW A MYOCARDIAL INFARCTION IS VENTRICULAR FIBRILLATION. WHAT ARE THE STRUCTURAL ELEMENTS OF THE HEART'S CONDUCTION SYSTEM?

The heart's conduction system is composed of modified cardiomyocytes. The modified cardiac muscle cells form the sinuatrial (SA) node, atrioventricular (AV) node, and atrioventricular bundles of His (common and right and left). The structural elements are described below:

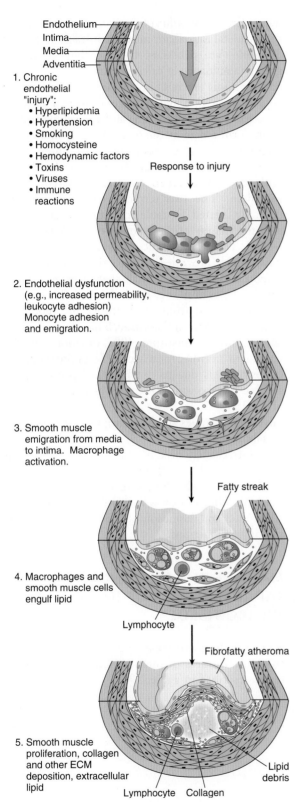

Endothelium
Intima
Media
Adventitia

1. Chronic
   endothelial
   "injury":
   • Hyperlipidemia
   • Hypertension
   • Smoking
   • Homocysteine
   • Hemodynamic factors
   • Toxins
   • Viruses
   • Immune
     reactions

Response to injury

2. Endothelial dysfunction
   (e.g., increased permeability,
   leukocyte adhesion)
   Monocyte adhesion
   and emigration.

3. Smooth muscle
   emigration from media
   to intima. Macrophage
   activation.

Fatty streak

4. Macrophages and
   smooth muscle cells
   engulf lipid

Lymphocyte

Fibrofatty atheroma

5. Smooth muscle
   proliferation, collagen
   and other ECM
   deposition, extracellular
   lipid

Lymphocyte   Collagen

Lipid
debris

FIGURE 2-31 Key events in the pathogenesis of athero-sclerosis. (Kumar V, Abbas A and Fausto N: *Robbins & Cotran Pathologic Basis of Disease*, 7e. WB Saunders, 2004. Fig. 11-11.)

● SA node. SA nodal cells are smaller than contractile atrial cells and contain fewer and more poorly arrayed myofibrils. The SA node lacks intercalated discs but other types of intercellular junctions exist.

● AV node. The cells of the AV node are similar to the SA nodal cells.

● AV bundles. Emerging from the AV node is a common bundle of specialized conducting cells. The common bundle bifurcates into right and left AV bundle branches that travel in the subendocardial layer of the endocardium on both sides of the interventricular septum. The specialized conducting cells in the proximal AV bundle appear similar to those in the AV node. Along the distal AV bundle branches, the cells distinguish themselves structurally. These cells are called Purkinje cells or fibers. Purkinje fibers are approximately 30 μm in diameter (twice the diameter of contractile ventricular myocytes) and contain one or two nuclei. Their cytoplasm contains abundant mitochondria and glycogen, but myofibrils are sparse. Purkinje fibers ultimately terminate on contractile ventricular myocytes residing in the endomyocardium (inner layer of the myocardium). Purkinje fibers are connected to one another and to contractile ventricular myocytes by gap junctions. Their large size and the presence of gap junctions propagate action potentials at high velocity.

Because Purkinje fibers reside in the inner layer of the heart wall, they are vulnerable to ischemic damage. Consequently, patients recovering from a myocardial infarction may experience ventricular arrhythmias due to Purkinje fiber injury.

WHAT ARE THE HISTOLOGIC CHARACTERISTICS OF THE HEART?

The heart is composed of three layers. From external to internal, the layers are the epicardium, myocardium, and endocardium. These layers are described below.

● Epicardium. The epicardium is composed of two layers: an outer layer of mesothelium supported by a basal lamina and an inner layer called the *subepicardium*. The subepicardium contains loose connective tissue, adipose tissue, coronary blood vessels, nerves, and ganglia.

● Myocardium. The myocardium is the middle and thickest layer of the heart. The layer contains contractile cardiac muscle cells and cardiac muscle cells specialized for controlling the heart's rhythmicity and secreting hormones. The hormone-secreting specialized cardiac muscle cells are chiefly located in the atria. The small peptide hormones secreted by the heart are atriopeptin, atrionatriuretic polypeptide, cardiodilatin, and cardionatrin. These hormones regulate blood volume, arterial pressure, and electrolyte concentration.

- Endocardium. The endocardium is composed of three layers: endothelium, subendothelium, and subendocardium. The subendothelium is endowed with collagen and elastic fibers, fibroblasts, and smooth muscle cells. The subendocardium is a loose connective tissue layer that contains blood vessels, nerves, and Purkinje fibers of the heart's conduction system.

WHAT ARE THE HISTOLOGIC CHARACTERISTICS OF CONTRACTILE CARDIOMYOCYTES (CARDIAC MUSCLE CELLS)?

The contractile cardiomyocytes exhibit the following characteristics at the level of the light microscope:

- The average diameter is 15 μm and average length is 80 μm.
- Most cells contain one large, oval nucleus that is centrally located. Some cardiac muscle cells may have two nuclei.
- Striated appearance due to the orderly array of thick and thin myofilaments.
- Intercalated disks.

The structural characteristics of cardiac muscle cells at the electron microscopic level are:

- The trilaminar-appearing sarcolemma is invested by an external lamina, a basal lamina-like structure
- T-tubules are extensions of the sarcolemma and its associated external lamina into the cell. T-tubules are 2 1/2 times larger in diameter than their counterparts in skeletal muscle. Cardiac muscle is more dependent on an influx of intracellular calcium ions than skeletal muscle for muscle contraction. Larger T-tubules are necessary because they contain a greater abundance of calcium ions.
- Sarcoplasmic reticulum is present and as it approaches a T-tubule, it dilates to form a terminal cisterna. A terminal cisterna and a T-tubule collectively form a diad at the level of the Z-line of the sarcomere. This contrasts with that observed in skeletal muscle where the T-tubule is abutted on both sides by terminal cisternae of sarcoplasmic reticulum. The two terminal cisternae and the centrally located T-tubule constitute a triad, which is in the vicinity of the junction of the A-band and I-band. The sarcoplasmic reticulum stores calcium ions, which are released into the sarcoplasm in response to action potentials that propagate along the T-tubules until they reach the diad. The release of calcium ions from the sarcoplasmic reticulum augments that from the extracellular fluid.
- Mitochondria constitute 40% or more of the volume of a cardiac muscle cell. The mitochondrial endowment is due to the heart's dependency on aerobic metabolism to meet its high consumption of ATP.
- Glycogen granules and lipid droplets are present as metabolic fuel.
- The intercalated disk is visualized as possessing transverse and lateral portions. The transverse portion must resist the vector of contractile force; therefore, this portion is well endowed with fasciae adherentes and desmosomes. The lateral portion is rich in gap junctions.

WHAT ARE THE MORPHOLOGIC CHARACTERISTICS OF INFARCTED CARDIAC TISSUE?

The gross, light microscopic (Fig. 2-32), and electron microscopic features of infarcted cardiac tissue over time are described in Table 2-9.

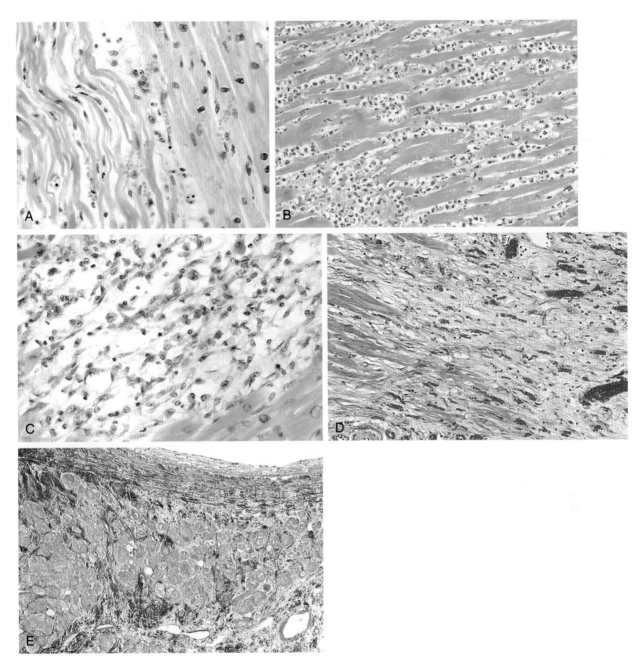

FIGURE 2-32 Microscopic changes of myocardial infarction and its repair. **A,** Coagulative necrosis of muscle fibers of a 1-day-old infarct. Normal muscles fibers are found to the right. **B,** Infiltration of neutrophils in the area of infarct that is 3 to 4 days old. **C,** Necrotic myocytes have nearly been cleared away by phagocytosis 7 to 10 days after the infarct. **D,** Granulation tissue is visible. **E,** Dense collagenous tissue has replaced the myocytes. (Kumar V, Abbas A and Fausto N: *Robbins & Cotran Pathologic Basis of Disease,* 7e. WB Saunders, 2004. Fig. 12-16.)

An 11-month-old female infant with cyanosis was driven to the emergency room by her parents. The physical examination revealed clubbing of the digits and that the infant was underdeveloped. Upon palpation, the physician detected a right ventricular impulse and thrill along the left sternal margin. Another finding was an audible systolic murmur over the pulmonary area. Hypoxemia and polycythemia were notable laboratory findings. Examination of the radiographs showed right ventricular hypertrophy, a narrow shadow of the great vessels, and a boot-shaped heart (coeur en sabot). Cardiac catheterization and angiocardiography showed stenosis of the right ventricular outflow track, right to left ventricular shunting of blood flow, diminished caliber of pulmonary trunk and pulmonary arteries, and normal morphology of the coronary arteries. The infant was diagnosed with tetralogy of Fallot and the congenital defects were surgically corrected.

WHAT ARE THE FOUR CARDINAL CARDIAC DEFECTS OF TETRALOGY OF FALLOT?

The four cardinal features of this congenital malformation are (Fig. 2-33):

- Overriding aorta
- Ventricular septal defect
- Pulmonary stenosis
- Right ventricular hypertrophy

WHAT IS THE EMBRYOLOGIC BASIS FOR THE CARDIAC DEFECTS SEEN IN THE TETRALOGY OF FALLOT?

Unequal division of the truncus arteriosus by the aorticopulmonary septum is responsible for the four cardinal cardiac defects that define the tetralogy of Fallot. Deviation of the aorticopulmonary septum toward the pulmonary trunk produces an aorta that is larger in diameter and a pulmonary outflow tract that is narrowed (stenotic). Because of the deviation, the aorticopulmonary septum no longer aligns with the interventricular septum. This causes the ventricular septal defect. The aorta, because it is larger in diameter than normal, overrides or straddles the interventricular septum. The pulmonary stenosis increases the pressure load on the right ventricle, which compensates by undergoing hypertrophy.

Truca Arteriosis

↑

Bulbur Cordis

↑

Vent

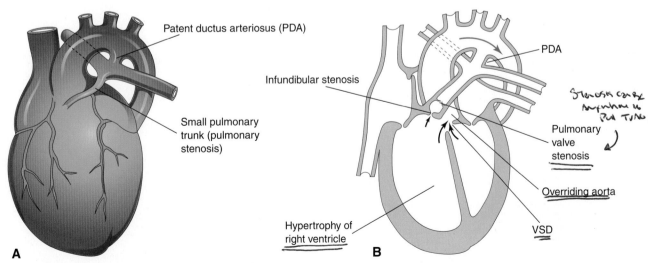

FIGURE 2-33 Cardinal features of tetralogy of Fallot. **A,** Illustration of an infant's affected heart. **B,** Coronal section of an infant's affected heart. (Moore K and Persaud TVN: *The Developing Human*, 7e. WB Saunders, 2003. Fig. 14-33.)

WHAT IS THE LOCATION OF THE PULMONARY (RIGHT VENTRICULAR) OUTFLOW TRACT OBSTRUCTION (STENOSIS) IN TETRALOGY OF FALLOT?

The pulmonary outflow may be obstructed in six different ways. The obstruction may involve or be located at:

- Inferior to the pulmonary semilunar valve
- Level of the pulmonary semilunar valve
- Pulmonary trunk

can occur @multiple levels

- Level of bifurcation of the pulmonary trunk into the right and left pulmonary arteries
- A branch of the pulmonary trunk
- All of the above levels may be stenotic

WHY WAS THERE A NARROW SHADOW OF THE GREAT VESSELS ON RADIOGRAPH?

The narrow shadow of the great vessels is produced by the diminished caliber of the pulmonary vessels.

SECTION III

Abdomen

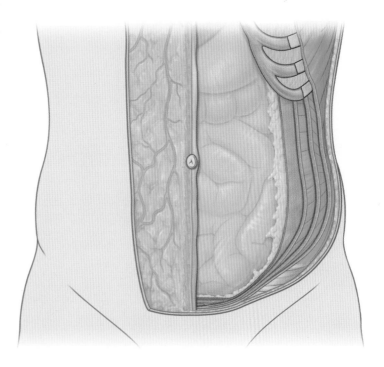

A 49-year-old man presented to his physician complaining of lower back pain. The pain has lasted for 3 days and is unaffected by movement, though the pain is alleviated somewhat when the patient's thighs are flexed. When the anterior abdominal wall was palpated, a tender pulsatile mass was detected just superior to the umbilicus. The physician also detected diminished pulses in the femoral and dorsalis pedis arteries, and bruits were heard over the palpable mass. Imaging studies showed an abdominal aortic aneurysm (Fig. 3-1) with atherosclerotic lesions of the common iliac arteries. The aneurysm was surgically repaired by the insertion of a synthetic prosthesis.

ANATOMICALLY, WHERE DO AORTIC ANEURYSMS COMMONLY OCCUR?

Most aortic aneurysms occur below the level of the renal arteries (Figs. 3-1 and 3-2). Less frequently the aneurysm involves the suprarenal abdominal aorta and thoracic aorta.

Patients with abdominal aneurysms frequently have involvement of the common iliac and internal iliac (hypogastric) arteries. Rarely are the external iliac arteries involved.

WHERE DO ABDOMINAL AORTIC ANEURYSMS MOST COMMONLY RUPTURE?

The abdominal aorta runs retroperitoneally in the abdomen. Consequently, abdominal aortic aneurysms most commonly rupture into the retroperitoneal space. Although rupture is a life-threatening condition, bleeding into the retroperitoneum may contain the rupture. Specifically, 80% rupture into the left retroperitoneal space. Most of the other 20% rupture into the peritoneal cavity. The rupture in this case is not contained, and massive bleeding leads to a rapid deterioration in circulatory function.

AT WHAT VERTEBRAL LEVELS DOES THE ABDOMINAL AORTA BEGIN AND END?

The abdominal aorta is a continuation of the thoracic aorta. The thoracic aorta passes through the aortic hiatus of the diaphragm at the level of the tenth T12 thoracic vertebra. The abdominal aorta continues its inferior course until it bifurcates into the common iliac arteries at the level of the fourth lumbar vertebra.

T12 → L4

WHAT ARE THE BRANCHES OF THE ABDOMINAL AORTA?

The abdominal aorta gives rise to visceral, parietal, and terminal branches that are either paired or unpaired. The branches of the abdominal aorta and the vertebral level at which they arise are:

- Inferior phrenic arteries (paired parietal) — T12
- Celiac trunk (unpaired visceral) — T12
- Superior mesenteric artery (unpaired visceral) — L1
- Middle suprarenal arteries (paired visceral) — L1
- Renal arteries (paired visceral) — L1
- Gonadal (ovarian or testicular) arteries (paired visceral) — L2
- Inferior mesenteric artery (unpaired visceral) — L3
- Lumbar arteries (paired parietal) — there are four pairs of lumbar arteries that spring from the abdominal aorta at L1-L4
- Median sacral artery (unpaired parietal) — this artery issues from the aorta at its bifurcation. The fifth pair of lumbar arteries branch from the median sacral artery.
- Common iliac arteries (paired terminal) — L4

WHAT ARE THE NORMAL HISTOLOGIC CHARACTERISTICS OF THE INFRARENAL ABDOMINAL AORTA?

The wall of the infrarenal abdominal aorta is composed of three tunics, as is the rest of the aorta. From internal to external, the tunics are:

- Tunica intima. This layer is composed of endothelium supported by a basal laminal. Deep to the basal laminal is the subendothelial layer, a layer of loose connective tissue harboring a few smooth muscle cells. External to the subendothelial layer is

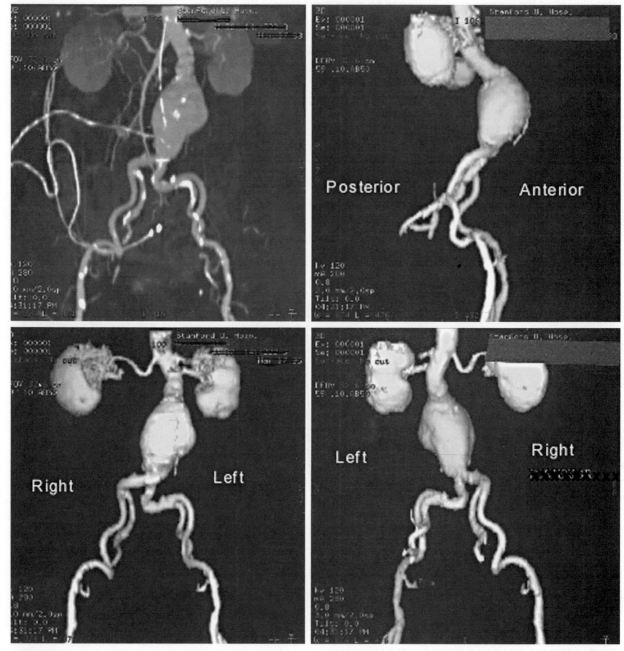

FIGURE 3-1 CT images of an infrarenal abdominal aortic aneurysm. *Upper right*, lateral view. *Upper left*, anterior view with intravenous contrast infusion. *Lower left*, anterior view. *Lower right*, posterior view. (Towsend C et al.: *Sabiston Textbook of Surgery, 17e.* WB Saunders, 2004. Fig. 64-4.)

a fenestrated elastic sheet, the internal elastic lamina (membrane). Because of the numerous elastic lamellae of the tunica media, the internal elastic lamina is not prominent.

● Tunica media. The media is chiefly composed of fenestrated elastic lamellae (Fig. 3-3). In the adult, these may number up to 70 in the thoracic aorta, decreasing to about 30 in the abdominal aorta. The smooth cells of the media are responsible for the deposition of extracellular matrix: glycosaminoglycans, of which chondroitin sulfate is a major constituent, elastin, and elastic, reticular, and collagen fibers. An indistinct external elastic lamina is also present.

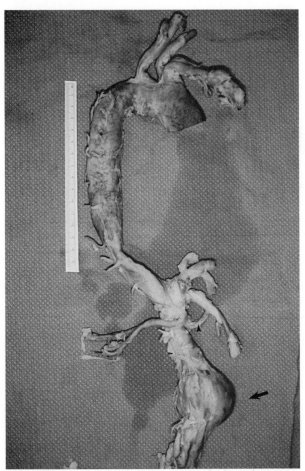

FIGURE 3-2 Human aorta showing an infrarenal abdominal aortic aneurysm at the arrow. (Towsend C et al.: *Sabiston Textbook of Surgery, 17e.* WB Saunders, 2004. Fig. 64-2.)

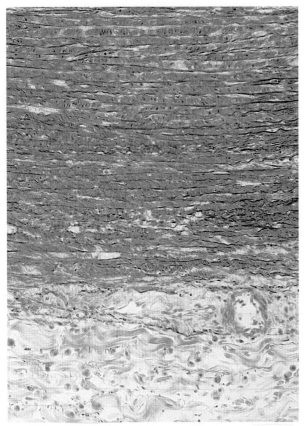

FIGURE 3-3 Light micrograph of the aorta (x132). Note the presence of elastic elements in the tunica media and tunica adventitia. (Gartner L and Hiatt J: *Color Textbook of Histology, 2e.* WB Saunders, 2001. Fig. 11-2.)

Media → intima & change the
phentyne

- Tunica adventitia (also known as the tunica externa). The relatively thin adventitial layer is composed of loosely arranged elastic and collagen fibers (Fig. 3-3). Scattered fibroblasts, vasa vasorum (see below), and nerve fibers also are found in this layer.

Vasa vasorum (vessels of the vessels) are found in the tunica adventitia of the aorta where they are important in preserving normal structure and function. The vessels ramify in the adventitia, sending penetrating branches into the outer media of most aortic segments. The vasa vasorum nourish the outer wall, whereas the inner wall is nourished by diffusion from the blood conveyed in the lumen.

WHAT IS THE SIGNIFICANCE OF SMOOTH MUSCLE CELLS IN THE SUBENDOTHELIAL LAYER OF THE TUNICA INTIMA?

In response to vascular injury, smooth muscle cells migrate from the tunica media to the subendothelium by passing through the fenestrae of the internal elastic lamina (Fig. 3-4). Once in the subendothelium, smooth muscle cells undergo a phenotypic transformation from contractile to proliferative-synthetic. Smooth muscle cells of the latter phenotype undergo mitosis and elaborate extracellular matrix in the subendothelial layer. The net result is thickening of the tunica intima.

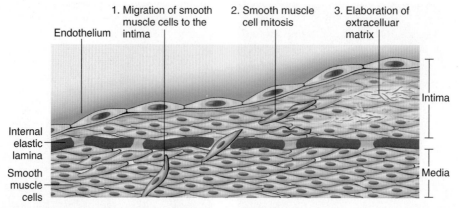

1. Migration of smooth muscle cells to the intima

2. Smooth muscle cell mitosis

3. Elaboration of extracelluar matrix

Endothelium

Internal elastic lamina

Smooth muscle cells

Intima

Media

FIGURE 3-4 Illustration of intimal thickening due to smooth muscle cell migration. (Kumar V, Abbas A and Fausto N: *Robbins & Cotran Pathologic Basis of Disease*, 7e. WB Saunders, 2004. Fig. 11-3. Modified and redrawn from Schoen FJ: *Interventional and Surgical Cardiovascular Pathology: Clinical Correlations and Basic Principles*. Philadelphia, WB Saunders Co., 1989, p. 254.)

WHY DO MOST ABDOMINAL AORTIC ANEURYSMS OCCUR BELOW THE LEVEL OF THE RENAL ARTERIES?

The vasa vasorum located in the tunica adventitia do not penetrate the tunica media of the infrarenal aorta. This means that most of its wall is dependent on diffusion of oxygen and transport of nutrients from luminal blood flow. If this delivery mechanism becomes compromised, as in atherosclerosis, which causes a thickening of the tunica intima, the media is subject to ischemic injury. Ischemic injury causes degeneration of the structural elements in the media leading to a weakening of its wall.

In addition to atherosclerosis, genetic and cellular factors also play roles in the pathogenesis of abdominal aortic aneurysms. Aneurysms (thoracic and abdominal) occur in 10% to 20% of first-degree relatives. Genetic abnormalities in these patients generally lead to defective synthesis of type III collagen (reticular fibers).

It has been shown that cellular events also contribute to the pathogenesis of aortic aneurysms. The release of proteolytic enzymes leads to a deterioration of the tunica media as collagen and elastin are enzymatically degraded. Specific elastases also are active in aneurysmal aortae compared to normal. Invasion of inflammatory cells and the subsequent release of their cytokines may also lead to an erosion of structural matrix elements in the tunica media. In another cellular mechanism, normal endothelial cells synthesize and release nitric oxide. Nitric oxide is not only a vasodilator, it also reduces inflammation by preventing leukocyte rolling and adhesion to the endothelium. In atherosclerosis, a derangement in nitric oxide synthesis promotes the emigration of inflammatory cells into the subendothelial layer.

A 20-year-old woman presents to the emergency room with complaints of right lower abdominal pain, nausea, and loss of appetite. When questioned about the pain, she stated that it was general in nature. But since then it moved to just under the sternum (epigastrium) then to the belly button, and now the patient felt it in her right lower abdominal area. Examination of her abdomen revealed diminished bowel sounds and rebound tenderness with muscle spasms in the right lower abdominal quadrant. Rovsing's, psoas, and obturator signs were also observed. Laboratory studies were unremarkable save for mild leukocytosis with increased neutrophils. The patient was diagnosed with appendicitis and a laparoscopic appendectomy was performed.

WHAT ARE ROVSING'S, PSOAS, AND OBTURATOR SIGNS?

The Rovsing's, psoas, and obturator signs are described in Table 3-1.

WHAT IS MCBURNEY'S POINT AND WHERE IS IT LOCATED?

McBurney's point is the surface landmark that indicates the approximate location of the appendix (Fig. 3-5). To locate McBurney's point, a line can be drawn from the right anterior superior iliac spine to the umbilicus. McBurney's point is one-third of the way along this line from the anterior superior iliac spine.

WHAT ARE THE LAYERS OF THE ABDOMINAL WALL THAT ARE INCISED OVER MCBURNEY'S POINT TO GAIN ACCESS TO THE ABDOMINAL CAVITY?

An incision of the abdominal wall over McBurney's point would cut through the following layers (Fig. 3-6):

- Skin (epidermis and dermis)
- Camper's fascia. This is the most external layer of the superficial fascia. Camper's fascia contains variable amounts of adipose tissue.
- Scarpa's fascia (stratum membranosum telae subcutaneae abdominis). This is the internal layer of the superficial fascia. Scarpa's fascia is a thin fibrous layer. Blood vessels and nerves are found between Camper's and Scarpa's fasciae.
- Deep fascia. This is a thin, tough, fibrous layer that is firmly adherent to the underlying musculature.
- External abdominal oblique muscle
- Internal abdominal oblique muscle
- Transversus abdominis muscle
- Transversalis fascia. This is a thin layer that lines most of the internal surface of the abdominal wall. The transversalis fascia that covers the iliacus muscle is the iliac fascia, that covering the psoas muscle is the psoas fascia, that covering the abdominal surface of the diaphragm is the diaphragmatic fascia, and that covering the pelvis is the pelvic fascia. The femoral sheath is an extension of the transversalis fascia and the iliacus fascia into the femoral triangle of the thigh.
- Extraperitoneal fat layer. This layer contains variable amounts of adipose tissue.
- Parietal peritoneum

TABLE 3-1 Description of Rovsing's, Psoas, and Obturator Signs	
Sign	Description
Rovsing's	Pressure on the left lower abdominal quadrant produces pain in the right lower quadrant.
Psoas	Extension of the right thigh stretches the psoas major muscle. The presence of pain during this procedure suggests an inflamed appendix contacting the stretched muscle.
Obturator	Passive medial rotation of the flexed thigh elicits pain when the inflamed appendix contacts the obturator internus muscle.

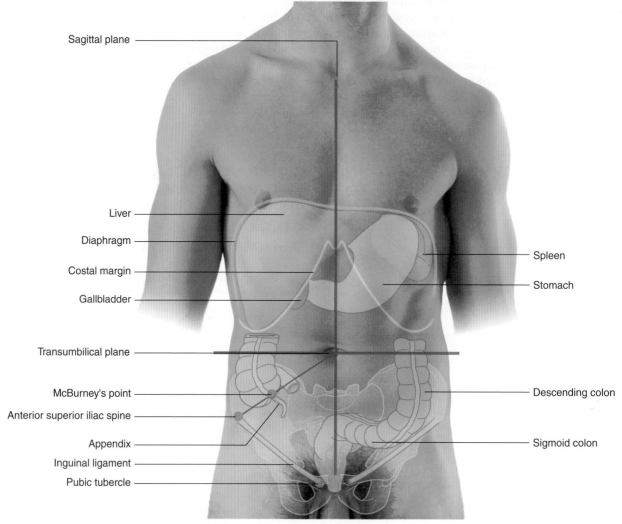

Sagittal plane

Liver

Diaphragm

Costal margin

Gallbladder

Transumbilical plane

McBurney's point

Anterior superior iliac spine

Appendix

Inguinal ligament

Pubic tubercle

Spleen

Stomach

Descending colon

Sigmoid colon

FIGURE 3-5 Abdominal quadrants demonstrating the surface topography of various viscera. Note McBurney's point indicating the position of the vermiform appendix. (Drake R, Vogl W and Mitchell A: *Gray's Anatomy for Students*. Churchill Livingstone, 2004. Fig. 4-150.)

WHAT ARE THE GROSS MORPHOLOGIC CHARACTERISTICS OF THE VERMIFORM APPENDIX?

The vermiform appendix is a worm-like muscular tube that attaches to the cecum at a point where the three teniae coli converge. The appendix averages 7 to 8 cm in length though this varies from 2 to 20 cm . An appendix measuring 33 cm (13 inches) has been documented. The appendix is suspended from the ileum by its own mesentery, the mesoappendix.

The location of the appendix is variable. Locations of the appendix are (Fig. 3-7):

- Retrocecal and retrocolic (most common location)
- Pelvic or descending. Here the appendix simply descends into the pelvis minor.
- Subcecal
- Preileal (anterior to the ileum)
- Postileal (posterior to the ileum)

Infrequently, the appendix can assume a subhepatic position if it adheres to the inferior surface of the liver following the return of the midgut loop into the abdomen.

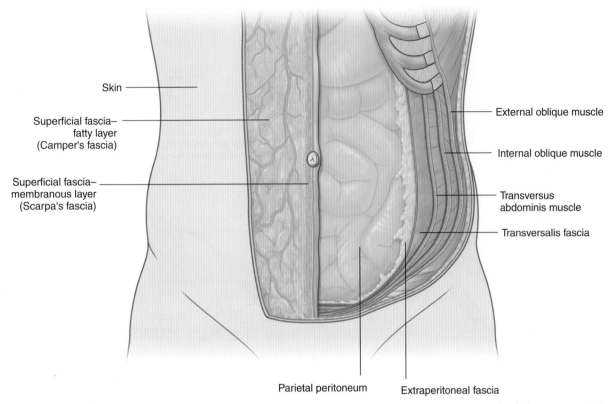

Skin

Superficial fascia–
fatty layer
(Camper's fascia)

Superficial fascia–
membranous layer
(Scarpa's fascia)

External oblique muscle

Internal oblique muscle

Transversus
abdominis muscle

Transversalis fascia

Parietal peritoneum

Extraperitoneal fascia

FIGURE 3-6 Layers of the abdominal wall. (Drake R, Vogl W and Mitchell A: *Gray's Anatomy for Students*. Churchill Livingstone, 2004. Fig. 4-24.)

WHAT IS THE BLOOD SUPPLY TO THE VERMIFORM APPENDIX?

The appendicular artery supplies the vermiform appendix. The artery branches from the ileocolic artery, a branch of the superior mesenteric artery, and travels within the mesoappendix to reach the organ. Accessory arteries to the appendix are common.

WHAT IS THE VENOUS DRAINAGE OF THE VERMIFORM APPENDIX?

Venous drainage of the appendix occurs along the following route: appendicular vein (there may be more than one) to the ileocolic vein. The ileocolic vein empties into the superior mesenteric vein. In turn, the superior mesenteric vein unites with the splenic vein to form the portal vein.

WHAT IS THE LYMPHATIC DRAINAGE OF THE VERMIFORM APPENDIX?

Lymph flows parallel to the branches of blood vessels. Lymph first drains to lymph nodes in the mesoappendix. From these nodes, lymph drains into ileocolic lymph nodes and then into superior mesenteric lymph nodes.

WHAT IS THE NERVE SUPPLY OF THE VERMIFORM APPENDIX?

Sympathetic and parasympathetic fibers from the superior mesenteric plexus supply the vermiform appendix. Sympathetic preganglionic fibers originate from the lateral gray horns of the inferior thoracic spinal cord level. The vagus nerves contribute the parasympathetic fibers to this plexus. The autonomic

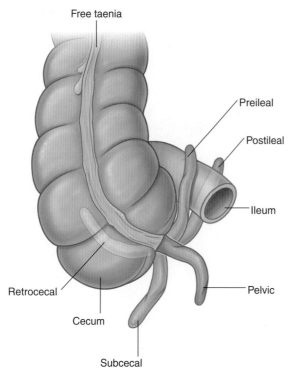

FIGURE 3-7 Locations of the vermiform appendix. (Drake R, Vogl W and Mitchell A: *Gray's Anatomy for Students*. Churchill Livingstone, 2004. Fig. 4-75.)

fibers accompany the superior mesenteric artery and its branches to the vermiform appendix.

IN APPENDICITIS, REFERRED PAIN IS REFERRED TO WHAT DERMATOME?

Visceral sensory fibers from the appendix enter the tenth thoracic spinal cord level in the company of sympathetic fibers (Fig. 3-8). Consequently, pain is referred to the dermatome of T10. The T10 dermatome is at the level of the umbilicus.

WHAT IS THE HISTOLOGIC ARCHITECTURE OF THE VERMIFORM APPENDIX?

The histologic architecture of the appendix is described as being the large intestine in miniature. The layers of the appendix are the:

● Mucosa. The mucosa contains simple columnar epithelium with goblet cells and M cells resting on a basal lamina, lamina propria, and muscularis

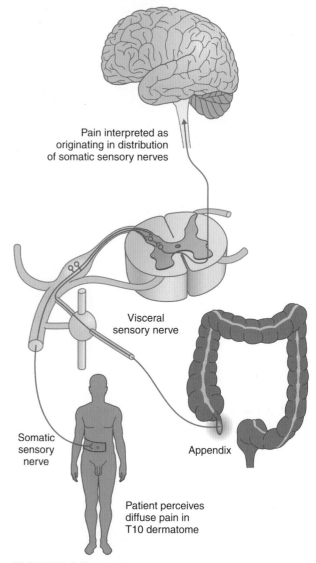

FIGURE 3-8 Mechanism for referred pain from appendicitis to the T10 dermatome. (Drake R, Vogl W and Mitchell A: *Gray's Anatomy for Students*. Churchill Livingstone, 2004. Fig. 2-82.)

mucosae. Intestinal glands (crypts of Lieberkuhn) are few and short in length. The glands contain columnar absorptive cells, goblet cells, regenerative cells, and enteroendocrine cells. The lamina propria is distinguished by numerous lymphoid nodules that extend into the underlying submucosa. The muscularis mucosae contains an inner circular layer and an outer longitudinal layer of smooth muscle.

● Submucosa. This connective tissue layer is distinguished by the presence of numerous lymphoid nodules.

- Muscularis externa. This layer contains two complete layers of smooth muscle. The inner layer is circular, whereas the outer layer is longitudinal. Teniae coli begin at the base of the appendix where it attaches to the cecum.
- Serosa

WHAT ARE M CELLS?

M cells, also known as microfold cells, are specialized cells found in the epithelium overlying Peyer's patches. M cells possess a few short microvilli on their luminal surface. The basal domain of the M cell is deeply invaginated. The deep recesses of these basal invaginations harbor lymphocytes and macrophages. Functionally, M cells play a pivotal role in the immunologic response of the intestinal system. Specifically, M cells continuously sample the contents of the lumen of the intestine for the presence of an antigenic challenge. If antigens are present, they are endocytosed by the M cells and transported to the underlying immune cells, which initiate an immune response.

A 52-year-old man presented to the physician with complaints of loss of appetite, weight loss, and weakness. The patient commented during the history that he drinks six to ten beers a day and more on weekends. The physical examination showed the following: jaundice, peripheral edema, distended abdomen, ascites, caput medusae, and wasted extremities. Laboratory tests revealed hypoproteinemia, hyperbilirubinemia, anemia, increased prothrombin time and elevated levels of serum aminotransferase and serum alkaline phosphatase. A liver biopsy confirmed the diagnosis of alcoholic cirrhosis.

WHAT IS THE BLOOD SUPPLY TO THE LIVER?

The liver has a dual blood supply. The liver receives 70% of its blood supply from the portal vein, which forms at the confluence of the superior mesenteric and splenic veins. The other 30% of its supply is from the hepatic artery proper. The celiac trunk, which springs from the abdominal aorta, gives rise to the common hepatic artery. The common hepatic artery projects to the right and bifurcates into the gastroduodenal artery and hepatic artery proper. In turn, the hepatic artery proper divides into right and left hepatic arteries, which enter the liver at the porta hepatis. The right and left hepatic arteries branch into interlobar arteries, and these then branch into interlobular arteries. Some of the interlobular arteries reach the portal triads as hepatic arterioles. The blood flowing through the portal vein is low in oxygen but rich in nutrients (i.e., monosaccharides and amino acids) absorbed from the small intestine. The hepatic artery proper contains blood that is well saturated with oxygen.

WHAT IS THE VENOUS DRAINAGE OF THE LIVER?

The sinusoids of the liver lobule convey blood to the central vein (aka, terminal hepatic venule or centrilobular venule), which is located in the center of the lobule. Sublobular veins then collect venous blood from the central veins. The sublobular veins converge to form two groups (upper and lower) of hepatic veins that empty into the inferior vena cava.

WHERE ARE THE PORTOSYSTEMIC ANASTOMOSES AND WHAT RESULTS IF THEY BECOME DISTENDED?

When the pressure is normal in the hepatic portal system, all the blood following to the liver is delivered to the hepatic veins that empty into the inferior vena cava. However, when portal venous blood flow is obstructed, as in the later stage of alcoholic cirrhosis, the ensuing elevated portal pressure shunts blood into collateral veins that empty into the systemic venous circulation. The largest of these portosystemic anastomoses occur at the following locations (Fig. 3-9):

- Gastroesophageal
- Anorectal
- Paraumbilical
- Retroperitoneal

These portosystemic anastomoses are further described in Table 3-2.

HOW CAN PORTAL HYPERTENSION BE RELIEVED SURGICALLY?

As venous flow to the liver through the portal system is impeded by the cirrhotic liver, blood flow must be partially diverted to other venous routes to relieve the portal hypertension. This can be accomplished by:

- Creating an anastomosis between the portal vein and the inferior vena cava
- Connecting the splenic vein to the renal vein following a splenectomy

WHAT IS THE INNERVATION OF THE LIVER?

The parenchyma of the liver is supplied from sympathetic and parasympathetic nerve fibers from the hepatic plexus, the largest derivative of the celiac plexus. The plexus is formed from sympathetic fibers that originate from spinal levels T6-T9 and from parasympathetic fibers from the vagus nerves. Nerve fibers accompany the hepatic artery, hepatic portal vein, and their branches to the liver. The fibers are vasomotor and innervate hepatocytes directly.

T6-T9 = sympathetic levels

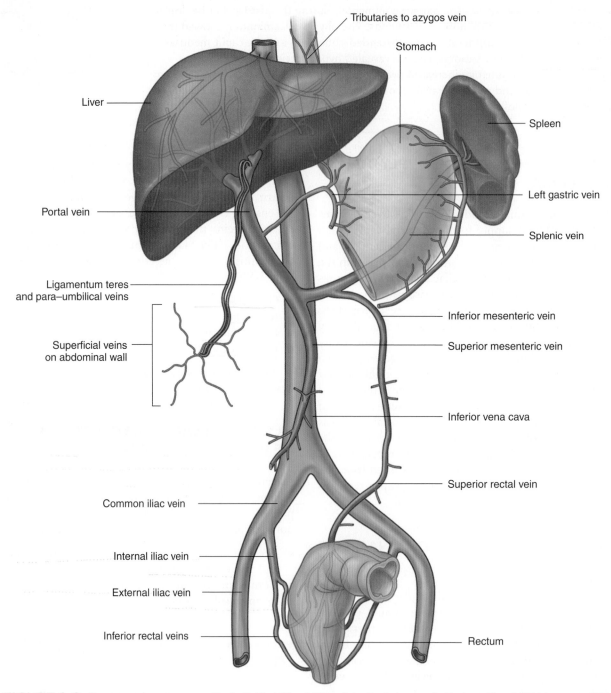

FIGURE 3-9   Portosystemic anastomoses. (Drake R, Vogl W and Mitchell A: *Gray's Anatomy for Students*. Churchill Livingstone, 2004. Fig. 4-106.)

Visceral afferent fibers accompany the sympathetic fibers. Pain from the liver is referred to the epigastric region and thence to the right hypochondriac region and posterior region of right back. If the diaphragm is irritated by liver disease, pain is referred to the right shoulder and/or posterior thoracic wall.

WHAT IS THE LYMPHATIC DRAINAGE OF THE LIVER?

Lymph from the liver is drained by superficial and deep lymph vessels. Most of the deep lymph vessels leave the porta hepatis and terminate in the hepatic

TABLE 3-2 Portosystemic Anastomoses		
Location	**Description**	**Clinical Significance**
Gastroesophageal	Esophageal veins that empty into the left gastric vein of the portal system anastomose with esophageal veins that drain into the azygos vein of the systemic venous system.	Esophageal varices form at the gastroesophageal junction.
Anorectal	Superior rectal vein, which empties into the portal system, anastomoses with the middle and inferior rectal veins. The middle and inferior rectal veins drain into the internal iliac and internal veins of the systemic venous system, respectively.	Hemorrhoids occur at the anorectal junction.
Paraumbilical	Paraumbilical veins, which accompany the ligamentum teres and median umbilical ligament, anastomose with subcutaneous veins of the anterior abdominal wall (e.g., superficial epigastric vein, which empties into the great saphenous vein).	Caput medusae forms around the umbilicus.
Retroperitoneal	Veins that empty into the splenic and pancreatic veins anastomose with the left renal vein. Anastomoses also occur between the splenic and colic veins and the lumbar veins.	Anastomoses occur between the veins of the bare area of the liver and veins of the diaphragm and right internal thoracic vein.

lymph nodes that accompany the hepatic vessels and ducts. Efferent lymph vessels then convey the lymph to the celiac lymph nodes. From the celiac lymph nodes, lymph empties into the thoracic duct. The remaining deep lymph vessels follow the hepatic veins, pass through the vena caval foramen in the diaphragm, and terminate in the middle group of phrenic nodes. From the phrenic nodes, efferent vessels drain to the parasternal nodes.

Most of the superficial lymph vessels join the deep lymph vessels in the porta hepatis to end in the hepatic lymph nodes. From these nodes, lymph flows through efferent lymph vessels to the celiac nodes and then to the thoracic duct. Superficial lymph vessels from the bare area of the liver take a different route. These vessels end in the phrenic and mediastinal nodes in the thoracic cavity. This is accomplished by their passage through the sternocostal hiatus and vena caval foramen in the diaphragm.

HOW DOES THE LIVER DEVELOP?

The first sign of development of the liver is the formation of the hepatic diverticulum (liver bud), a ventral outgrowth of endoderm from the distal foregut during the fourth week of development. The hepatic diverticulum enlarges and divides into a larger cranial part, the primordium of the liver, and a smaller caudal part, which becomes the gallbladder. The rapidly dividing endodermal cells in the hepatic diverticulum differentiate into the hepatocytes and epithelial cells lining the biliary ducts within the liver. Mesenchyme from the septum transversum is responsible for the connective and hemopoietic tissue and macrophages (Kupffer cells). Hemopoiesis by the liver begins during the sixth week and the hepatic cells begin to produce bile during the twelfth week.

HOW IS A LIVER BIOPSY OBTAINED?

Liver biopsies are commonly obtained by a needle puncture that penetrates the tenth intercostal space in the right midaxillary line. To avoid injury to an inflated lung, the patient is asked to forcefully exhale.

WHAT ARE THE THREE HISTOLOGIC ARCHITECTURES THAT CAN DESCRIBE THE LIVER?

The liver can be histologically described as having three histologic patterns: liver lobule, hepatic acinus (of Rappaport), and the portal lobule (Fig. 3-10). The liver lobule is a polygonal structure with three to six portal spaces at its periphery. Portal spaces contain the structures of the portal triad (branch of the hepatic portal vein, branch of the hepatic artery proper, and bile duct), lymphatic vessels, and nerves. The center of

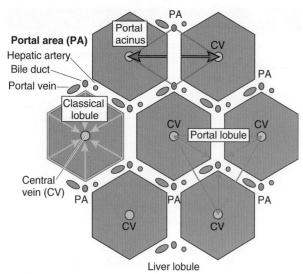

FIGURE 3-10 Illustrations of the hepatic lobule, hepatic acinus, and portal lobule. (Gartner L and Hiatt J: *Color Textbook of Histology, 2e.* WB Saunders, 2001. Fig. 18-11.)

the lobule contains the central vein (also called the *terminal hepatic vein*). Running from the periphery of the lobule to the central vein are cords of hepatocytes. Sinusoids are located between the cords of hepatocytes.

The hepatic acinus is a diamond-shaped structure that is defined within two adjacent liver lobules. The acinus is defined by starting at the central vein of one lobule and drawing a line to a portal space between the two liver lobules. The line is continued to the central vein of the neighboring lobule. From this central vein, the line is drawn to the portal space opposite the previous one and then back to the starting point. The hepatic acinus is supplied by blood vessels that run between the two hepatic lobules. The hepatocytes that reside next to the blood supply are in zone 1 (periportal region), the hepatocytes closest to the central vein are in zone 3 (centrilobular region), and the hepatocytes between these two zones are in zone 2 (midzonal region). Injury and cell death of hepatocytes typically exhibit a zonal pattern. Cells in zone 3 (perilobular region) are more vulnerable to injury from ischemia and drug and toxic reactions.

The portal lobule is a triangle-shaped region of hepatocytes formed within three adjacent liver lobules. The triangle is defined by connecting the three dots represented by the central veins of each lobule. The portal lobule defines the area of parenchyma that drains into the portal space in the center of the triangle.

WHAT ARE THE CHARACTERISTICS OF HEPATOCYTES AND HOW DO THESE FEATURES DIFFER IN THE THREE ZONES OF THE HEPATIC ACINUS?

Hepatocytes exhibit the following attributes:

- Polygonal in shape
- Each cell contains one centrally located nucleus, although about 25% of the hepatocytes are binucleate. Chromatin is principally in the form of euchromatin with clumps of heterochromatin at the periphery of the nucleus.
- One or two prominent nucleoli reside in each nucleus.
- Cytoplasm is basophilic.
- Free ribosomes are numerous. Polysomes (polyribosomes) form when free ribosomes attach to mRNA. Polysomes synthesize proteins that are used internally by the cell.
- Rough endoplasmic reticulum is well developed.
- Smooth endoplasmic reticulum varies in its abundance. Hepatocytes in zone 1 (periportal region) of the hepatic acinus contain poorly developed smooth endoplasmic reticulum, whereas cells residing in zone 3 (centrilobular region) are well endowed with this organelle.
- Glycogen deposits are found in the cytoplasm. Glycogen is found in large deposits proximate to smooth endoplasmic reticulum in hepatocytes of zone 3 of the hepatic acinus. In zone 1 of the acinus, glycogen exists as diffuse deposits. The abundance of glycogen is dependent on the nutritional status of the individual: glycogen is abundant after a meal and less abundant after fasting.
- A large complement of mitochondria with hepatocytes containing as many as 2,000 of these ATP-generating organelles. Mitochondria are larger and fewer in number in cells of zone 1 of the hepatic acinus. In zone 3, mitochondria are more numerous and smaller.
- Multiple Golgi complexes are found in each cell proximate to the bile canaliculi.
- Endosomes, lysosomes, and peroxisomes are numerous.
- Microvilli are present on the sinusoidal domains of the hepatocytes. Microvilli project into the perisinusoidal space (of Disse) and are estimated to increase surface area by sixfold. This important structural endowment increases the rate of exchange between the hepatocyte and sinusoidal blood.

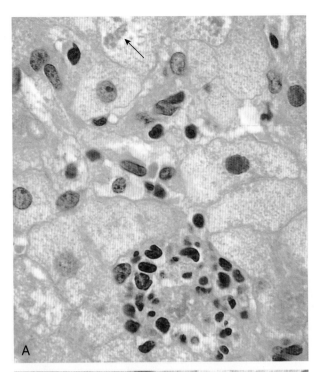

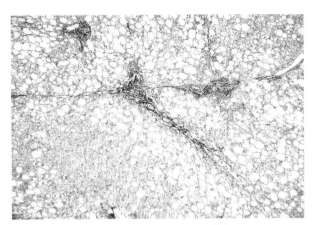

FIGURE 3-12 Alcoholic liver showing the immense accumulation of lipid in the hepatocytes. Observe the early signs of fibrosis (blue staining elements stained by Masson Trichrome). (Kumar V, Abbas A and Fausto N: *Robbins & Cotran Pathologic Basis of Disease*, 7e. WB Saunders, 2004. Fig. 18-24.)

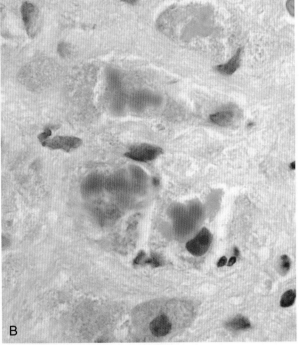

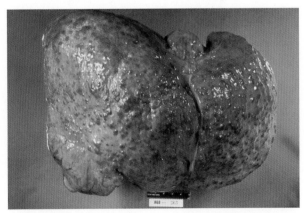

FIGURE 3-13 Alcoholic cirrhosis showing the nodules on the surface of the liver. (Kumar V, Abbas A and Fausto N: *Robbins & Cotran Pathologic Basis of Disease*, 7e. WB Saunders, 2004. Fig. 18-26.)

FIGURE 3-11 Alcoholic hepatitis. **A,** Inflammatory cells are surrounding the location of a necrotic hepatocyte (lower part of micrograph). Note eosinophilic Mallory body in hepatocyte at arrow. **B,** Eosinophilic Mallory bodies are observed in hepatocytes. (Kumar V, Abbas A and Fausto N: *Robbins & Cotran Pathologic Basis of Disease*, 7e. WB Saunders, 2004. Fig. 18-25.)

● Bile canaliculi are located along the lateral domains of the hepatocytes.

WHAT ARE MALLORY BODIES?

Mallory bodies (alcoholic hyalin) are intracytoplasmic inclusions found in hepatocytes damaged by alcohol. The bodies appear eosinophilic and are composed principally of keratin, an intermediate filament (Fig. 3-11).

HOW DOES THE CIRRHOTIC LIVER ATTEMPT TO HEAL ITSELF?

With alcoholic liver disease, the hepatocytes accumulate large lipid droplets in the cytoplasm (Fig. 3-12). The fatty liver enlarges to a mass of up to 4 to 6 kg compared with a normal mass of 1.4 to 1.8 kg in males and 1.2 to 1.4 kg in females. Alcohol abuse also results in the formation of fibrous septa that are thin and delicate initially. Later, the fibrous elements become more prominent and begin to surround and wall off nests of hepatocytes. The proliferation of the entrapped hepatocytes forms a nodular pattern to the liver (Fig. 3-13). As this process continues, the liver progressively shrinks. Persinusoidal (stellate) cells are important players in this remodeling process.

in they layDow ECM (collagen)

The parents brought their 4-week-old son to the pediatrician complaining that he suffered episodes of projectile vomiting. It was learned from the history that the vomitus was nonbilious and that the infant had a voracious appetite between vomiting episodes. The physical examination revealed peristaltic waves in the epigastrium, and a palpable mass was detected in this area as well. Imaging studies (ultrasound and radiologic) revealed a thickened pyloric sphincter (Fig. 3-14). The infant was diagnosed with congenital hypertrophic pyloric stenosis and was treated by pyloromyotomy.

WHAT LAYER OF THE GASTRIC WALL IS RESPONSIBLE FOR THE CONSTRICTION OF THE PYLORUS?

Congenital hypertrophic pyloric stenosis is caused by a thickening, and possibly hyperplasia, of the inner circular layer of the muscularis externa. Although the etiology of the condition is unknown, a genetic basis has been established as identical twins have a high concordance rate.

HOW IS A PYLOROMYOTOMY PERFORMED?

The pylorus is surgically accessed by an incision in the right upper abdominal quadrant or a periumbilical incision. A pyloromyotomy can also be performed laparoscopically. Once the pylorus is located, an incision is made across the pyloric muscularis externa while preserving the integrity of the inner mucosal lining (Fig. 3-15).

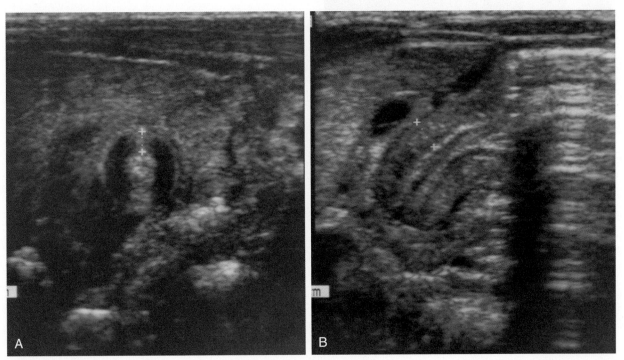

A   B

FIGURE 3-14 Hypertrophic pyloric sphincter. **A**, Transverse abdominal sonogram showing a pyloric sphincter thickness greater than 4 mm (distance between the two crosses). **B**, Horizontal sonogram showing a pyloric channel length greater than 14 mm.

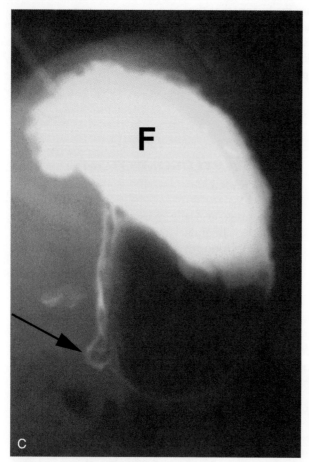

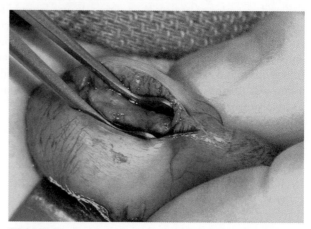

FIGURE 3-15 Pyloromyotomy for hypertrophic pyloric stenosis. The hypertrophied pyloric muscle has been reflected to show the mucosa. (Towsend C et al.: *Sabiston Textbook of Surgery, 17e.* WB Saunders, 2004. Fig. 70-8.)

FIGURE 3-14, cont'd C, Radiograph of stomach showing a stenotic pylorus (*arrow*) and a distended fundus (*F*). (Moore K and Persaud TVN: *The Developing Human, 7e.* WB Saunders, 2003. Fig. 12-4. **Part B**: From Wyllie R: Pyloric stenosis and other congenital anomalies of the stomach. In Behman RE, Kliegman RM, Arvin AM [eds]: *Nelson Textbook of Pediatrics, 15e.* Philadelphia, WB Saunders, 1996. **Part C**: Courtesy of Dr. Prem S. Sahni, Department of Radiology, Children's Hospital, Winnipeg, Manitoba, Canada.)

A 21-year-old woman presented to her physician with complaints of diarrhea and abdominal pain. During the history, the patient stated that she suffered from these symptoms for a period of 2 to 3 weeks about 1 year ago and that her mother suffers from similar symptoms. A mass in the right lower abdominal quadrant was detected upon palpation. Laboratory tests showed that the patient's leukocyte count was slightly elevated and stool culture was negative for pathogenic organisms. Radiologic studies revealed a narrowed distal ileum accompanied by dilation of the segment proximal to the obstructive lesion and mucosal cobblestoning ulcerations. Abscesses and fistulae were not observed radiologically. Endoscopic examination showed areas of ulceration in the colon (the rectum was normal) interspersed with normal mucosa as well as the cobblestoning ulcerations of the distal ileum. The patient was diagnosed with Crohn's disease and treated with Pentasa, an oral 5-aminosalicylic acid, and folic acid supplementation.

WHAT IS THE ARTERIAL SUPPLY TO THE ILEUM AND THE COLON?

The ileum being a midgut derivative is supplied by the superior mesenteric artery. The colon is dually derived from the midgut and the hindgut. The cecum, vermiform appendix, ascending colon, and the right half to right two-thirds of the transverse colon are supplied by the superior mesenteric artery. The branches of the superior mesenteric artery that supply these segments of the large intestine are the ileocecal, right colic, and middle colic arteries.

The remaining distal colon formed from the hindgut is supplied by the inferior mesenteric artery. The middle rectal and the inferior rectal arteries provide blood in the inferior rectum and anal canal. The middle rectal is a branch of the internal iliac artery and the inferior rectal artery springs from the internal pudendal artery. The internal pudendal artery issues from the internal iliac artery.

COMPARE AND CONTRAST THE HISTOLOGIC CHARACTERISTICS OF THE ILEUM AND COLON

The histologic characteristics of the wall of the ileum and colon are described in Table 3-3.

WHAT ARE THE DISTINGUISHING RADIOLOGIC FEATURES OF THE JEJUNUM, ILEUM, AND COLON?

The jejunum exhibits plicae circulares that are well developed. This structural modification confers a "feathery" appearance to the jejunum (Fig. 3-16). As you proceed distally, the plicae circulares become less prominent in the ileum. Consequently, this segment of the gastrointestinal tract does not exhibit a "feathery" pattern (Fig. 3-16). The large intestine is readily identified on radiographic examination by its large diameter and by the presence of its hallmark feature, haustra (Fig. 3-17).

COMPARE AND CONTRAST THE MORPHOLOGIC CHARACTERISTICS OF CROHN'S DISEASE AND ULCERATIVE COLITIS.

The morphologic characteristics of Crohn's disease and ulcerative colitis are summarized in Table 3-4 and Figure 3-18.

TABLE 3-3 Histologic Characteristics of the Ileum and Colon

Wall Layer	Ileum	Colon
Mucosa	Plicae circulares (valves of Kerckring) are present proximally, but progressively diminish in height until they disappear in the terminal ileum. Villi are present. Absorptive cells exhibit well-developed microvilli (brush border). Intestinal glands (crypts of Lieberkuhn) contain Paneth cells.	Plicae circulares are absent. Villi are absent. Absorptive cells possess poorly developed microvilli. Intestinal glands are more numerous and longer and Paneth cells are absent.
Submucosa	Peyer's patches are distinguishing features. The patches extend into the lamina propria of the mucosa.	Lymphoid nodules are typically seen.
Muscularis externa	Inner circular layer and outer longitudinal layer of smooth muscle.	Inner layer circular layer of smooth muscle; outer layer is composed of three bands of smooth muscle called *teniae coli*. These bands splay as they enter the rectum.
Serosa/adventitia	Serosa (visceral peritoneum) is present.	Serosal and adventitial layers are found in various segments of the colon.

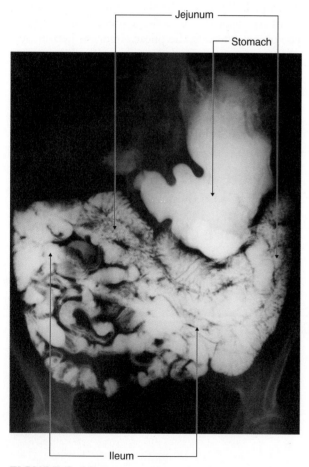

FIGURE 3-16 Barium contrast radiograph showing jejunum (has a feathery appearance) and ileum. (Drake R, Vogl W and Mitchell A: *Gray's Anatomy for Students*. Churchill Livingstone, 2004. Fig. 4-63.)

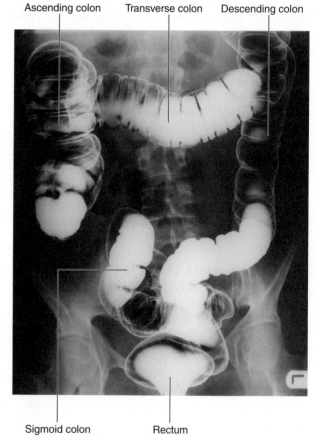

FIGURE 3-17 Barium contrast radiograph showing the segmented appearance of the large intestine. (Drake R, Vogl W and Mitchell A: *Gray's Anatomy for Students*. Churchill Livingstone, 2004. Fig. 4-71.)

TABLE 3-4 Characteristics of Crohn's Disease and Ulcerative Colitis

Feature	Crohn's	Ulcerative Colitis
Location of lesions	Small intestine alone in 40% of cases Small intestine and colon in 30% of cases Colon alone in 30% of cases Rarely, the mouth, esophagus, stomach, and duodenum may be involved	Rectum extending proximally to involve entire colon May backwash into distal ileum

Wall involvement	All four layers are involved
	Muscularis mucosae exhibits reduplication,
	  hypertrophy, and irregularity
	Hypertrophy of muscularis externa
	Fibrosis of mucosa, submucosa, and muscularis
	  externa ultimately leads to strictures
		Mucosa is ulcerated
		Fibrosis in submucosa represents healing
		Muscularis external is normal except in severe cases

Intestinal glands
  (crypts of Lieberkuhn)
	Distortion of intestinal glands is less severe than
	  that of ulcerative colitis
		Intestinal glands branch and are irregular.

Metaplasia	Gastric pyloric metaplasia
	Paneth cell metaplasia in distal colon
	  (normally absent)
		Gastric pyloric metaplasia
		Paneth cell metaplasia in distal colon
		  (normally absent)

Continuity of lesions	Intervening normal-appearing intestine appears
	  between lesions (skip lesions)
		Lesions are continuous beginning in the rectum.
		  In severe cases, the lesions spread along the
		  entire length of the colon and may backwash
		  into the distal ileum.

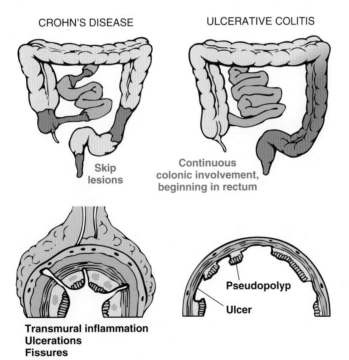

CROHN'S DISEASE   ULCERATIVE COLITIS

Skip
lesions

Continuous
colonic involvement,
beginning in rectum

Pseudopolyp

Ulcer

Transmural inflammation
Ulcerations
Fissures

FIGURE 3-18 Morphologic comparison of Crohn's disease and ulcerative colitis. (Kumar V, Abbas A and Fausto N: *Robbins & Cotran Pathologic Basis of Disease*, 7e. WB Saunders, 2004. Fig. 17-43.)

A 32-year-old Native American woman presented to her physician with mild complaints of fatigue, weakness, and dizziness. The patient was 62 inches in height and weighed 190 lb. During the history she indicated that her mother, who is still alive, is a diabetic. She also stated that she had increased thirst and more frequent urination. Laboratory tests later indicated a normal fasting insulin level and hyperglycemia (220 mg/dL). She was diagnosed with type II diabetes mellitus.

WHAT ARE THE CELLULAR CHARACTERISTICS OF INSULIN-SECRETING CELLS?

Although several cell types exist in the pancreatic islets (of Langerhans), it is the beta cell that is responsible for the synthesis and secretion of insulin. The beta cell is the most numerous cell type in the islet, comprising about 70% of its mass. The beta cells reside in the core of the islet.

The beta cells contain the usual constellation of organelles found in cells that synthesize proteins. These are:

- Euchromatic nucleus, which indicates active transcription of mRNA
- Rough endoplasmic reticulum that is well developed for the translation of mRNA to preproinsulin, a single polypeptide. Preproinsulin is then enzymatically cleaved within the cisterna of the rER.
- Juxtanuclear Golgi apparatus for the sorting and packaging of proinsulin into clathrin-coated vesicles. The clathrin is quickly shed as the secretory vesicle migrates toward the plasma membrane.
- Mitochondria with shelflike cristae.

- Secretory vesicles contain one or more dense crystals in a lighter amorphous matrix.

WHAT ARE THE MORPHOLOGIC CHARACTERISTICS OF THE PANCREATIC ISLETS IN TYPE I AND TYPE II DIABETES MELLITUS?

In type I diabetes mellitus, the pancreatic islets have the following morphologic characteristics:

- Pancreatic islets decrease in number and there is a reduction in their size.
- Inflammation of the islets, which is referred to as insulitis (Fig. 3-19). T lymphocytes are the main type of leukocyte that infiltrates the islets.
- Beta cells lack secretory granules of insulin. This is observed earlier in the course of the disease when beta cells are still present.

In type II diabetes mellitus, the pancreatic islets have the following morphologic characteristics:

- Islet cell mass may be reduced.
- Amyloid deposition is observed. The amyloid slowly replaces the pancreatic islets (Fig. 3-19).

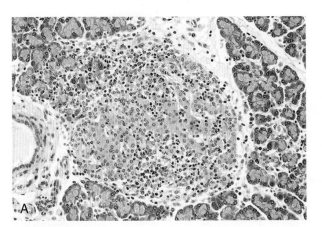
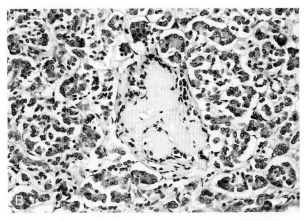

FIGURE 3-19 **A**, Insulitis in a rat model of diabetes mellitus. **B**, Deposition of amyloid in diabetes mellitus. (Kumar V, Abbas A and Fausto N: *Robbins & Cotran Pathologic Basis of Disease*, 7e. WB Saunders, 2004. Fig. 24-35. Part A Courtesy of Dr. Arthur Like, University of Massachusetts, Worchester, MA.)

- Fibrosis of the pancreatic islets may be seen in advanced stages.
- In contrast to type I, insulitis is not present.

WHAT ROLES DO GLUCOSE TRANSPORTER PROTEINS PLAY IN REGULATING INSULIN SECRETION AND INSULIN ACTION ON THE TARGET CELLS?

There are two glucose transporter proteins that regulate the flow of glucose into beta cells and target cells. GLUT-2 is an insulin-independent glucose transporter found in beta cells and hepatocytes. It allows an influx of glucose that is used by the beta cell to generate ATP (Fig. 3-20). ATP inhibits a K^+ channel protein causing depolarization of the membrane. Membrane depolarization opens Ca^{2+} channels. The subsequent influx of Ca^{2+} triggers a cascade of events that cause secretion of insulin. Insulin then enters the microvasculature and is transported in the bloodstream to exert its effects on target cells.

When insulin binds to its receptor on the plasma membrane of the target cell, it activates the phosphatidylinositol-3-kinase pathway (Fig. 3-21). One of the effects of activating this pathway is that it causes vesicles containing GLUT-4 to translocate to the cell surface. GLUT-4 is an insulin-dependent glucose transport protein. This translocation increases the number of GLUT-4 molecules embedded in the plasma membrane. The influx of glucose is increased by this action of insulin as glucose influx is proportional to the number of GLUT-4 receptors.

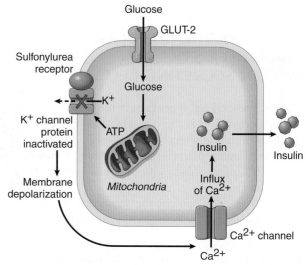

FIGURE 3-20 Insulin synthesis and secretion in a ß-cell. Glucose transport into the ß-cell is mediated by GLUT-2, an insulin-independent glucose transporter. Glucose is metabolized to generate ATP, which inhibits the efflux of potassium ions. Inhibition of the potassium ion channel depolarizes the membrane which causes an influx of calcium ions. Calcium ions trigger the release of insulin. (Kumar V, Abbas A and Fausto N: *Robbins & Cotran Pathologic Basis of Disease*, 7e. WB Saunders, 2004. Fig. 24-28.)

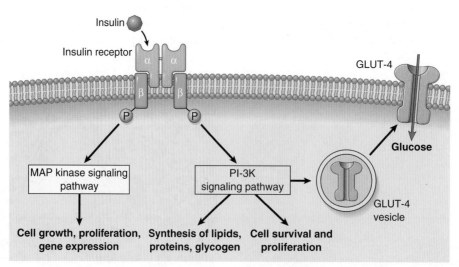

FIGURE 3-21 Mechanism of insulin's action on a target cell in increasing glucose uptake. Insulin binds to its receptor leading to a series of phosphorylations. Activation of the PI-3K signaling pathway causes GLUT-4, an insulin-dependent glucose transporter, to be translocated to the plasma membrane. GLUT-4 is responsible for the influx of glucose in the target cell. (Kumar V, Abbas A and Fausto N: *Robbins & Cotran Pathologic Basis of Disease*, 7e. WB Saunders, 2004. Fig. 24-30.)

WHAT ROLE DO INSULIN RECEPTORS AND GLUT-2 AND GLUT-4 TRANSPORTERS PLAY IN THE DEVELOPMENT OF TYPE II DIABETES MELLITUS?

Type II diabetes mellitus is characterized by cell resistance to insulin. Theoretically, defects in insulin receptors and the glucose transporters (GLUT-2 and GLUT-4) could have a hand in the development of insulin resistance. Although mutations in the insulin receptors are rare, defects in the post-receptor signaling pathways have been implicated as playing a significant role in reducing the target cells' responsiveness to insulin.

The GLUT-4 transporter is a coconspirator in the case of muscle. In type II diabetes mellitus, muscle cells have a reduced capacity to translocate GLUT-4 transporters to the sacrolemma. The net effect of this defect is a decrease in the uptake of glucose by muscle cells. Therefore, defective GLUT-4 translocation can also cause insulin resistance.

A 52-year-old woman presents in the emergency room with complaints of sudden right upper quadrant pain, nausea, and vomiting. The patient weighed 170 lb, height was 60 inches, and she had a mild fever. Tenderness and guarding inferior to the right costal margin and a positive Murphy's sign were noted during the physical examination. Laboratory results showed slightly elevated levels of serum bilirubin, alkaline phosphatase, and leukocytes. Ultrasound imaging detected gallstones (Fig. 3-22) and a thickened wall of the gallbladder. The patient was diagnosed with acute calculous cholecystitis. She was placed on intravenous antibiotics and nonsteroidal analgesics to alleviate the pain. Laparoscopic cholecystectomy was performed 2 days later.

WHAT ARE THE GROSS MORPHOLOGIC CHARACTERISTICS OF THE GALLBLADDER?

The gallbladder is a pear-shaped organ that occupies a fossa on the inferior surface of the right lobe of the liver. The superior surface of the gallbladder is attached to the fossa by connective tissue (adventitia), whereas its inferior surface is covered by the peritoneum that is continuous with the hepatic surface. The gallbladder is 7 to 10 cm long and has a capacity of about 50 mL. The gallbladder has three anatomical regions: fundus, body, and neck. The fundus, the dilated cap of the gallbladder, contacts the anterior abdominal wall at the ninth right costal cartilage. The body of the organ projects up,

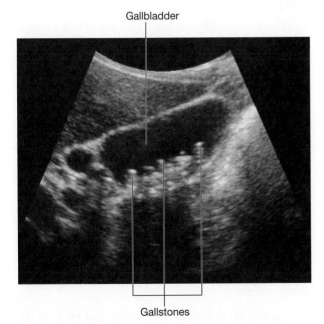

Gallbladder

Gallstones

FIGURE 3-22 Ultrasound demonstrating stones in the gallbladder. (Drake R, Vogl W and Mitchell A: *Gray's Anatomy for Students.* Churchill Livingstone, 2004. Fig. 4-94.)

posteriorly, and to the left, where it narrows to form the neck. The neck is continuous with the cystic duct.

WHAT ARE THE BORDERS OF THE HEPATOCYSTIC TRIANGLE (OF CALOT)?

The hepatocystic triangle has three borders: superior, medial, and lateral. The borders are formed as follows (Fig. 3-23):

- The superior border is defined by the cystic artery.
- The medial border by the common hepatic duct.
- The lateral border by the cystic duct.

The triangle of Calot is a useful anatomical landmark in identifying the arterial supply to the gallbladder prior to its surgical removal.

WHAT IS THE ARTERIAL SUPPLY TO THE GALLBLADDER?

The gallbladder is supplied by the cystic artery, which commonly springs from the right hepatic artery. The cystic artery usually courses posteriorly in the hepatocystic triangle along the medial side of the cystic duct and bifurcates into superficial and deep branches prior to penetrating the wall of the gallbladder.

WHAT ARTERIAL VARIATIONS MUST THE SURGEON ACCOUNT FOR BEFORE PERFORMING A CHOLECYSTECTOMY?

Before dividing the cystic artery, the surgeon should rule out the presence of a variant cystic artery and an accessory cystic artery. A variant cystic artery supplies an arterial branch to the liver. If this hepatic feeder is

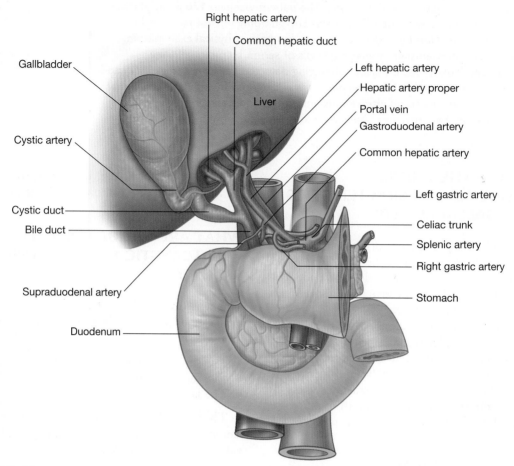

FIGURE 3-23 Triangle of Calot is bordered by the cystic artery, common hepatic duct, and cystic duct. (Drake R, Vogl W and Mitchell A: *Gray's Anatomy for Students*. Churchill Livingstone, 2004. Fig. 4-99.)

present, the variant cystic artery must be divided distal to this branch to preserve blood flow to the liver.

An accessory cystic artery may spring from one of three sources:

- Hepatic artery proper
- Gastroduodenal artery
- Celiac trunk

If the accessory cystic artery is present and not identified, removal of the gallbladder results in hemorrhaging.

Other variations include:

- Originates from the hepatic artery proper coursing outside of the hepatocystic triangle anterior to the common bile duct
- Issues from the right hepatic artery coursing outside of the hepatocystic triangle anterior to the common hepatic and cystic ducts

- Springs from the left gastric artery coursing anteriorly in the hepatocystic triangle anterior to the common hepatic and cystic ducts
- Branches from the gastroduodenal artery or the celiac trunk
- Cystic artery replaces the right hepatic artery

WHAT IS THE VENOUS DRAINAGE OF THE GALLBLADDER?

The venous drainage of the gallbladder occurs via several routes:

- Cystic veins that drain the fundus and body of the gallbladder drain into the liver
- Veins from the neck of the gallbladder and the biliary ducts empty directly or indirectly into the hepatic portal vein or directly into the liver

WHAT IS THE LYMPHATIC DRAINAGE OF THE GALLBLADDER AND CYSTIC DUCT?

Lymph draining the gallbladder and cystic duct passes through the cystic lymph node before filtering through the hepatic lymph nodes. Lymph then flows from the hepatic nodes to celiac nodes.

WHAT IS THE INNERVATION OF THE GALLBLADDER AND HOW DOES THIS RELATE TO WHERE PAIN IS REFERRED?

Sympathetic fibers, from the lateral gray horns of spinal cord segments T7 to T9, travel in the greater splanchnic nerves to the celiac plexus, thence to the gallbladder along the branches of the hepatic artery. Parasympathetic fibers from the vagus accompany the sympathetic fibers to supply the gallbladder.

Referred pain is based on the above dermatomes. This means that the visceral afferents, which are principally from the right, will refer pain to the right upper abdominal quadrant. If the gallbladder irritates the visceral peritoneum of the diaphragm, pain may refer to the right shoulder. This occurs because the visceral peritoneum of the diaphragm is innervated by the phrenic nerve (C3-C5).

HOW CAN A GALLSTONE LEAD TO PANCREATITIS?

A gallstone can be propelled along the biliary tree to the hepatopancreatic ampulla (of Vater). If the gallstone is large enough, it will plug the ampulla and prevent pancreatic juice from flowing into the duodenum. This damming effect causes an increase in the pressure within the ductal system of the pancreas, which leads to interstitial edema. In turn, interstitial edema compresses the blood vessels, causing ischemia. The injurious stimulus of ischemia evokes damage of the acinar cells and a subsequent activation of the pancreatic enzymes. The activated enzymes begin to digest the pancreas, which leads to the development of pancreatitis.

A COMPLICATION OF ACUTE CALCULOUS CHOLECYSTITIS IS PERFORATION OF THE GALLBLADDER. WHAT ARE THE LAYERS OF THE WALL OF THE GALLBLADDER THAT WOULD BE PERFORATED?

The wall of the gallbladder is composed of four layers. From internal to external, the layers are the:

- Mucosa. This layer contains simple columnar epithelium supported by a basal lamina and underlying connective tissue, the lamina propria. Near the neck of the gallbladder, the lamina propria contains simple tubuloalveolar glands. These glands extend into the fibromuscular layer and secrete mucus.
- Fibromuscular layer or muscularis. This layer contains an irregular, loose array of smooth muscle fibers and collagen and elastic fibers. The smooth muscle fibers run longitudinally, transversely, and obliquely. The collagen and elastic fibers reside in the spaces between the smooth muscle fibers.
- Perimuscular connective tissue layer. This is a dense connective layer of collagen and elastic fibers. Also occupying this layer are macrophages, fibroblasts, adipose cells, and the nerves, blood vessels, and lymphatics that supply the organ.
- Serosa and adventitia. A serosa covers the part of the gallbladder facing the abdominal cavity. The part facing the liver is coated by adventitia.

HOW DOES THE GALLBLADDER DEVELOP?

The gallbladder develops from the distal part of the foregut. The first visible sign is the development of a hepatic diverticulum during the fourth week of development (Fig. 3-24). The diverticulum divides into a large cranial part and a small caudal part. The small caudal part is the primordium of the gallbladder. The cystic duct develops from the stalk that connects the diverticulum to the foregut.

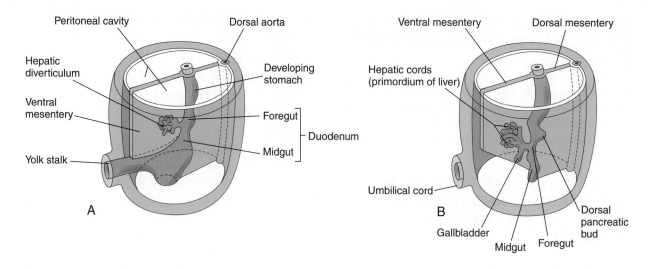

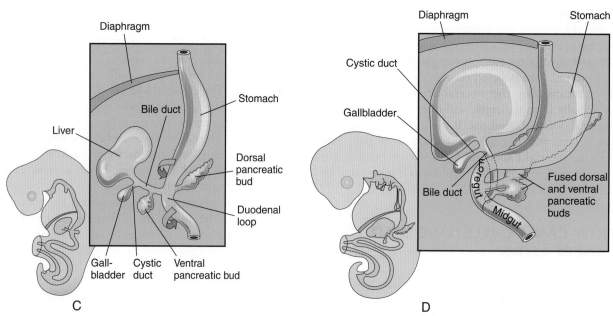

FIGURE 3-24 Illustrations showing the progressive development of the gallbladder. Note that the gallbladder develops from the smaller, caudal portion of the hepatic diverticulum. (Moore K and Persaud TVN: *The Developing Human*, 7e. WB Saunders, 2003. Fig. 12-5.)

A 46-year-old man presented to his physician with complaints of difficulty swallowing (dysphagia) and persistent heartburn of moderate discomfort. Because of the manifestation of dysphagia, a barium swallow was ordered that revealed a stricture at the distal end of the esophagus. Next, an endoscopic examination demonstrated esophagitis, and a biopsy showed the presence of Barrett's esophagus (Fig. 3-25B, C and Fig. 3-26). The patient was diagnosed with gastroesophageal reflux disease (GERD) and managed with the proton-pump inhibitor, omeprazole. After 6 months of medical management with omeprazole, the patient still had not achieved good results. He then underwent a fundoplication procedure to restore the competency of the lower esophageal sphincter (LES).

A FUNDOPLICATION INVOLVES WRAPPING THE DISTAL END OF THE ESOPHAGUS WITH THE FUNDUS OF THE STOMACH. TO PERFORM THIS SURGICAL PROCEDURE, THE ARTERIAL SUPPLY AND VENOUS DRAINAGE OF THE FUNDUS MUST BE DIVIDED. WHICH VESSELS WOULD THE SURGEON HAVE TO DIVIDE TO PERFORM THE FUNDOPLICATION? WHAT IS THE PARENT VESSEL OF THESE ARTERIES?

A fundoplication is the wrapping of the fundus of the stomach around the intra-abdominal esophagus. To perform a fundoplication, the fundus most be mobilized. This requires that the vessels that supply and drain the fundus be divided. The surgeon, therefore, divides the short gastric arteries (Fig. 3-27), which issue from the splenic artery, a branch of the celiac trunk, and the short gastric veins.

IS SIMPLE COLUMNAR EPITHELIUM WITH GOBLET CELLS NORMALLY FOUND IN THE ESOPHAGUS? IF NOT, WHAT TYPE OF EPITHELIUM NORMALLY LINES THE ESOPHAGUS?

No. The esophagus is normally lined by stratified squamous, nonkeratinized epithelium to protect it against the abrasive forces of the bolus of food. This type of epithelium, however, does not confer protection against the persistent insult of acid splashing into the distal esophagus in GERD. Consequently, the normal epithelium must undergo an adaptive transformation into an epithelial type, such as that found in the stomach or small intestine, which protects it against the injurious effects of acid reflux (Figs. 3-25 and 3-26). The mucosa of the stomach and duodenum is protected by the presence of simple columnar epithelium that secretes alkaline mucus. In the stomach these are mucus cells, whereas in the duodenum and the rest of the intestines, these are goblet cells. This transformation from one type of epithelium to another is called metaplasia, a process that is reversible if the injurious stimulus is removed. Although metaplasia is an adaptive response to an adverse environment, it is also a precancerous change that can lead to the generation of cancer.

WHAT DRIVES THE METAPLASIA OBSERVED IN BARRETT'S ESOPHAGUS?

It is postulated that the local injury and inflammation due to reflux of gastric acid causes an upregulation of the Wnt receptors, thereby increasing Wnt signaling. Signals from the Wnt receptors are communicated to the nucleus by the action of ß-catenin, an intracellular protein. The conveyed signal then switches on new genes. The cells with these activated new genes morph into intestinal progenitor cells.

IS THE LOWER ESOPHAGEAL SPHINCTER A TRUE ANATOMICAL SPHINCTER?

No. To be a true anatomical sphincter, the muscle fibers must form a thickening that encircles the tubular structure. One example is the pyloric sphincter, which can be palpated in the cadaver as a thickened ring of smooth muscle of the inner circular layer of the muscularis externa. The LES does demonstrate circularly arranged smooth muscle fibers in the muscularis externa that extend from the esophageal hiatus to the cardia of the

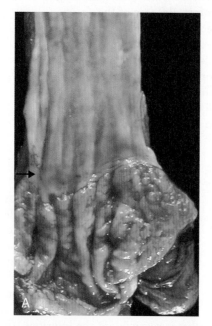

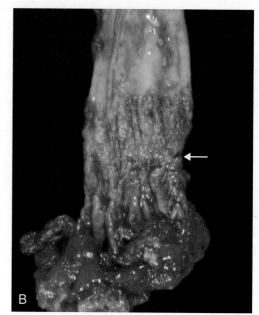

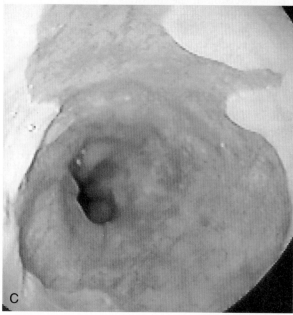

FIGURE 3-25 Barrett's esophagus. **A,** Arrow is pointing to the gastroesophageal junction of a normal esophagus. Esophagus is above the arrow and the stomach is below the arrow. **B,** The arrow is denoting the granular Barrett's esophagus. **C,** Endoscopic view of Barrett's esophagus. Pale areas represent normal stratified squamous epithelium, whereas the red areas represent gastrointestinal epithelium. (Kumar V, Abbas A and Fausto N: *Robbins & Cotran Pathologic Basis of Disease,* 7e. WB Saunders, 2004. Fig. 17-6.)

stomach, but they do not form a thickened collar around the esophagus. Therefore, the LES is a functional sphincter that normally remains tonically contracted until it dilates in response to the advancing peristaltic waves propelling the bolus of food toward the stomach.

A second sphincter mechanism also exists for the esophagus. This is provided by the skeletal muscle fibers of the right crus of the diaphragm, which wraps around the esophagus as it descends through the diaphragm.

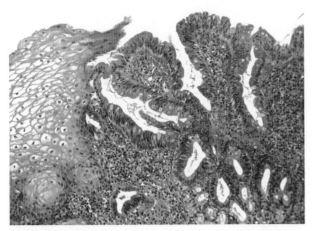

FIGURE3-26 Micrograph of Barrett's esophagus. Stratified squamous epithelium is observed at the left and simple columnar epithelium with goblet cells is seen to the right. (Kumar V, Abbas A and Fausto N: *Robbins & Cotran Pathologic Basis of Disease, 7e.* WB Saunders, 2004. Fig. 17-7.)

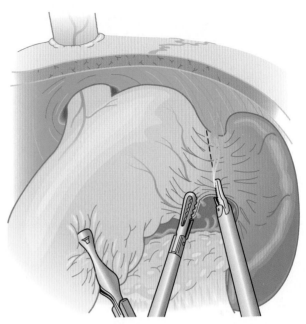

FIGURE 3-27 Mobilization of the fundus of the stomach by dividing the short gastric vessels. (Towsend C et al.: *Sabiston Textbook of Surgery, 17e.* WB Saunders, 2004. Fig. 40-8.)

A 54-year-old man presented to his physician with complaints of decreased urine output and dark-colored urine. His arterial pressure was 150/90. The results of urinalysis were positive for the presence of erythrocytes, leukocytes, and casts. It also showed that specific gravity was above normal and that proteins were elevated. The laboratory result for renin showed that its secretion was suppressed. The patient's glomerular filtration rate, as measured by radionuclide clearance, was decreased. The patient was diagnosed with glomerulonephritis.

WHAT IS THE ARTERIAL SUPPLY TO THE KIDNEY?

Each kidney is supplied by a renal artery that issues from the aorta at the level of the first lumbar vertebra inferior to the superior mesenteric artery. The right renal artery arises just inferior to its fellow. As the artery approaches the hilum of the kidney, it divides into anterior and posterior divisions. Each of these divisions branches into five segmental arteries. The first vessels to spring from the segmental arteries are lobar arteries, which supply the lobes. From these branch interlobar arteries that pass between the renal pyramids in the medulla to the corticomedullary junction. The interlobar arteries then arch over the bases of the pyramids to become arcuate arteries. Springing from these are interlobular arteries that travel through the interstitial spaces between renal lobules. Afferent arterioles branch from the interlobular vessels to supply the glomerular capillaries of the renal corpuscles. The glomerular capillaries are drained by efferent arterioles.

HOW IS THE RENAL CORPUSCLE DESCRIBED HISTOLOGICALLY?

Each kidney contains 1 million to 4 million renal corpuscles. Renal corpuscles are composed of an outer epithelial capsule, which is called the *parietal layer of the glomerular (Bowman's) capsule* (Fig. 3-28). Inside the capsule, a tuft of capillaries, the glomerulus, is covered by an inner epithelial layer, called the *visceral layer* of

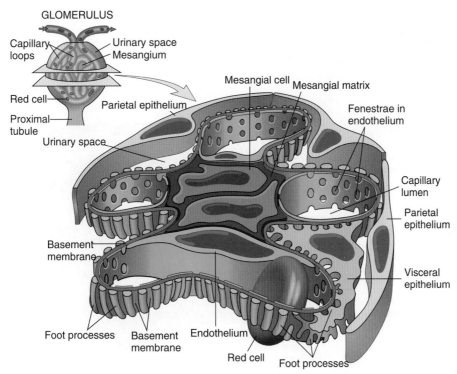

FIGURE 3-28 Illustration of a renal corpuscle. (Kumar V, Abbas A and Fausto N: *Robbins & Cotran Pathologic Basis of Disease*, 7e. WB Saunders, 2004. Fig. 20-1.)

the glomerular capsule. The visceral layer is composed of cells called *podocytes*. The podocytes and glomerular capillaries constitute the filtration barrier (see below). The space between the parietal and visceral layers is the capsular (Bowman's) space. This space receives the ultrafiltrate from the blood flowing through the glomerulus. The renal corpuscle possesses two poles: vascular and urinary. The vascular pole receives the afferent arteriole, which delivers arterial blood to the glomerulus, and an efferent arteriole, which conveys blood away from the glomerulus. The urinary pole is the end of the renal corpuscle that is continuous with the proximal convoluted tubule.

Located between the glomerular capillaries are intraglomerular mesangial cells. These cells are phagocytic and are responsible for vacuuming the basal lamina trapped particulate matter. Mesangial cells are also contractile; thus, they are capable of altering the blood flow through the glomerular capillaries.

NORMALLY, THE GLOMERULAR FILTRATION BARRIER PREVENTS THE FILTRATION OF CELLS AND PROTEINS WITH THE EXCEPTION OF THOSE OF SMALL MOLECULAR WEIGHT. WHAT STRUCTURES FORM THE FILTRATION APPARATUS IN THE KIDNEY?

The filtration barrier is composed of glomerular capillary endothelium, basal lamina of the endothelium, basal lamina of podocytes, and specialized epithelial cells called podocytes (Fig. 3-29). The endothelium of the glomerular capillaries is specialized for filtration by the presence of fenestrae (pores). The fenestrae are not spanned by a diaphragm and range in size between 70 and 90 nm. The pore size excludes blood cells and macromolecules, such as albumin, of 69,000 daltons

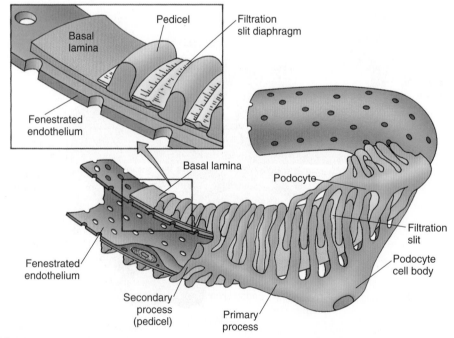

FIGURE 3-29 Illustration of the structural components of the glomerular filtration apparatus. (Gartner L and Hiatt J: *Color Textbook of Histology*, *2e*. WB Saunders, 2001. Fig. 19-7.)

and greater from the ultrafiltrate that forms in the capsular (Bowman's) space of the renal corpuscle.

The fused basal laminae of the endothelium and podocytes have a trilaminar organization that is 300 nm thick. The middle layer, lamina densa, has an electron-dense appearance and is 100 nm thick. The lamina densa contains type IV collagen. Located on both sides of the lamina densa are the laminae rarae. These 100 nm thick laminae are less electron dense and contain laminin, fibronectin, and proteoglycans rich in heparan sulfate, a glycosaminoglycan. The basal lamina is another barrier to filtration for two reasons. First, the basal lamina contains many molecules with negative charges, which act to repel similarly charged molecules in the blood from being filtered. The second reason is that the molecular organization of the basal lamina serves as a trap for macromolecules larger than 69,000 daltons. To prevent clogging of this molecular trap, the basal lamina and snared macromolecules are cleared by intraglomerular mesangial cells. The removed basal lamina is replaced by new basal lamina elements secreted by endothelial cells and podocytes.

The third component of the filtration barrier is formed by podocytes, which constitute the visceral layer of Bowman's capsule. Podocytes assume an intimate relationship with the glomerular capillaries. Podocytes have several primary cytoplasmic processes that follow the length of the capillaries. Springing from the primary processes are secondary processes (pedicels) that envelop the circumference of the capillaries. The secondary processes of one podocyte interdigitate with secondary processes of another podocyte (Fig. 3-29). The clefts that exist between these interdigitations are called *filtration slits*. The filtration slits are 20 to 40 nm wide and are spanned by a porous, thin-slit diaphragm.

WHAT ARE THE HISTOLOGIC ALTERATIONS IN GLOMERULONEPHRITIS?

Glomerulonephritis is characterized by one or more of the following tissue alterations:

- Hypercellularity (Fig. 3-30). Several different cell types can contribute to the increase in cell number observed in the glomerular capillaries: endothelial cells, mesangial cells, neutrophils, monocytes, lymphocytes, and parietal epithelial cells. In rapidly progressive glomerulonephritis, the hypercellularity forms a crescent-shaped mass of cells (Fig. 3-31).
- Basal lamina thickening typically due to the deposition of immune complexes
- Effacement and detachment of podocyte processes (Fig. 3-32)
- Hyalinization and sclerosis. As a result of endothelial cell or capillary wall injury, the vessel becomes leakier than normal. Consequently, there is an increased exudate of plasma proteins into the structures of the glomerulus. This plasm protein exudate is referred to as *hyalin*. Accumulation of hyalin contributes to the obliteration of glomerular capillaries, which is a characteristic of sclerosis.

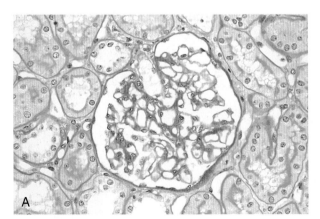
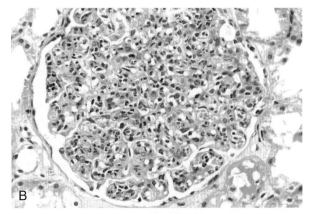

FIGURE 3-30 Acute proliferative glomerulonephritis. **A**, Normal glomerulus. **B**, Note the hypercellularity of the glomerulus due to an infiltration of leukocytes and proliferation of cells associated with the glomerulus. (Kumar V, Abbas A and Fausto N: *Robbins & Cotran Pathologic Basis of Disease*, 7e. WB Saunders, 2004. Fig. 20-16. Courtesy of Dr. H. Rennke, Brigham and Women's Hospital, Boston, MA.)

WHAT CELLS SECRETE RENIN AND WHAT ARE THEIR ULTRASTRUCTURAL CHARACTERISTICS?

The juxtaglomerular apparatus is located at the vascular pole of the renal corpuscle (Fig. 3-33). The apparatus is composed of the macula densa, juxtaglomerular cells, and extraglomerular mesangial cells. Of these structures, it is the juxtaglomerular cells that synthesize and release renin. These cells are specialized smooth muscle cells in the tunica media of the afferent arteriole and are rarely found in the efferent arteriole.

Ultrastructurally, juxtaglomerular cells vary in their differences, with some cells having features of typical smooth muscle cells to cells with very few or no myofilaments and a large number of secretory vesicles. The latter cells possess the usual complement of organelles found in protein-secreting cells.

The macula densa (Latin for dense spot) is a region of closely packed columnar cells in the distal convoluted tubule that abuts the afferent arteriole and the juxtaglomerular cells. The macula densa cells are specialized for measuring the ionic and water content of the ultrafiltrate as it flows through the distal convoluted tubule. If sodium and chloride ion concentrations are too low, the macula densa signals the juxtaglomerular cells to release renin. Renin initiates an enzymatic cascade that culminates in the formation of angiotensin II. Angiotensin II preferentially constricts the efferent arteriole, thereby increasing the glomerular filtration rate. The increase in filtration rate increases the concentration of sodium and chloride in the ultrafiltrate. The macula densa also increases the glomerular filtration rate by dilating the afferent arteriole.

The functional significance of the extraglomerular mesangial cells has not been elucidated.

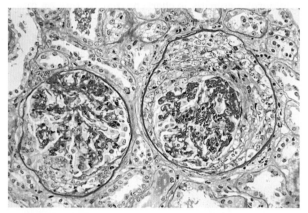

FIGURE 3-31 Crescentic glomerulonephritis (PAS stain). Observe the crescent mass of cells in each renal corpuscle. The mass of cells is caused by an infiltration of leukocytes and a proliferation of cells. (Kumar V, Abbas A and Fausto N: *Robbins & Cotran Pathologic Basis of Disease*, 7e. WB Saunders, 2004. Fig. 20-17. Courtesy of Dr. M.A. Venkatachalam, University of Texas Health Sciences Center, San Aantonio, TX.)

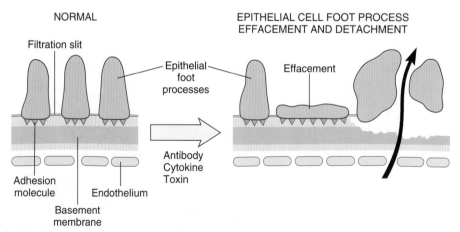

FIGURE 3-32 Effacement and detachment of podocyte foot processes in response to injurious stimuli. (Kumar V, Abbas A and Fausto N: *Robbins & Cotran Pathologic Basis of Disease*, 7e. WB Saunders, 2004. Fig. 20-12.)

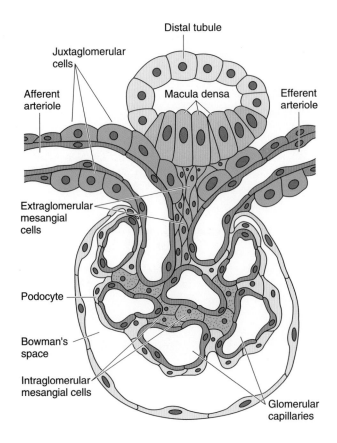

FIGURE 3-33 Illustration of the juxtaglomerular apparatus. (Gartner L and Hiatt J: *Color Textbook of Histology*, *2e*. WB Saunders, 2001. Fig. 19-14.)

A 16-year-old boy, requiring a sports physical examination, was brought to the physician's office by his father. When the physician performed the examination for an inguinal hernia, he felt an impulse against his fingertip at the superficial inguinal ring. This finding was consistent with an inguinal hernia.

WHAT ARE THE STRUCTURES THAT FORM THE ANTERIOR AND POSTERIOR WALLS, ROOF, AND FLOOR OF THE INGUINAL CANAL?

- The anterior wall is formed principally by the aponeurosis of the external abdominal oblique muscle. The internal abdominal oblique muscles contributes by enhancing the structural integrity of the lateral margin of the anterior wall.
- The posterior wall is formed principally by the transversalis fascia. The conjoint tendon reinforces the medial margin of the posterior wall. The conjoint tendon represents the convergence of the internal abdominal oblique and transversus abdominis tendons as it attaches to the pecten pubis.
- The roof is formed by the internal abdominal oblique and transversus abdominis muscles.
- The floor is chiefly formed by the inguinal ligament and medially by the lacunar ligament. The lacunar ligament is formed by the reflected fibers of the inguinal ligament to the pectineal line of the pecten pubis.

WHAT STRUCTURES DEFINE THE BOUNDARIES OF THE INGUINAL (HESSELBACH'S) TRIANGLE?

The three structures that define the boundaries of the inguinal triangle are (Fig. 3-34):

- The inguinal ligament (of Poupart) forms the inferior border.
- The inferior epigastric artery defines the lateral boundary.
- The rectus abdominis muscle forms the medial border.

WHAT LANDMARK OF THE INGUINAL TRIANGLE IS USED TO DIFFERENTIATE A DIRECT INGUINAL HERNIA FROM AN INDIRECT?

The inferior epigastric artery and vein are the landmarks. Direct inguinal hernias protrude through the inguinal canal medial to the inferior epigastric vessels, whereas indirect inguinal hernias pass lateral to these vessels.

IF THE PATIENT HAD A FEMORAL HERNIA RATHER THAN AN INGUINAL DEFECT, WHAT ARTERY, IF PRESENT, COULD BE MISTAKENLY SEVERED DURING ITS SURGICAL REPAIR, CAUSING UNCONTROLLED HEMORRHAGING?

An aberrant obturator artery replaces the obturator artery in 20% to 30% of the population. The normal parent vessel of the obturator artery is the internal iliac artery, but when an aberrant obturator artery is present, it springs from the inferior epigastric artery and may curve around the lacunar ligament. If the presence or absence of this vessel is not confirmed, the surgeon risks dividing this artery during repair of the femoral hernia.

WHAT NERVES ARE VULNERABLE TO INJURY DURING A SURGICAL REPAIR OF AN INGUINAL HERNIA?

Because of their anatomical relationships, several nerves are at risk for injury during repair of the inguinal hernia (Fig. 3-35). The three most commonly injured nerves during an open repair procedure are:

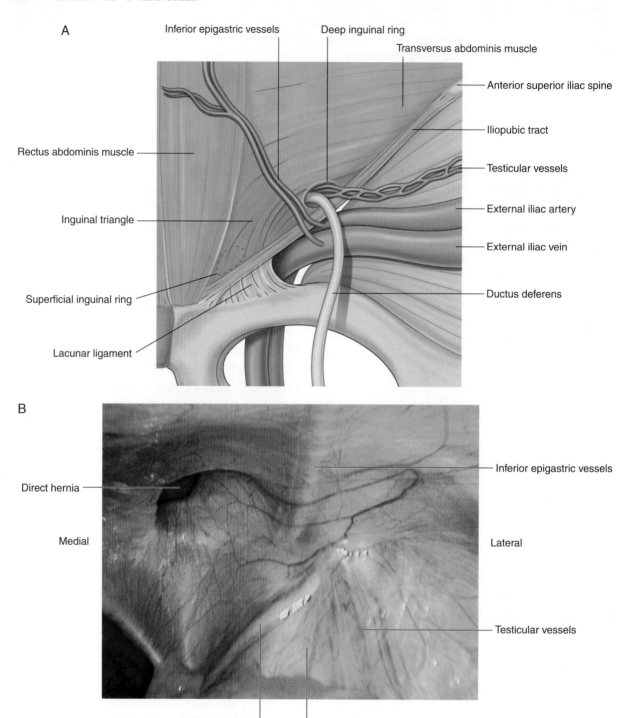

A

Inferior epigastric vessels

Deep inguinal ring

Transversus abdominis muscle

Anterior superior iliac spine

Iliopubic tract

Testicular vessels

External iliac artery

External iliac vein

Ductus deferens

Rectus abdominis muscle

Inguinal triangle

Superficial inguinal ring

Lacunar ligament

B

Direct hernia

Medial

Inferior epigastric vessels

Lateral

Testicular vessels

Ductus deferens

External iliac vessels

FIGURE 3-34   Right inguinal (Hesselbach's) triangle. **A,** Internal view. **B,** Laparoscopic view. (Drake R, Vogl W and Mitchell A: *Gray's Anatomy for Students.* Churchill Livingstone, 2004. Fig. 4-50.)

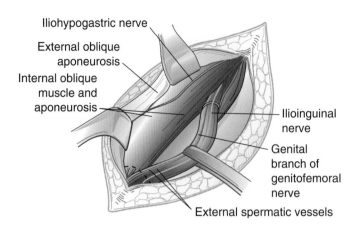

Iliohypogastric nerve

External oblique aponeurosis

Internal oblique muscle and aponeurosis

Ilioinguinal nerve

Genital branch of genitofemoral nerve

External spermatic vessels

FIGURE 3-35 Relationships of the ilioinguinal and genito-femoral nerves in the inguinal canal during surgical repair. (Arregui M, Nagan R: *Inguinal Hernia: Advances or Controversies?* © 1994. Radcliffe Medical Press Ltd. Reproduced with permission of the copyright holder.)

TABLE 3-5 Distribution of the Iliohypogastric, Ilioinguinal, and Genital Branch of Genitofemoral Nerves

Nerve	Sensory Distribution	Motor Distribution
Iliohypogastric (L1)	Skin overlying iliac crest, and hypogastric and suprapubic regions	Internal abdominal oblique Transversus abdominis
Ilioinguinal (L1)	Scrotal skin or skin of labium majus, mons pubis, and medial thigh	Internal abdominal oblique Transversus abdominis
Genital branch of genitofemoral (L1 and L2)	Scrotal skin or skin of mons pubis and labium majus	Cremaster muscle

- Iliohypogastric (L1)
- Ilioinguinal (L1)
- Genital branch of the genitofemoral nerve (L1-L2)

If the hernia is repaired laparoscopically, the lateral femoral cutaneous (L2-L3) and genitofemoral (L1-L2) nerves may be damaged.

WHAT BLOOD VESSELS MUST BE RETRACTED OR LIGATED DURING AN ANTERIOR APPROACH TO HERNIAL REPAIR?

In an anterior approach, the surgeon will encounter several superficial blood vessels. These are:

- Superficial circumflex iliac artery and vein
- Superficial epigastric artery and vein
- External pudendal (superficial and deep) arteries and veins

The arteries above spring from the femoral artery and the veins drain into the great saphenous vein.

WHAT ARE THE MOTOR AND SENSORY DISTRIBUTIONS OF THE ILIOINGUINAL, ILIOHYPOGASTRIC, AND GENITAL BRANCH OF THE GENITOFEMORAL NERVE?

The sensory and motor distributions of these nerves are described in the Table 3-5.

HOW CAN THE PHYSICIAN ASSESS INJURY TO THE GENITAL BRANCH OF THE GENITOFEMORAL NERVE?

The physician would assess the function of the genital branch of the genitofemoral by testing the cremasteric reflex. This reflex is evoked by stroking the upper medial thigh. This region of skin is innervated by the ilioinguinal nerve (L1). The sensation is conveyed by afferent fibers in L1 to the spinal cord. Efferent fibers of this reflex arc leave the cord to enter the genitofemoral nerve. If the genital branch is intact, the ipsilateral testis will be elevated by contraction of the cremaster muscle.

A mother rushed her 2-year-old son to the emergency department. She had earlier changed his diaper before bedtime and noticed that his stool and diaper were colored with bright red blood. The doctor asked her if she had previously noticed anything unusual about her son's soiled diaper. She said, "This was the first time I noticed the blood. Last week one of his diapers contained black-appearing stool, but I did not think that there was anything wrong at the time." Lab results showed that hematocrit and hemoglobin were on the low end of normal. A technetium (Tc 99m)-pertechnetate scan showed a hot spot along the boy's ileum (Fig. 3-36). He was diagnosed with Meckel's (ileal) diverticulum. The lesion was surgically resected.

WHAT IS THE PURPOSE OF THE TC 99M-PERTECHNETATE SCAN?

The purpose of Tc 99m-pertechnetate is to label the heterotopic gastric mucosa. Specifically, Tc 99m-pertechnetate is taken up by mucus-secreting cells causing a hot spot to appear with the scan.

WHAT IS THE EMBRYOLOGIC BASIS OF A MECKEL'S DIVERTICULUM?

A Meckel's diverticulum is a congenital outpouching of the ileum that occurs in 2% to 4% of the population, with males more commonly affected than females. During development, the primitive midgut destined to become the ileum communicates with the yolk sac through the vitelline duct (yolk stalk). Ultimately, the entire vitelline duct degenerates. If the proximal segment of the vitelline duct persists, it forms an outpouching of the ileum at its antimesen-teric border 40 to 50 cm (16 to 20 inches) from the ileocecal junction (Fig. 3-37). In some cases, the Meckel's diverticulum is connected by a fibrous cord to the umbilicus or by a tissue pipe called an *omphaloenteric fistula* (Latin for pipe).

A MECKEL'S DIVERTICULUM IS CLASSIFIED AS A TRUE DIVERTICULUM. WHAT DISTINGUISHES A TRUE DIVERTICULUM FROM A FALSE DIVERTICULUM?

A true diverticulum involves all four layers of the wall of the tubular structure. In the case of the ileum, the diverticulum involved the mucosa, submucosa,

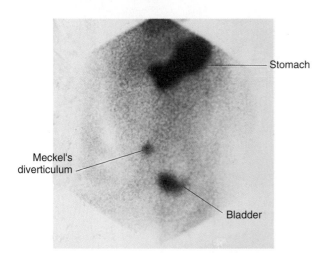

FIGURE 3-36 Tc 99m-pertechnetate scintigraphy demonstrating heterotopic gastric mucosa in a Meckel's diverticulum. (Towsend C et al.: *Sabiston Textbook of Surgery, 17e.* WB Saunders, 2004. Fig. 46-45. Courtesy of Melvyn H. Schreiber, M.D., The University of Texas Medical Branch.)

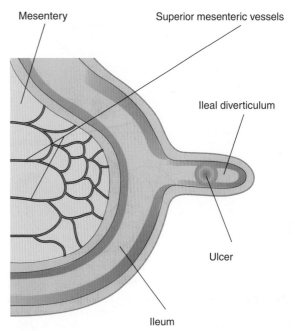

FIGURE 3-37 Illustration of a Meckel's diverticulum containing heterotopic gastric mucosa. (Moore K and Persaud TVN: *The Developing Human, 7e.* WB Saunders, 2003. Fig. 12-22.)

muscularis externa (sometimes referred to as the *muscularis propria*), and serosa. In contrast, a false diverticulum (pseudodiverticulum) only involves the two innermost layers: mucosa and submucosa.

WHY DO SOME MECKEL'S DIVERTICULA ULCERATE?

Heterotopic gastric mucosa is present in 50% of Meckel's diverticula. The gastric mucosa is derived from pluripotent cells lining the yolk stalk (vitelline duct). Ulcers develop if the heterotopic gastric mucosa harbors acid-secreting parietal cells. Nidi of gastric

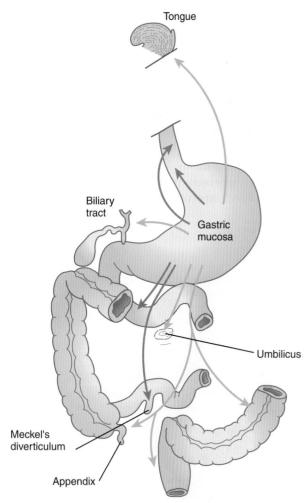

FIGURE 3-38 Structures that may harbor gastric tissue. The red arrows show sites of most frequent occurrence. The pink arrows indicate less common sites of occurrence. (Carlson B: *Human Embryology and Developmental Biology, 3e*. Mosby, 2004. Fig. 15-7. Based on Gray SW, Skandalakis JE: *Embryology for surgeons*, Philadelphia, 1972, WB Saunders.)

mucosa may also occur with relative frequency in the duodenum and abdominal esophagus and less commonly in the appendix, rectum, sigmoid colon, umbilical region, biliary tract, and at the base of the tongue (Fig. 3-38). In some cases (5%), Meckel's diverticula contain pancreatic tissue and, less frequently, colonic mucosa is found.

WHERE DO DIVERTICULA COMMONLY FORM IN THE SMALL AND LARGE INTESTINES?

The most common sites of diverticula are in the large intestine. The sigmoid colon is most frequently involved, followed by the descending colon. These diverticula are classified as pseudodiverticula, as only the mucosa and submucosa protrude through a weakness in the colonic wall.

After the colon, the duodenum has the greatest incidence of diverticulum formation. These pseudo-

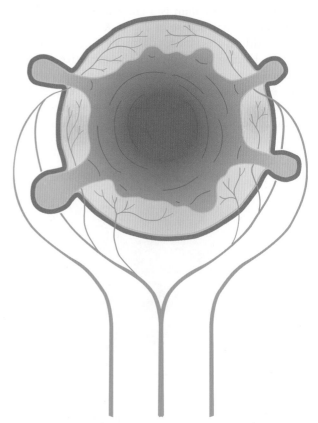

FIGURE 3-39 Development of diverticula. Diverticula form at weak points in the wall of the large intestine. These weak points occur where blood vessels penetrate the wall. (Towsend C et al.: *Sabiston Textbook of Surgery, 17e*. WB Saunders, 2004. Fig. 48-15.)

diverticula occur in the descending (second) segment of the duodenum 67% to 75% of the time. The horizontal (third) segment is the second most commonly affected duodenal part, and the superior (first) segment is the least involved.

WHY DO DIVERTICULA COMMONLY OCCUR IN THE LARGE INTESTINE?

The development of diverticula is dependent on two factors: (1) areas of weakness in the colonic wall and (2) increased intraluminal pressure. Histologically, the wall of the colon is distinctive because of the absence of a complete longitudinal layer of smooth muscle in its muscularis externa. In its place are three longitudinal bands of smooth muscle called teniae coli. Points of weakness in the colon are created by the penetration of wall by vasa recta and nerves. Because the neurovascular structures penetrate the colonic wall between the mesenteric tenia coli and the lateral teniae coli, diverticula are confined to the mesenteric wall of the colon and do not occur on the antimesenteric side of the wall (Fig. 3-39).

A 55-year-old man with a history of alcohol abuse presents to the emergency department with chronic epigastric pain radiating to the back and jaundice. He comments that the pain is aggravated after eating and after an evening of alcohol consumption, and he also complains of nausea and vomiting and feeling full after consuming small amounts of food (early satiety). An abdominal CT scan revealed a dilated main pancreatic duct and several pseudocysts of the pancreas. Ultimately, a diagnosis of chronic pancreatitis was made.

WHAT ARE THE PARTS OF THE PANCREAS?

The pancreas, which resembles a sea horse lying transversely, has the following parts (Fig. 3-40):

- Head. The hooklike prolongation of the head is called the *uncinate process.*
- Neck
- Body
- Tail

WHAT ARE THE ANATOMICAL RELATIONSHIPS OF THE PANCREAS?

The pancreas has the following anatomical relationships (Fig. 3-41):

- Rests in the epigastric and left hypochondriac regions along the posterior abdominal wall
- Lies across the vertebral bodies of L1-L3
- Lies posterior to the stomach
- Transverse colon attaches to its anterior border

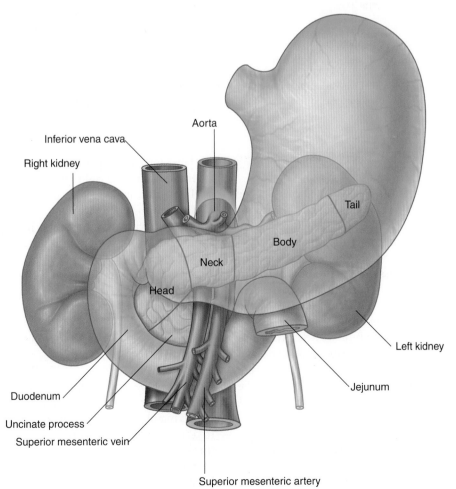

FIGURE 3-40 Pancreas. (Drake R, Vogl W and Mitchell A: *Gray's Anatomy for Students.* Churchill Livingstone, 2004. Fig. 4-87.)

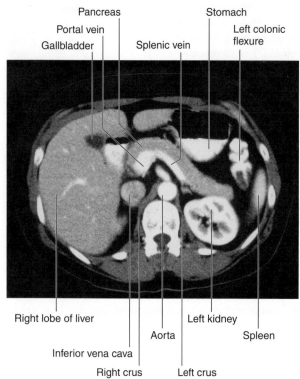

Pancreas
Portal vein
Gallbladder
Splenic vein
Stomach
Left colonic flexure

Right lobe of liver
Inferior vena cava
Right crus
Aorta
Left crus
Left kidney
Spleen

FIGURE 3-41 Abdominal CT scan showing the anatomical relationships of the pancreas. (Drake R, Vogl W and Mitchell A: *Gray's Anatomy for Students.* Churchill Livingstone, 2004. Fig. 4-88.)

The four regions of the pancreas have the following anatomical relationships:

● Head. The head fits into the C-shaped curve of the duodenum. Its posterior surface lies on the inferior vena cava, right renal vessels, and the left renal vein as it empties into the inferior vena cava. The uncinate process hooks around the superior mesenteric vessels to assume its position posterior to these vessels. The common bile duct passes in a groove along the posterosuperior surface of the head and may be embedded in it.
● Neck. The superior mesenteric vessels groove its posterior surface and the superior mesenteric and splenic veins converge to form the portal vein posterior to the neck. The neck lies next to the pylorus of the stomach, and its anterior surface is covered by peritoneum.
● Body. The peritoneum lines its anterior surface. Its posterior surface contacts the aorta, superior mesenteric artery, left adrenal gland, left kidney, and the left renal vessels. The splenic vein also is in

contact with its posterior surface and may even penetrate the gland.
● Tail. The end of the tail usually comes into contact with the hilum of the spleen. As the tail approaches the spleen, it is surrounded by the layers of the hepatorenal ligament. The splenic vessels accompany the tail within this ligament. Because of the anatomic relationship of the pancreatic tail with the hilum of the spleen, care must be exercised during a splenectomy to avoid damaging the pancreas.

WHAT IS THE BLOOD SUPPLY TO THE PANCREAS?

The blood supply to the pancreas is from the:

● Anterior and posterior superior pancreaticoduodenal arteries, branches of the gastroduodenal artery
● Anterior and posterior inferior pancreaticoduodenal arteries, branches of the superior mesenteric artery
● Branches of the splenic artery, i.e., dorsal pancreatic, great pancreatic, caudal pancreatic, and several unnamed twigs.

WHAT IS THE VENOUS DRAINAGE OF THE PANCREAS?

The pancreas is drained by the following veins:

● The anterior superior pancreaticoduodenal vein empties into the right gastro-omental vein.
● The posterior superior pancreaticoduodenal vein drains into the portal vein.
● The anterior and posterior inferior pancreaticoduodenal veins empty into the superior mesenteric vein.
● Several small unnamed veins drain into the splenic vein.

WHAT IS THE LYMPHATIC DRAINAGE OF THE PANCREAS?

The lymph vessels accompany the blood vessels that supply and drain the spleen. The lymph vessels convey lymph mainly to the pancreaticosplenic nodes and some to the pyloric nodes. From these nodes, lymph is transported by efferent lymphatic vessels to three sets of additional nodes: celiac, superior mesenteric, and hepatic.

WHAT IS THE NERVE SUPPLY TO THE PANCREAS?

Preganglionic sympathetic fibers originate from the lateral gray horns of spinal cord levels T6 to T10 and travel in the thoracic splanchnic nerves to the celiac and superior mesenteric ganglia. Postganglionic sympathetic fibers leave the ganglia and become commingled with parasympathetic fibers from the vagus in the celiac and superior mesenteric plexuses. The autonomic nerve fibers accompany blood vessels that supply the pancreas to reach the gland. Visceral afferent fibers are conveyed in the sympathetic fibers. Pain from the pancreatic head is referred to the lower epigastrium (e.g., pancreatitis).

WHAT IS THE NORMAL HISTOLOGIC APPEARANCE OF THE EXOCRINE PANCREAS?

The exocrine pancreas is classified as a compound acinar gland. It is surrounded by a delicate connective tissue capsule. Extensions of the capsule called septa divide the gland into lobules. The lobules contain spherical structures called acini. An acinus is a collection of 40 to 50 serous (acinar) cells. The acinus is separated from neighboring acini by a basal lamina. The center of the acinus contains a lumen that receives secretions from the acinar cells. This lumen represents the initial duct segment (intra-acinar intercalated duct) of the gland and is lined by centroacinar cells. The intra-acinar intercalated duct continues outside of the acinus as an intercalated duct that ultimately empties into an intralobular duct. Several intralobular ducts then converge to form an interlobular duct that empties into the main or accessory pancreatic duct.

WHAT ARE THE CELLULAR FEATURES OF ACINAR CELLS?

The acinar cell exhibits the following cellular features:

- Shaped like a pyramid with its base supported by a basal lamina. The apex points toward the lumen in the central part of the acinus.
- At the light microscopic level, the acinar cell clearly demonstrates polarity. The base of the cell is basophilic, whereas the apex is acidophilic.

- The basophilia is caused by the presence of the nucleus, polyribosomes, and abundant rough endoplasmic reticulum.
- The acidophilia, on the other hand, is imparted by a large number of secretory vesicles (granules).
- Mitochondria are numerous in the basal region of the acinar cell, but their acidophilia is obscured by the intense basophilia.
- A well-developed Golgi apparatus is also found in these cells.

WHAT IS A PSEUDOCYST?

A pseudocyst is a cavity filled with fluid and necrotic debris, but it is not lined by epithelium.

HOW DOES THE PANCREAS PROTECT ITSELF FROM SELF DIGESTION BY MANY OF ITS SYNTHESIZED ENZYMES?

To protect itself against self digestion, the acinar cells of the exocrine pancreas must synthesize its digestive enzymes in an inactive form. These inactive enzymes are called *proenzymes* and they are packaged by the Golgi complex into zymogen (secretory) granules. Intracellular activation of these enzymes by injurious stimuli causes autodigestion of the pancreas. This is the basis of pancreatitis.

WHAT ARE THE MORPHOLOGIC ALTERATIONS OF CHRONIC PANCREATITIS?

The morphologic alterations that accompany chronic pancreatitis (Fig. 3-42) are:

- Pancreas is hard. Dilated ducts and calcified concretions may be present.
- Fibrosis of the parenchyma
- Acini are reduced in number and size.
- Epithelium of the pancreatic ducts may atrophy, hypertrophy, or undergo squamous metaplasia.
- Concretions may be present in the ducts.
- Pancreatic islets (of Langerhans) become enveloped by sclerotic tissue and are eventually reduced in number

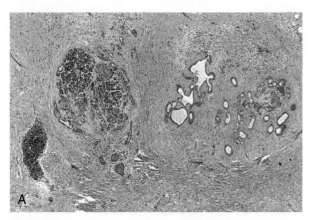

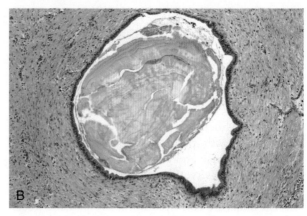

FIGURE 3-42 Chronic pancreatitis. **A**, Extensive fibrosis and atrophy of the glands is evident. **B**, Dilated pancreatic ducts with eosinophilic ductal concretions. (Kumar V, Abbas A and Fausto N: *Robbins & Cotran Pathologic Basis of Disease*, 7e. WB Saunders, 2004. Fig. 19-8.)

A 55-year-old man presented with complaints of epigastric pain that was of burning quality. He stated that the pain occurred on an empty stomach about 3 hours after meals and at bedtime. When prompted by the physician, he commented that the pain was relieved by meals and antacids. The ensuing endoscopic examination (Fig. 3-43) and biopsy revealed a peptic ulcer in the stomach that was positive for *Helicobacter pylori*. The physician prescribed amoxicillin and metronidazole to eradicate the *H. pylori* and omeprazole, a proton-pump inhibitor.

WHAT IS THE ARTERIAL SUPPLY TO THE STOMACH?

The stomach is richly supplied with arterial vessels. These vessels are the:

- Left gastric artery, a branch of the celiac trunk. The left gastric artery courses along the lesser curvature of the stomach. In some individuals, a branch from the left gastric artery is the primary or secondary supply of the left lobe of the liver. A surgeon must evaluate this potential supply to the liver before ligating the left gastric artery.
- Right gastric artery, a branch of the common hepatic artery. The right gastric artery travels along the lesser curvature of the stomach to anastomose with the left gastric artery.
- Right gastro-omental artery, springing from the gastroduodenal artery, passes along the greater curvature of the stomach.

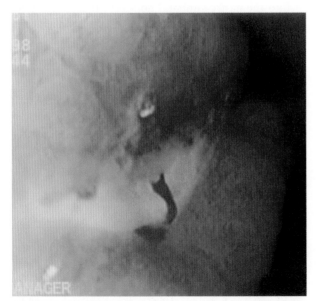

FIGURE 3-43 Gastric ulcer (appears white) with bleeding vessel. (Goldman L and Ausiello D: *Cecil Textbook of Medicine, 22e.* WB Saunders, 2004. Fig. 138-2.)

- Left gastro-omental artery, takes origin from the splenic artery and courses along the greater curvature of the stomach to anastomose with the right gastro-omental artery.
- Short gastric arteries, branches of the splenic artery. The short gastric arteries supply the fundus of the stomach and anastomose with the left gastric and left gastro-omental arteries.

IF A THROMBUS OR EMBOLUS OCCLUDED THE CELIAC TRUNK, WOULD THE STOMACH STILL RECEIVE ARTERIAL BLOOD?

If the celiac trunk was occluded, the stomach would become dependent on its collateral circulation from the superior mesenteric artery. Springing from the superior mesenteric artery or its first jejunal branch is the inferior pancreaticoduodenal artery. The inferior pancreaticoduodenal artery promptly divides into anterior and posterior branches that anastomose with the superior anterior and posterior pancreaticoduodenal branches of the gastroduodenal artery. The gastroduodenal artery issues from the common hepatic artery, a branch of the celiac trunk. Thus, the superior mesenteric artery, through its anastomoses, may supply the stomach with some blood flow even if the celiac trunk is occluded.

WHAT IS THE VENOUS DRAINAGE OF THE STOMACH?

The veins of the stomach are the:

- Left gastric vein, which empties directly into hepatic portal vein
- Right gastric vein, which also drains directly into the hepatic portal vein
- Right gastro-omental vein empties into the superior mesenteric vein or it may join the splenic vein or hepatic portal vein

- Left gastro-omental vein usually empties into the splenic vein
- Short gastric veins drain into the splenic vein

WHAT IS THE INNERVATION OF THE STOMACH?

The stomach is innervated by parasympathetic nerve fibers from the vagus and sympathetic nerve fibers that originate from the lateral gray horns of spinal cord segments T6 to T9 or T10.

The left and right vagus nerves become the anterior and posterior vagal trunks as they descend through the thoracic cavity. The vagal innervation of the stomach is depicted in Figure 3-44. The anterior (left) vagal trunk divides near the gastroesophageal junction into the hepatic branch, which supplies the liver and the pylorus by the pyloric branch. The other branch follows the ventral surface of the stomach along its lesser curvature as the anterior nerve of Latarjet. The posterior (right) trunk of the vagus gives rise to a celiac branch and the criminal nerve of Grassi. The criminal nerve of Grassi supplies the gastric glands in the fundus. If this nerve is left undivided after a vagotomy to surgically treat ulcers, the procedure may prove to be ineffective as ulcers are likely to recur. After issuing these branches, the nerve continues on the dorsal surface of the stomach along the lesser curvature

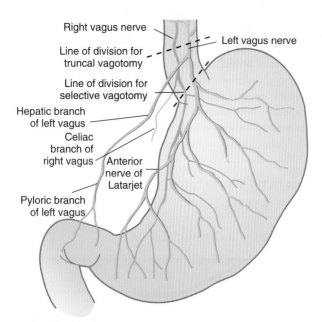

Right vagus nerve

Left vagus nerve

Line of division for truncal vagotomy

Line of division for selective vagotomy

Hepatic branch of left vagus

Celiac branch of right vagus

Anterior nerve of Latarjet

Pyloric branch of left vagus

FIGURE 3-44 Vagal branches innervating the stomach. (Towsend C et al.: *Sabiston Textbook of Surgery, 17e.* WB Saunders, 2004. Fig. 45-4.)

as the posterior nerve of Latarjet. Functionally, parasympathetic stimulation increases glandular secretions and contraction of the stomach.

The sympathetic preganglionic fibers travel in the greater and lesser splanchnic nerves to the celiac plexus. The preganglionic sympathetic fibers primarily terminate in the celiac ganglia. From here, postganglionic fibers accompany the gastric and gastro-omental arteries to innervate the stomach. The fibers then penetrate the wall of the stomach to reach their destinations in the myenteric (Auerbach) and submucosal (Meissner) enteric plexuses. The postganglionic sympathetic fibers are joined by preganglionic parasympathetic fibers, which synapse with postganglionic parasympathetic neurons in these plexuses. Sympathetic fibers are vasomotor to the blood vessels supplying the stomach, convey visceral pain, and are motor to the pyloric sphincter.

WHAT IS THE LYMPHATIC DRAINAGE OF THE STOMACH?

The stomach has four principal lymphatic watersheds. These drainage areas are (Fig. 3-45):

- Lymph drains into the left gastric nodes from the lesser curvature of the stomach and most of its body. Left gastric lymph nodes receive lymph from the largest area of the stomach.
- Gastro-omental nodes receive lymph from the second largest area of the stomach. Lymph drains into the gastro-omental nodes from the right portion of the greater curvature of the stomach and most of the pylorus. Lymph vessels from this region also drain directly into pyloric lymph nodes. The gastro-omental nodes also receive lymph from the left portion of the greater curvature.
- Pancreaticosplenic lymph nodes receive lymph from the fundus and a portion of the body.
- Pyloric lymph nodes receive lymph from the lesser curvature over the pylorus part of the stomach.

HOW DOES THE STOMACH DEVELOP?

The events that occur in the development of the stomach are as follows:

- The primordium of the stomach begins as a slight dilatation of the caudal foregut during the middle of the fourth week. This dilatation occurs in the median plane.

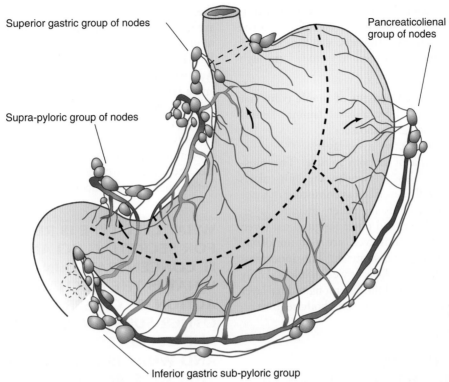

Superior gastric group of nodes

Pancreaticolienal group of nodes

Supra-pyloric group of nodes

Inferior gastric sub-pyloric group

FIGURE 3-45 Lymphatic drainage of the stomach. Left gastric nodes-superior gastric group; pyloric nodes-suprapyloric and infrapyloric nodes; pancreaticolienal-pancreaticosplenic; and gastroomental (unlabeled) follow greater curvature of stomach. (Towsend C et al.: *Sabiston Textbook of Surgery, 17e*. WB Saunders, 2004. Fig. 45-3.)

- The dilatation then begins to enlarge in the ventro-dorsal plane. The dorsal surface grows more rapidly, creating a convex border, whereas the slowly expanding ventral surface creates a concave border. The convex and concave borders are the future greater and lesser curvatures of the stomach, respectively.

- The stomach next undergoes concomitant rotations about two axes. One rotation occurs 90 degrees in a clockwise direction about the longitudinal axis. As a result the left side of the stomach becomes its ventral surface and the right side becomes its posterior surface. The second rotation occurs about the ventrodorsal axis, which causes the pyloric end of the stomach to shift cranially and to the right and the cranial end to move caudally and to the left.

- The stomach now assumes its final position in the abdominal cavity.

ANATOMICALLY, WHERE DO MOST GASTRIC ULCERS OCCUR?

The majority of gastric ulcers occur along the lesser curvature of the stomach at or near the incisura angularis. The incisura angularis is an important anatomical landmark to delineate the pyloric antrum from the corpus of the stomach.

IF THE PATIENT HAD DELAYED TREATMENT AND THE ULCER PERFORATED THE WALL OF THE STOMACH, THROUGH WHICH LAYERS WOULD IT ERODE?

Peptic ulcers are defined as tissue defects in the mucosal lining of stomach (in this case) or duodenum that have at least penetrated into the submucosal connective tissue layer. Lesions that are confined to the mucosa are known as erosions. In the case of perforation, the mucosal defect has eroded through the following layers:

- Mucosa. The mucosa consists of simple columnar epithelium supported by a basal lamina, lamina propria, and muscularis mucosae.
- Submucosa (a connective tissue layer)
- Muscularis externa of smooth muscle. The muscularis externa, also known as the muscularis propria, is generally described as consisting of three layers of smooth muscle: inner oblique layer, middle circular layer, and outer longitudinal layer. These three layers, however, are not uniformly evident throughout the stomach. The innermost oblique smooth muscle layer is well developed only in the cardiac region, and the outer longitudinal layer is best observed in the cardiac and body regions.
- Serosa

WHAT ARE THE HALLMARK HISTOLOGIC CHARACTERISTICS OF THE MUCOSA OF THE PYLORIC ANTRUM THAT DIFFERENTIATE IT FROM THE CARDIAC AND FUNDUS AND BODY REGIONS OF THE STOMACH?

Histologically, the mucosa of the stomach exhibits three regional differences that can be distinguished from one another based on the following characteristics: length of tubular glands relative to gastric pits (foveolae) and cellular diversity. The three histologic regions of the stomach are the cardiac mucosa, pyloric mucosa, and the mucosa of the fundus and body.

The mucosa of the fundus and body displays short pits and long tubular glands called *gastric glands*. The gastric glands contain the most diverse cell population of the three regions. This cellular diversity imparts a palette of colors with typical hematoxylin and eosin (H & E) staining. Cell types common to this region but not to the cardiac or pyloric regions are chief (zymogenic) and parietal (oxyntic) cells. Chief cells are basophilic, whereas parietal cells are acidophilic. The light-staining to clear-staining cells are mucous (surface and neck), regenerative (stem), and occasional endocrine-secreting (enteroendocrine) cells.

The cardiac mucosa exhibits gastric pits that are shorter than those of the fundus/body and the base of the cardiac tubular glands is more coiled. Parietal cells are infrequent and chief cells are absent, resulting in a monochromatic, clear-staining appearance with H & E. The mucous surface cell is the predominate cell type with some mucous neck cells, regenerative cells, and a few enteroendocrine cells.

The pyloric mucosa is characterized by deep gastric pits and short pyloric tubular glands that branch and are coiled. Like the cardiac glands, the pyloric glands have a monochromatic appearance because they contain the same cell types; however, mucous neck cells outnumber surface mucous cells in pyloric glands.

WHAT CELL TYPE IS RESPONSIBLE FOR SECRETING HCl AND WHERE IS IT CONCENTRATED IN THE MUCOSA? WHAT IS THE MECHANISM OF ACTION OF OMEPRAZOLE? WHAT OTHER SUBSTANCE IS SYNTHESIZED AND SECRETED BY THIS CELL TYPE AND WHAT IS THE SIGNIFICANCE OF THIS SUBSTANCE?

The parietal (oxyntic) cell is responsible for secreting HCl into the lumen of the stomach. The acidophilic parietal cells are principally located in the neck region of gastric glands. By definition, gastric glands are located in the mucosa associated with the fundus and body of the stomach. A distinguishing feature of parietal cells is intracellular canaliculi. These structures are formed by invaginations of the plasma membrane and are lined by microvilli. Intracellular canaliculi and microvilli increase the surface area for acid secretion.

The parietal cell membrane contains a hydrogen-potassium ATPase (pump), an integral protein. The hydrogen-potassium pump is driven by the expenditure of energy in the form of ATP to move hydrogen protons from the intracellular environment of the parietal cell to the gastric lumen in exchange for movement of potassium protons from the gastric lumen to the intracellular milieu of the parietal cell. Proton-pump inhibitors, such as omeprazole, inhibit the hydrogen-potassium pump, thus reducing its ability to acidify the juice of the gastric lumen.

Parietal cells are also responsible for the synthesis and secretion of intrinsic factor, a glycoprotein. Intrinsic factor is required for adequate absorption of vitamin B_{12} in the ileum. A vitamin B_{12} deficiency, as a result of insufficient intrinsic factor, leads to pernicious anemia.

WHAT IS THE ANATOMICAL BASIS OF THE REFERRED PAIN TO THE EPIGASTRIUM?

Visceral pain afferent fibers from the stomach are conveyed by the greater splanchnic nerves (mainly the left), components of the sympathetic nervous system, to the sympathetic trunk. The visceral pain afferent fibers enter spinal cord levels T6-T9 or T10 and converge with somatic afferents from the epigastrium and hypochondriac regions of the body wall. Because the body is accustomed to sensing pain from somatic regions, the visceral pain from the stomach is referred to the epigastrium and can be referred to the left hypochondriac region, as the left greater splanchnic nerve is the principal nerve conveying the visceral pain afferents.

WHAT EMBRYONIC GERM LAYER GIVES RISE TO THE GASTRIC EPITHELIUM AND GLANDS? WHEN CAN GASTRIC PITS BE FIRST OBSERVED? WHEN DO PARIETAL CELLS BEGIN TO SECRETE HYDROCHLORIC ACID?

The epithelium and glands of the stomach are derived from the endoderm of the midgut segment of the primitive gut tube. Histologically, parietal cells first appear at 11 weeks. Parietal cells begin to secrete hydrochloric acid in earnest within a few hours after birth.

A 42-year-old man presented to his primary care provider with complaints of headache, sweating (diaphoresis), and a sense of his heart pounding in his chest (palpitation). He stated that these attacks would begin suddenly (paroxysmal symptoms) and subside gradually. The attacks would last for perhaps 10 minutes and occur about two to three times per week. An initial arterial pressure measurement was normal, 124/82. Ten minutes after this initial recording, the patient complained that he was experiencing an abrupt onset of headache, sweating, and palpitation. Another arterial pressure measurement was obtained, which was recorded as 165/94. Laboratory findings indicated that the patient had a pheochromocytoma, a neoplasm of chromaffin cells.

WHAT GERM LAYER GIVES RISE TO CHROMAFFIN CELLS?

The cortex and medulla of the adrenal gland have separate origins. The mesothelium (derived from mesoderm) lining the posterior abdominal wall differentiates into the cortex, and the medulla forms from neural crest cells, which are derived from neuroectoderm.

WHERE ARE CHROMAFFIN CELLS FOUND IN THE HUMAN BODY?

Although chromaffin cells are chiefly located in the adrenal medullae, they are also widely distributed extra-adrenally. Some of these extra-adrenal sites of chromaffin (Fig. 3-46) cells are:

- Organ of Zuckerkandl. This aggregation of chromaffin cells is located near the bifurcation of the aorta.
- Along the paravertebral ganglia of the sympathetic trunk.
- Carotid bodies
- Urogenital system. Chromaffin cells may be located along the kidneys, ureters, epididymis, prostate, and ovary.

These extra-adrenal sites are clinically important as 10% of pheochromocytomas occur here.

ONE OF THE LABORATORY FINDINGS IN THIS PATIENT WAS ELEVATED PLASMA CHROMOGRANIN A. WHAT IS THE ROLE OF CHROMOGRANIN A AND WHY WOULD IT BE ELEVATED IN A PATIENT WITH A PHEOCHROMOCYTOMA?

Chromogranin A is one of a family of chromogranin proteins. These proteins are synthesized by the chromaffin cells and packaged by the Golgi complex, along with catecholamines, into secretory vesicles. It is believed that chromogranins serve as binding proteins for catecholamines. Consequently, chromogranins and catecholamines would be elevated in a patient with a pheochromocytoma. Chromogranins (A and B) also are secreted in nonfunctional pancreatic endocrine tumors.

IN CHROMAFFIN CELLS, WHY IS CORTISOL REQUIRED FOR THE SYNTHESIS OF EPINEPHRINE?

Cortisol is required to stimulate phenylethanolamine-N-methyltransferase (PNMT), the enzyme that

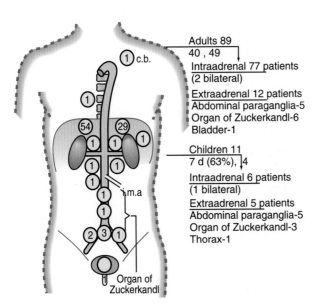

Adults 89
40 , 49
Intraadrenal 77 patients
(2 bilateral)
Extraadrenal 12 patients
Abdominal paraganglia-5
Organ of Zuckerkandl-6
Bladder-1

Children 11
7 d (63%), 4
Intraadrenal 6 patients
(1 bilateral)
Extraadrenal 5 patients
Abdominal paraganglia-5
Organ of Zuckerkandl-3
Thorax-1

FIGURE 3-46 Locations of chromaffin tissue as quantitated by the presence of pheochromocytomas. Numbers based on 100 patients. (Towsend C et al.: *Sabiston Textbook of Surgery, 17e.* WB Saunders, 2004. Fig. 37-22. From Manger WM, Gifford RW, Melicow MM: *Pheochromocytoma.* New York, Springer-Verlag, 1977, p. 45.)

converts norepinephrine to epinephrine. In order for cortisol to exert its regulatory effect, the medulla must have a unique dual blood supply. It has an arterial supply from the long cortical arteries and a venous supply from short cortical arteries. The long cortical arteries arise from the subcapsular arterial plexus, travel through the cortex without branching, and empty into the capillary network of the medulla. The short cortical arteries also arise from the subcapsular plexus, but these vessels feed sinusoidal capillaries that supply the cortical cells with arterial blood. The sinusoidal capillaries possess fenestrae that progressively get larger in diameter as the capillaries penetrate into the deep cortex. The sinusoidal capillaries of the zona reticularis empty into a venous plexus at the interface of the reticularis and medulla. Small venules spring from this plexus and penetrate into the medulla. Cortisol is delivered to the chromaffin cells via the sinusoidal capillaries.

WHERE IN THE CELL ARE THE ENZYMES LOCATED FOR THE CONVERSION OF TYROSINE TO DOPAMINE, CONVERSION OF DOPAMINE TO NOREPINEPHRINE, AND NOREPINEPHRINE TO EPINEPHRINE?

Chromaffin cells secrete primarily epinephrine and some norepinephrine. The precursor molecule for catecholamines is the amino acid tyrosine. Tyrosine is enzymatically converted to DOPA by the enzyme *tyrosine hydroxylase*. The enzyme *DOPA decarboxylase* then forms dopamine from DOPA. These two synthetic steps occur in the cytoplasm. After its formation in the cytoplasm, dopamine is translocated into the secretory vesicle and converted by the enzyme, *dopamine beta-hydroxylase*, to norepinephrine. To synthesize epinephrine, norepinephrine is transported out of the secretory vesicle into the cytoplasm where it is converted to epinephrine by PNMT, an enzyme activated by cortisol. Epinephrine is then transported into the secretory vesicle.

SYMPATHETIC OUTFLOW (PREGANGLIONIC FIBERS) TO THE ADRENAL MEDULLA ARISES FROM WHICH SPINAL CORD SEGMENTS?

Sympathetic preganglionic neurons reside in the lateral gray horns of spinal cord segments T8 to L1. Their fibers are conveyed in the thoracic and lumbar splanchnic nerves to the chromaffin cells.

WHILE CONDUCTING IMAGING STUDIES TO ASSESS EXTRA-ADRENAL INVOLVEMENT, A DOUBLE INFERIOR VENA CAVA WAS AN INCIDENTAL FINDING. WHAT IS THE EMBRYOLOGIC BASIS OF THIS DEVELOPMENTAL CURIOSITY?

A double inferior vena cava is typically discovered as an incidental finding during imaging studies to assess unrelated conditions. The variation is asymptomatic, although it may be associated with an obstruction of the pelvic ureter. To understand the embryologic basis of the variation, one must first be grounded in the developmental processes that contribute to the formation of a normal inferior vena cava.

The inferior vena cava develops from a system of various cardinal veins and the right vitelline vein. The various paired cardinal veins that participate in this development are (Fig. 3-47):

● Right and left posterior cardinal veins
● Right and left subcardinal veins
● Right and left supracardinal veins

Three anastomoses between the cardinal system of veins also contribute:

● The subcardinal anastomosis between the right and left subcardinal veins
● The iliac venous anastomosis between the posterior cardinal veins
● The subsupracardinal anastomosis between the right and left supracardinal veins

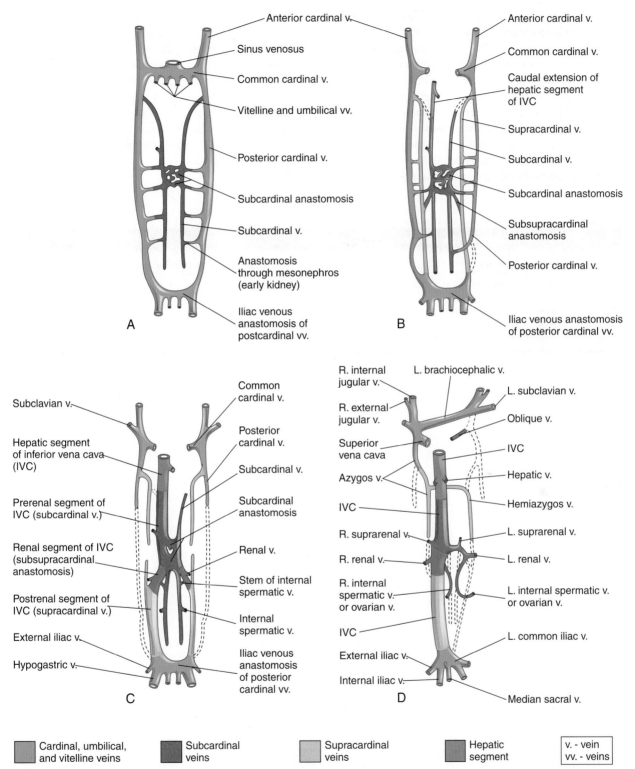

Cardinal, umbilical, and vitelline veins

Subcardinal veins

Supracardinal veins

Hepatic segment

v. - vein
vv. - veins

FIGURE 3-47 Development of the inferior vena cava. (Moore K and Persaud TVN: *The Developing Human, 7e.* WB Saunders, 2003. Fig. 14-4. Modified from Arey LB: *Developmental Anatomy, revised 7th ed.* Philadelphia, WB Saunders, 1974.)

As seen in Figure 3-47, the left side of the venous system undergoes regression, whereas the right side continues to develop. This asymmetrical venous remodeling process results in the formation of the inferior vena cava to the right of the vertebral column. The primordial venous structures and their contribution to the adult inferior vena cava are summarized in Table 3-6.

A double inferior vena cava occurs in 0.2% to 3% of the cases. Its development is due to the persistence of the left supracardinal vein. When this variation occurs, the left (duplicated) inferior vena cava is described thus:

- Being smaller, being larger, or equal in diameter when compared to its fellow
- Receiving the left gonadal vein just as the right gonadal vein empties into the inferior vena cava
- After receiving the left renal vein, its superior course ultimately joins it to the right inferior vena cava.
- The common iliac veins are typically connected by a persistent iliac venous anastomosis of the posterior cardinal veins.

TABLE 3-6 Derivatives of the Inferior Vena Cava	
Embryonic Venous Structure	**Adult Derivative of Inferior Vena Cava**
Cranial segment of the right vitelline vein and hepatic sinusoids	Hepatic segment
Right subcardinal vein	Prerenal segment
Subcardinal-supracardinal anastomosis	Renal segment
Right supracardinal vein	Postrenal segment
Iliac venous anastomosis of posterior cardinal veins	Common iliac veins

SECTION IV

Pelvis and Perineum

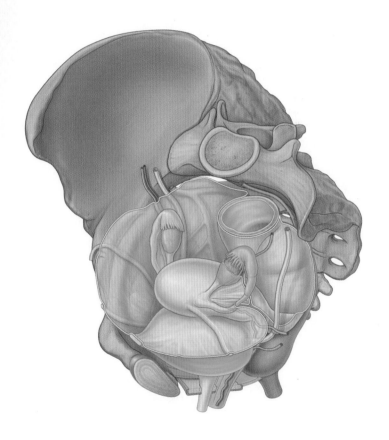

A 20-year-old female college student presented to the University Student Health Clinic with a complaint of a painful lump in her external genitalia. The physical examination confirmed the presence of a tender mass. The patient was diagnosed with a Bartholin gland abscess that was surgically drained.

WHAT ARE BARTHOLIN GLANDS?

Bartholin glands, also known as greater vestibular glands, are small (about 1 cm in diameter) paired glands located on either side of the vaginal orifice. The glands lie in the superficial perineal pouch (Fig. 4-1) and are partly covered by the posterior portions of the bulbs of the vestibule and by the bulbospongiosus muscles. The duct of each gland opens into the vestibule between the hymen and the labium minus (Fig. 4-2).

Histologically, the paired bodies are classified as tubuloalveolar glands and their ducts are lined by transitional epithelium. The glandular cells are stimulated by sexual arousal to secrete mucus that lubricates the introitus. Recent studies have identified endocrine cells in the greater vestibular glands. The endocrine cells secrete several hormones, such as bombesin, serotonin, calcitonin, and human chorionic gonadotropin. The functional significance of these hormones remains to be elucidated.

HOW DO BARTHOLIN GLANDS DEVELOP?

Endodermal outgrowths from the urogenital sinus develop into the functional cells of the glands. The surrounding mesenchyme forms the stroma of the glands (Fig. 4-3). The greater vestibular glands are homologues of the bulbourethral (Cowper's) glands in the male.

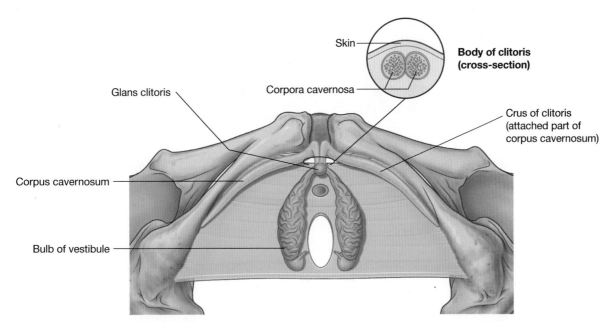

FIGURE 4-1 Greater vestibular (Bartholin) gland. (Drake R, Vogl W and Mitchell A: *Gray's Anatomy for Students*. Churchill Livingstone, 2004. Fig. 5-71.)

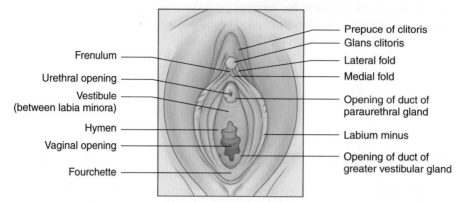

Prepuce of clitoris
Glans clitoris
Lateral fold
Medial fold
Opening of duct of paraurethral gland
Labium minus
Opening of duct of greater vestibular gland

Frenulum
Urethral opening
Vestibule (between labia minora)
Hymen
Vaginal opening
Fourchette

FIGURE 4-2 Opening of the duct of the greater vestibular gland into the vestibule. (Drake R, Vogl W and Mitchell A: *Gray's Anatomy for Students*. Churchill Livingstone, 2004. Fig. 5-73.)

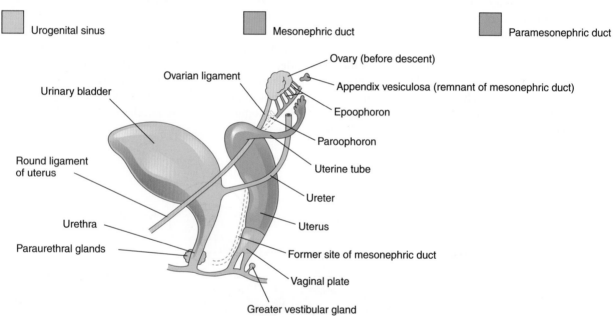

Urogenital sinus

Mesonephric duct

Paramesonephric duct

Ovary (before descent)
Ovarian ligament
Appendix vesiculosa (remnant of mesonephric duct)
Urinary bladder
Epoophoron
Paroophoron
Uterine tube
Round ligament of uterus
Ureter
Urethra
Uterus
Paraurethral glands
Former site of mesonephric duct
Vaginal plate
Greater vestibular gland

FIGURE 4-3 Development of the greater vestibular glands. (Moore K and Persaud TVN: *The Developing Human*, 7e. WB Saunders, 2003. Fig. 13-32B.)

During the examination of a full-term male infant, it was discovered that his right testis did not descend into the scrotum. One year later the testis remained undescended. The infant was diagnosed with cryptorchidism and an orchiopexy was performed.

WHAT IS THE MOST LIKELY LOCATION OF A CRYPTORCHID TESTIS?

The most frequent location of an undescended testis is in the inguinal canal (Fig. 4-4). Other locations are anywhere along the pathway that the testis travels to descend into the scrotum. Cryptorchidism is slightly more common with the right testis than the left and occurs bilaterally in 25% of cases.

WHY DID THE PHYSICIAN WAIT 1 YEAR BEFORE PERFORMING AN ORCHIOPEXY?

An orchiopexy is a surgical procedure that moves and fixes an undescended testis in the scrotum. The physician waited 1 year to see if the cryptorchid testis would spontaneously descend into the scrotum. Surgical correction is necessary before 2 years of age to stave off histologic deterioration.

WHAT ARE THE MORPHOLOGIC CHARACTERISTICS OF A CRYPTORCHID TESTIS?

A cryptorchid testis exhibits the following morphologic characteristics:

- The basal laminae of the seminiferous tubules become thickened.
- The seminiferous tubules become dense cords of connective tissue.
- The interstitial cells (of Leydig) are unaffected.
- The testis atrophies.
- Interestingly, a patient with unilateral cryptorchidism will experience deterioration of germ cells in the contralateral descended testis.

HOW DO THE TESTES DEVELOP?

Development of the testes requires primordial germ cells and the SRY gene located on the short arm of the Y chromosome. The SRY gene encodes the protein, *testis-determining factor (TDF)*.

The primordial germ cells originate from the endoderm that lines the dorsal area of the yolk sac during the fourth week of development. As the lateral folds develop and fuse in the ventral midline of the embryo, the dorsal part of the yolk sac is sequestered within the embryo. Concomitant with the folding is the migration of the primordial germ cells from the dorsal yolk sac to the gonadal (genital) ridges, the indifferent gonad (Fig. 4-5). This cellular march occurs through the mesentery of the hindgut. When the primordial germ cells enter the gonadal ridges, they become incorporated into primary sex cords. Primary sex cords are epithelial structures of the gonadal ridge that extend into the underlying mesenchyme. Next, the indifferent gonad develops an outer cortex and an inner medulla. In the XY complement of chromosomes, the medulla is stimulated to differentiate into the seminiferous tubules of the testis, whereas the cortex is destined to regress through the apoptotic pathway of cell death,

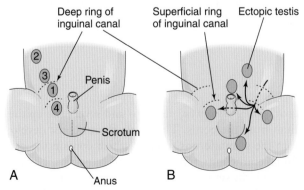

FIGURE 4-4 Sites of cryptorchid testes, numbered in order of frequency. (Moore K and Persaud TVN: *The Developing Human*, 7e. WB Saunders, 2003. Fig. 13-47.)

137

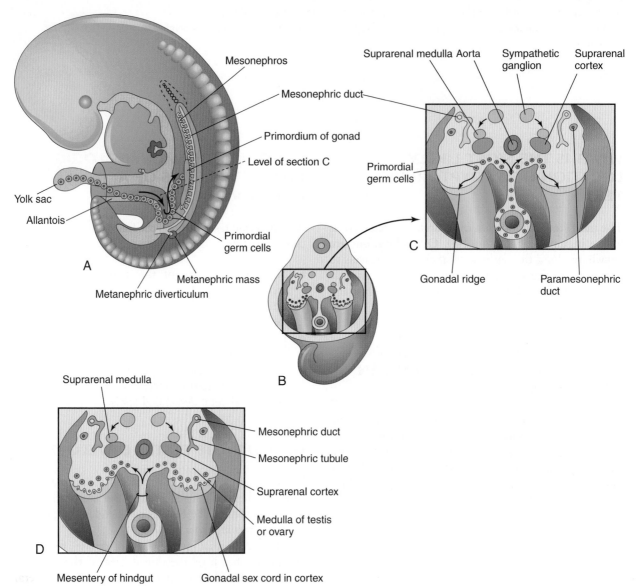

FIGURE 4-5 **A**, Illustration showing the migration of primordial germ cells from the yolk sac to the 5-week-old embryo. **B**, Illustration showing the location of the gonadal ridges. **C**, Transverse section showing the migration of primordial germ cells into the developing gonads. **D**, Transverse section of a 6-week-old embryo showing gonadal cords. (Moore K and Persaud TVN: *The Developing Human*, 7e. WB Saunders, 2003. Fig. 13-28.)

save for vestigial remnants that form the rete testis, a segment of the male genital duct system.

Stimulation of the primary sex cords, containing the primordial germ cells, by TDF causes the cords to extend into the medulla (Fig. 4-6). The cords, now called *seminiferous (testicular) cords*, eventually lose their connection with the surface epithelium of the gonadal ridge. This occurs when the fibrous connective tissue coat, *tunica albuginea*, develops and severs the epithelium from the cords. The seminiferous cords develop into the seminiferous tubules, which contain the germinal epithelium, tubuli recti, and rete testis. Located between the seminiferous tubules is mesenchyme. The mesenchyme gives rise to the connective elements between the tubules and to the interstitial cells (of Leydig).

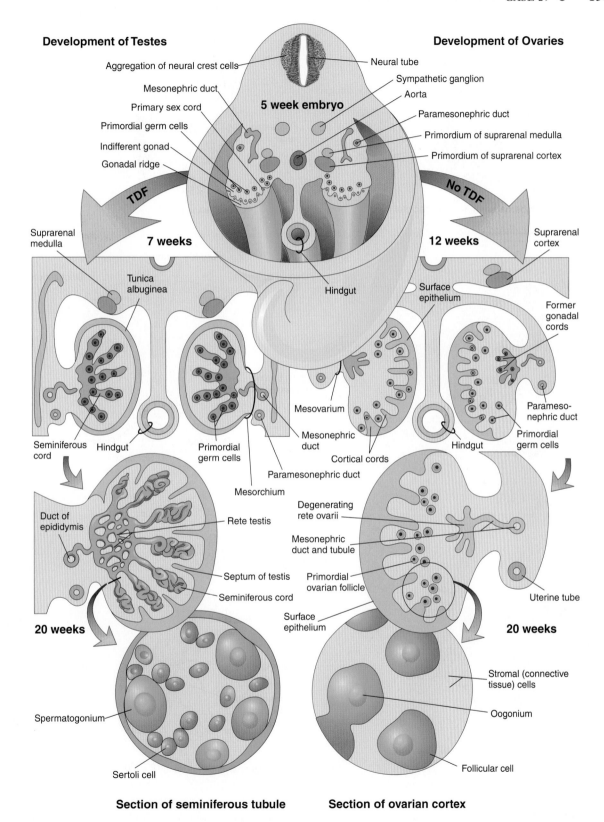

Development of Testes

Development of Ovaries

Aggregation of neural crest cells

Neural tube

Mesonephric duct

Sympathetic ganglion

Primary sex cord

Aorta

5 week embryo

Primordial germ cells

Paramesonephric duct

Indifferent gonad

Primordium of suprarenal medulla

Gonadal ridge

Primordium of suprarenal cortex

TDF

No TDF

Suprarenal medulla

7 weeks

12 weeks

Suprarenal cortex

Tunica albuginea

Surface epithelium

Former gonadal cords

Hindgut

Mesovarium

Paramesonephric duct

Seminiferous cord

Hindgut

Primordial germ cells

Mesonephric duct

Cortical cords

Hindgut

Primordial germ cells

Paramesonephric duct

Mesorchium

Duct of epididymis

Rete testis

Degenerating rete ovarii

Mesonephric duct and tubule

Primordial ovarian follicle

Uterine tube

Septum of testis

Seminiferous cord

Surface epithelium

20 weeks

20 weeks

Stromal (connective tissue) cells

Spermatogonium

Oogonium

Sertoli cell

Follicular cell

Section of seminiferous tubule

Section of ovarian cortex

FIGURE 4-6 Illustrations of the development of the indifferent gonads. Development of the testes in response to testis-determining factor is shown on the left. (Moore K and Persaud TVN: *The Developing Human*, 7e. WB Saunders, 2003. Fig. 13-30.)

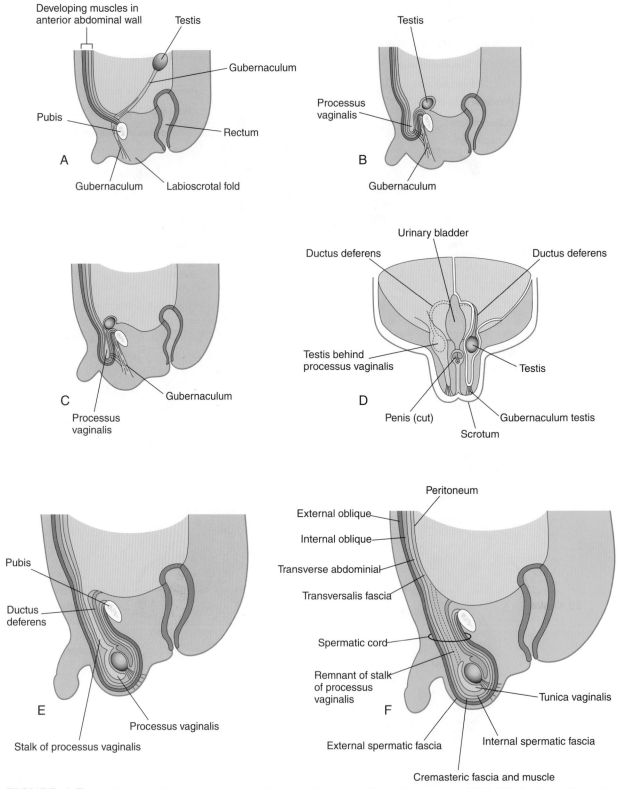

FIGURE 4-7   Development of the inguinal canals and descent of the testes. (Moore K and Persaud TVN: *The Developing Human*, 7e. WB Saunders, 2003. Fig. 13-46.)

HOW DO THE TESTES DESCEND INTO THE SCROTUM?

Because testicular descent includes passage through the inguinal canals, it is essential to include inguinal canal development in the response to this question.

The first structure to consider in the development of the inguinal canals is the gubernaculum (Fig. 4-7). The gubernaculum is a ligament that develops at the inferior border of the testis as the mesonephros degenerates. The gubernaculum descends along the posterior abdominal wall and then courses obliquely though the future site of the inguinal canal. The descent ends when the gubernaculum attaches to the inferior portion of the labioscrotal swelling. The role of the gubernaculum in testicular descent is subject to scientific debate. Some authorities postulate that as the gubernaculum shortens, it pulls the testis into the scrotum. Others posit that the gubernaculum merely serves as a guide wire that the testis follows into the scrotum. Regardless of its role in testicular descent, it does serve to anchor the testes into the scrotum.

The second structure of import is the processus vaginalis. The processus vaginalis is an extension of peritoneum that follows the path blazed by the gubernaculum. As the processus vaginalis follows along the ventral surface of the gubernaculum, it pushes the layers of the abdominal wall ahead of it. These abdominal wall components form the walls of the inguinal canal and the layers of the spermatic cord and are described in cases 23 and 24. The path of the processus vaginalis creates an opening in the transversalis fascia, the deep (internal) inguinal ring, and an opening upon its exit through the aponeurosis of the external abdominal oblique, the superficial (external) inguinal ring. The descent of the testis involves three phases:

- The first phase of testicular descent involves testicular hypertrophy and regression of the mesonephros, which, if present, would limit descent. The testis must also be released from the cranial suspensory ligament. This is accomplished by androgens that cause regression of the ligament and the subsequent release of the testis. Release from the ligament provides some inferior migration of the testis.
- The second phase is the transabdominal descent. Regression of the paramesonephric ducts by mullerian-inhibiting hormone allows the testis to descend inferiorly to the deep (internal) inguinal ring. Testicular descent also involves Leydig insulin-like 3 hormone.
- The third phase is known as the inguinoscrotal phase. This phase requires the presence of androgens and also may require the calcitonin gene-related peptide, which is released by the genitofemoral nerve. During this phase, the testis follows the processus vaginalis through the inguinal canal and into the scrotum.

After his birth, a newborn was placed in the hospital's nursery. Within 24 hours of birth, the newborn developed abdominal distension and his vomitus contained bile. It was also noted that he had failed to pass meconium during this time. X-rays with a barium enema (Fig. 4-8) and a rectal biopsy lead to the diagnosis of Hirschsprung's disease (congenital megacolon).

C A S E

30

WHAT IS THE ARTERIAL SUPPLY TO THE RECTUM?

The rectum is supplied by the following arteries, which form an anastomotic network around the rectum:

- Superior rectal artery. The superior part of the rectum is supplied by the superior rectal artery, a branch of the inferior mesenteric artery. The superior rectal artery divides into two branches that descend along the lateral walls of the rectum.
- Middle rectal artery. The middle and inferior parts of the rectum are supplied by two middle rectal arteries. Each middle rectal artery issues from the anterior division of the internal iliac artery. These arteries are frequently absent.

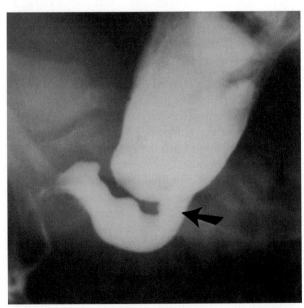

FIGURE 4-8 Barium contrast radiograph of Hirschsprung's disease. The aganglionic segment of the colon is constricted. The colon proximal to the stenosis is distended. The arrow is pointing to the zone of transition between the narrowed segment and the distended segment. (Moore K and Persaud TVN: *The Developing Human,* 7e. WB Saunders, 2003. Fig. 12-27. Courtesy of Dr. Martin H. Reed, Department of Radiology, University of Manitoba and Children's Hospital, Winnipeg, Manitoba, Canada.)

- Inferior rectal artery. The inferior part of the rectum is supplied by two inferior rectal arteries. Each inferior rectal artery springs from its respective internal pudendal artery, a branch of the internal iliac artery.

WHAT IS THE VENOUS DRAINAGE OF THE RECTUM?

The rectum contains an internal rectal venous plexus and an external rectal venous plexus that communicate with one another. The internal venous plexus is located in the submucosa, whereas the external venous plexus is external to the muscularis externa of the organ. The venous plexuses drain into the rectal veins as follows:

- The superior rectal vein receives venous blood from the internal venous plexus and the superior part of the external rectal venous plexus. The superior rectal vein is a tributary of the inferior mesenteric vein.
- The middle rectal veins receive venous blood from the middle portion of the external rectal venous plexus. The middle rectal veins then drain into the internal iliac veins.
- The inferior rectal veins receive venous blood from the inferior part of the external rectal venous plexus. The inferior rectal veins are tributaries of the internal pudendal veins.

WHAT IS THE LYMPHATIC DRAINAGE OF THE RECTUM?

Lymph is dually drained from the rectum. Lymphatic vessels from the proximal half of the rectum accompany the superior rectal artery to pararectal lymph nodes. From here they drain into lymph nodes in the mesentery associated with the sigmoid colon; they then empty into the inferior mesenteric and lumbar lymph nodes. Lymphatic vessels from the distal half of the rectum accompany the middle rectal vessels and empty into internal iliac lymph nodes.

143

WHAT IS THE INNERVATION OF THE RECTUM?

The rectum is innervated by sympathetic and parasympathetic fibers. The sympathetic fibers originate from the lateral gray horns of spinal cord levels L1-L2 and sometimes L3. The fibers leave the sympathetic trunk through lumbar splanchnic nerves that reach the superior hypogastric plexus. From here they travel to the inferior hypogastric plexus where they commingle with parasympathetic fibers derived from the pelvis splanchnic nerves (S2-S4). Sympathetic and parasympathetic fibers from the inferior hypogastric plexus supply the rectum.

WHAT IS THE PATHOGENESIS OF HIRSCHSPRUNG'S DISEASE?

Hirschsprung's disease is characterized by the absence of parasympathetic ganglion cells in the myenteric and submucosal plexuses. This absence results from the failure of neural crest cells (derived from neuroectoderm) to migrate into the wall of the large intestine. This migration of neural crest cells normally occurs during the fifth to seventh weeks of development.

WHAT IS THE RADIOLOGIC APPEARANCE OF THE BOWEL IN A PATIENT WITH HIRSCHSPRUNG'S DISEASE?

The aganglionic segments of the colon are constricted due to contraction of the smooth muscle. The normal, proximal ganglionic segments are distended by the accumulating fecal mass (Fig. 4-8).

IN HIRSCHSPRUNG'S DISEASE, WHICH SEGMENTS OF THE INTESTINES CAN BE AGANGLIONIC?

The intestinal segments that can exhibit aganglionosis are:

● The distal rectum is always involved.
● Extends proximally from the distal rectum to the rectosigmoid junction in about 75% of patients

● Extends proximally from the distal rectum to the splenic (left colic) flexure or transverse colon in about 17% of cases
● May involve the entire colon with variable involvement of the small intestine in only 8% of cases

WHAT ARE THE GROSS AND LIGHT MICROSCOPIC CHARACTERISTICS OF THE RECTUM?

The morphologic features of the rectum grossly are:

● The rectum begins at the rectosigmoid junction, which is anterior to the level of the third sacral vertebra.
● It ends just inferior to the tip of the coccyx.
● The inferior end of the rectum is dilated, forming the rectal ampulla.
● Contrary to its name, which means *straight*, the rectum possesses three flexures as its follows the concave surfaces of the sacrum and coccyx.
● As viewed by a sigmoidoscope, the rectum has three permanent shelf-like folds that extend into the lumen. These tissue shelves, called *transverse rectal folds* (plicae transversales recti or valves of Houston), help to support the fecal mass.

The histologic features of the rectum are similar to the colon. The differences are:

● The intestinal glands of the rectum are deeper but the density (number per surface area) is less.
● Goblet cells are especially abundant. The secreted mucus from the goblet cells lubricates the mucosa, thus protecting it from the abrasive frictional forces of the fecal mass.
● Temporary longitudinal folds of mucosa and submucosa are present in the rectum. These folds disappear with distending pressure and reappear after the pressure has been reduced.
● The transverse rectal folds (valves of Houston) are formed by mucosa, submucosa, and the inner circular layer of the muscularis externa.
● The teniae coli disappear in the rectum. As these three longitudinal bands of smooth muscle descend into the rectum, they splay out to form a complete outer longitudinal muscle layer (this can be seen grossly as well). This layer is thicker on the anterior and posterior rectal walls than its lateral walls.

WHAT ARE THE ANTERIOR AND POSTERIOR RELATIONSHIPS OF THE RECTUM?

The anterior and posterior relationships of the rectum in men and women are described in Table 4-1.

WHY IS IT IMPORTANT TO OBTAIN THE RECTAL BIOPSY AT LEAST 2 CM ABOVE THE PECTINATE (DENTATE) LINE?

The number of myenteric (Auerbach's) and submucosal (Meissner's) ganglia progressively decrease in number distally through the anal canal. A biopsy taken 2 cm superior to the pectinate line ensures that the tissue sample is taken from a region that would, in the absence of Hirschsprung's disease, contain ganglia.

TABLE 4-1 Relationships of the Rectum in Men and Women		
	Anterior	**Posterior**
Male	Fundus of urinary bladder	Sacral vertebrae 3–5
	Distal parts of ureters	Coccyx
	Ductus deferens	Anococcygeal ligament
	Seminal vesicles	Median sacral vessels
	Prostate	Superior rectal artery
		Inferior ends of sympathetic trunks
		Sacral plexuses
Female	Vagina	Same as male

WHAT IS THE DENTATE LINE?

The dentate (pectinate) line is a comb-shaped region of the anal canal (Fig. 4-9). Embryologically, it represents the former site of the anal membrane. This means that the dentate line is a dividing line between the superior two-thirds of the anal canal derived from hindgut and the inferior one-third of the anal canal derived from proctodeum.

WHAT ARE THE DIFFERENCES BETWEEN THE HINDGUT-DERIVED ANAL CANAL AND THAT DERIVED FROM THE PROCTODEUM?

The differences between the superior two-thirds and the inferior one-third of the anal canal center on epithelial type, arterial supply, venous and lymphatic drainage, and nerve supply.

The epithelium from the superior two-thirds is derived from the endoderm of the hindgut. This epithelium is simple columnar with goblet cells. The epithelial lining extending inferior to the dentate line is formed from ectoderm of the proctodeum. This epithelium is nonkeratinized stratified squamous proximally but becomes keratinized inferior to the anocutaneous line (white line of Hilton). The transition zone between the pectinate line and the anocutaneous line is known as the *anal pecten*.

The principal arterial supply to the superior two-thirds is from the superior rectal artery, a branch of the inferior mesenteric, the artery to the hindgut. The inferior segment receives its chief supply from the

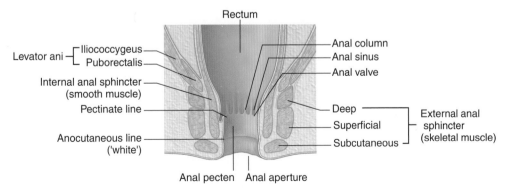

FIGURE 4-9 Rectum and anal canal. (Drake R, Vogl W and Mitchell A: *Gray's Anatomy for Students.* Churchill Livingstone, 2004. Fig. 5-38.)

inferior rectal artery, a branch of the internal pudendal artery, springing from the internal iliac artery.

Lymphatics superior to the deutate line drain into epirectal nodes. Lymph then flows superiorly into pararectal nodes and various nodal groups along the superior rectal artery. Below the dentate line, lymphatics ultimately empty into external iliac veins.

The nerve supply to the superior two-thirds is from fibers of the sympathetic and parasympathetic nervous divisions. The inferior third is innervated somatically by the inferior rectal branch of the pudendal nerve. The pudendal nerve is formed by the anterior divisions of ventral primary rami from spinal cord segments S2-S4.

A 40-year-old African-American woman presented to the gynecologist complaining of bleeding between her periods and of low back pain on examination. In response to the physician's questioning, the patient said her periods have been regular and the bleeding between her periods has gone on for 3 months. She also mentioned that her low back pain started about 6 weeks ago. The pelvic examination and an ultrasound study revealed multiple, medium-sized, firm masses in the uterus. The patient was diagnosed with a leiomyoma (fibroids) and she consented to a hysterectomy.

WHAT ARE THE LIGAMENTS THAT ATTACH TO THE UTERUS, UTERINE TUBES, AND OVARIES?

The internal organs of generation in the female have numerous ligaments that attach to them. The ligaments of the uterus are (Fig. 4-10):

- The broad ligament of the uterus, a double layer of peritoneum, attaches the lateral borders of the uterus to the lateral pelvic walls and pelvic floor. The broad ligament is divided into three parts: mesovarium, mesosalpinx, and mesometrium. The mesometrium is the largest division of the broad ligament and it attaches the body of the uterus, inferior to the ligament of the ovary, to the pelvic floor.
- The round ligaments of the uterus extend from the anterolateral borders of the uterine fundus. As they course anterolaterally in the pelvic cavity, they cross anterior to the ureters, branches of the internal iliac arteries, and external iliac arteries. They then enter the inguinal canals at the deep (internal) inguinal ring and leave at the superficial (external) inguinal ring to insert into the labia majora.
- The transverse cervical (cardinal) ligaments tether the cervix and vaginal fornix to the lateral walls of the pelvis. These are the most important ligaments supporting the uterus.
- The uterosacral ligaments attach the lateral walls of the cervix to the sacrum.
- The pubocervical ligaments extend from the anterior surfaces of the cervix and superior vagina to the pubic bones.

The ligaments of the ovary are (Fig. 4-10):

- The mesovarium. This extension of the broad ligament attaches to each ovary at its hilum.
- The suspensory ligaments of the ovary (infundibulopelvic ligaments) are lateral and superior continuations of the mesovarium of each ovary. The suspensory ligament of the ovary attaches to the lateral pelvic wall and transmits the ovarian vessels, nerves, and lymphatics. These neurovascular structures pass through the mesovarium to enter and leave the hilum of the ovary.
- The ligaments of the ovary (utero-ovarian ligaments) extend from the uterine ends of the ovaries to the uterus just inferior to the entry of the uterine tubes.

The ligament associated with each uterine tube is the mesosalpinx, one of the three parts of the broad ligament.

To perform a hysterectomy, the uterus has to be freed from its ligamentous attaches. The structures that are divided are the broad ligament, ligaments of the ovary, round ligaments of the uterus, and the cardinal, uterosacral, and pubocervical ligaments (Fig. 4-11). In addition, the uterine tubes must be divided.

WHAT BLOOD VESSELS WOULD HAVE TO BE DIVIDED TO REMOVE THE UTERUS?

The uterus is supplied by the following arteries, which must be divided to perform a hysterectomy:

- The uterine arteries provide the principal blood supply to the uterus. These arteries issue from the anterior division of the internal iliac arteries and anastomose with branches of the ovarian and vaginal arteries.
- The ovarian arteries, which originate from the abdominal aorta inferior to the renal arteries. The branches from the ovarian arteries to the uterus would be divided.

The uterus is drained by the uterine veins, which are tributaries of the internal iliac veins. These veins would also have to be divided.

WHAT IS THE INNERVATION OF THE UTERUS?

The uterus is innervated by the sympathetic and para-sympathetic divisions of the autonomic nervous

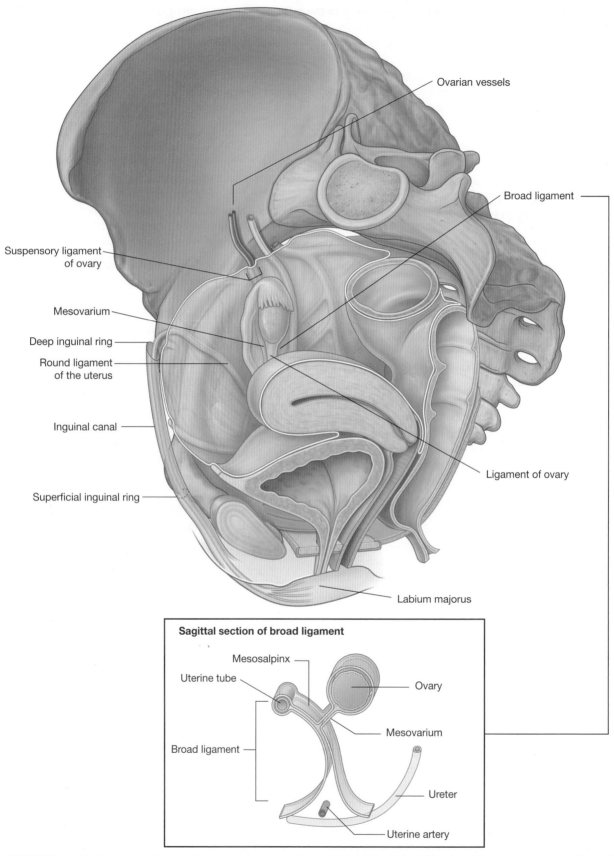

FIGURE 4-10 Ligaments of the female reproductive organs. (Drake R, Vogl W and Mitchell A: *Gray's Anatomy for Students*. Churchill Livingstone, 2004. Fig. 5-50.)

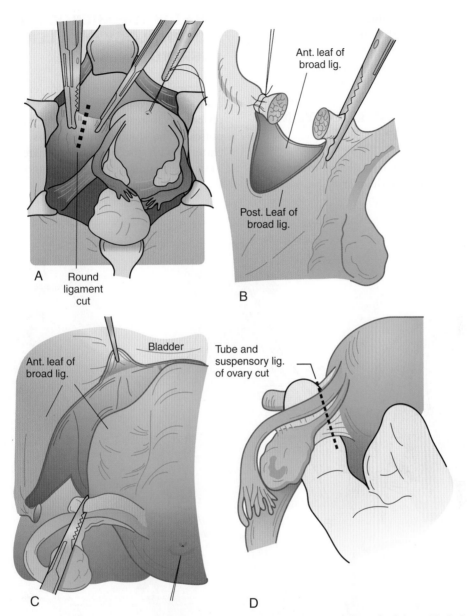

FIGURE 4-11 Dissection of ligaments and vessels during a hysterectomy. (Towsend C et al.: *Sabiston Textbook of Surgery, 17e.* WB Saunders, 2004. Fig. 74-12. Modified from Mitchell CW, Wheeless CR: *Atlas of Pelvic Surgery, 3rd ed.* Baltimore, Lippincott Williams & Wilkins, 1997.)

system. The sympathetic preganglionic fibers originate from the lateral gray horns of spinal cord segments T12 and L1. From the sympathetic trunk, sympathetic fibers are distributed to the ovarian (component of the celiac plexus) and uterovaginal (component of the inferior hypogastric plexus) plexuses. Sympathetic fibers leave these plexuses to supply the uterus.

Parasympathetic preganglionic fibers arise from sacral spinal cord segments S2 to S4. They then travel to and pass through the ovarian and uterovaginal plexuses to synapse with small ganglia proximate to the uterus. Postganglionic parasympathetic fibers then travel to the uterus.

HOW DOES THE UTERUS DEVELOP?

The uterus develops from the uterovaginal primordium, which is formed by the confluence of the paramesonephric (Müllerian) ducts (Fig. 4-12). The splanchnic mesenchyme that surrounds the utero-vaginal primordium develops into the myometrium and connective tissue of the endometrium.

WHERE ARE UTERINE LEIOMYOMAS TYPICALLY FOUND?

Uterine leiomyomas are almost always found in the myometrium of the body of the uterus.

WHAT IS THE MICROSCOPIC MORPHOLOGY OF A LEIOMYOMA (FIBROID)?

Contrary to the name *fibroid*, leiomyomas are not composed of connective tissue; thus, fibroid truly is a misnomer. Instead, they are benign tumors of smooth muscle. The smooth muscle cells exhibit a whorled pattern, with the well-differentiated cells having a similar appearance to the nontumor smooth cells in the myometrium (Fig. 4-13).

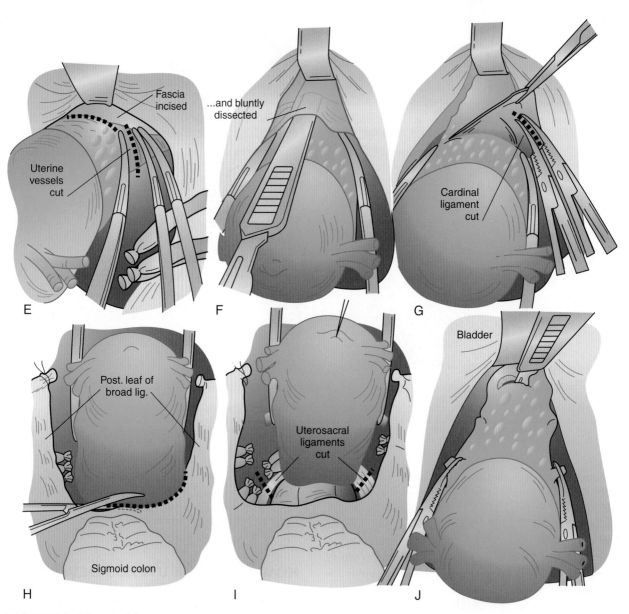

FIGURE 4-11, cont'd.

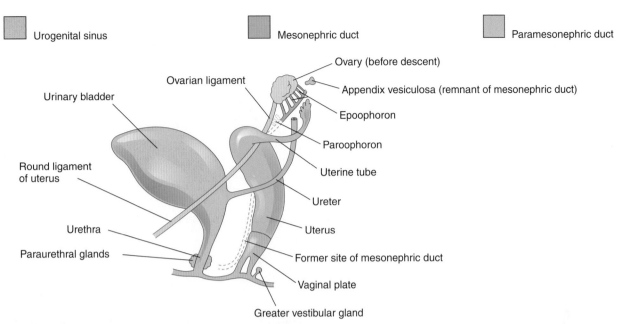

□ Urogenital sinus   □ Mesonephric duct   □ Paramesonephric duct

Ovary (before descent)

Appendix vesiculosa (remnant of mesonephric duct)

Ovarian ligament

Urinary bladder

Epoophoron

Paroophoron

Round ligament
of uterus

Uterine tube

Ureter

Urethra

Uterus

Paraurethral glands

Former site of mesonephric duct

Vaginal plate

Greater vestibular gland

FIGURE 4-12 Development of the uterus. (Moore K and Persaud TVN: *The Developing Human*, 7e. WB Saunders, 2003. Fig. 13-32B.)

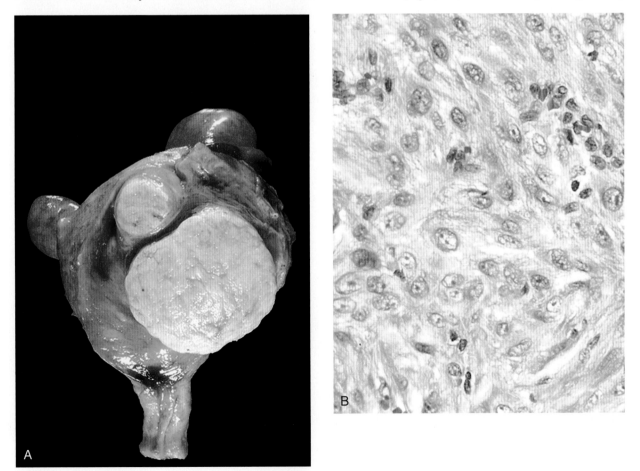

FIGURE 4-13 A, Leiomyoma of the myometrium. Note the white tumor. **B**, Leiomyoma displaying well-differentiated, spindle-shaped smooth cells. (Kumar V, Abbas A and Fausto N: *Robbins & Cotran Pathologic Basis of Disease*, 7e. WB Saunders, 2004. Fig. 22-34.)

A 55-year-old woman presented with complaints of pelvic fullness and vague gastrointestinal symptoms. Palpation detected a significant mass in the abdominopelvic region. Transvaginal ultrasonography revealed a mass in the left ovary. Lab results showed an elevated level of CA-125. Radiologic studies revealed metastases to the upper abdomen and the colon. A total hysterectomy and bilateral salpingo-oophorectomy were performed and the involved colon was resected. Pathologic examination of the removed ovaries led to a diagnosis of serous cystadenocarcinoma (Fig. 4-14). The patient was then placed on chemotherapy.

WHAT IS THE ARTERIAL SUPPLY TO THE OVARY?

The ovary is supplied solely by the ovarian artery. The ovarian artery springs from the aorta at the level of the second lumbar vertebra and descends retroperitoneally. It then enters the suspensory ligament, and arterial branches are distributed to the ovary within the mesovarium. The ovarian artery also supplies the uterine tube and anastomoses with the uterine artery (Fig. 4-15).

WHAT IS THE VENOUS DRAINAGE OF THE OVARY?

Veins leave the hilum of each ovary to empty into a pampiniform venous plexus. The pampiniform plexus communicates with the uterine venous plexus. Originating from each pampiniform plexus is the ovarian vein. The right ovarian vein empties into the infe-

rior vena cava, whereas its fellow drains into the left renal vein, which empties into the inferior vena cava.

WHAT IS THE LYMPHATIC DRAINAGE OF THE OVARY?

Lymphatic vessels from the ovary accompany the ovarian vessels superiorly. Lymph flows into the preaortic and lateral aortic lymph nodes.

WHAT IS THE NERVE SUPPLY TO THE OVARY?

The ovaries are innervated by sympathetic and parasympathetic fibers. The preganglionic sympathetic fibers originate from the lateral gray horns of spinal cord segments T10 and T11. Parasympathetic fibers are conveyed in the vagus nerves. The autonomic fibers are distributed along the ovarian vessels from the ovarian plexus. The ovarian plexus communicates with the uterine plexus.

WHAT IS THE MORPHOLOGY OF THE OVARY?

The ovary is covered by a simple cuboidal epithelium called *germinal epithelium*. Immediately deep to the epithelium is the tunica albuginea, a fibrous capsule composed of dense irregular collagenous connective tissue. The ovary is divided into an outer cortex and inner medulla. The cortex of the adult ovary contains follicles in various stages of development (Fig. 4-16). A corpus luteum and corpus albicans also may be found in the cortex. The medulla is a connective tissue core that houses blood vessels that are continuous with the ovarian artery and vein. The medulla also harbors hilar cells that secrete androgens.

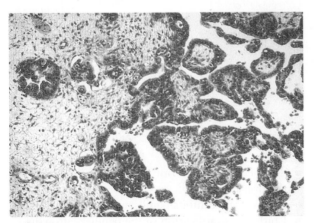

FIGURE 4-14 Micrograph of papillary serous cystadenocarcinoma of the ovary. Note the cancer's invasion of the stroma. (Kumar V, Abbas A and Fausto N: *Robbins & Cotran Pathologic Basis of Disease, 7e.* WB Saunders, 2004. Fig. 22-42.)

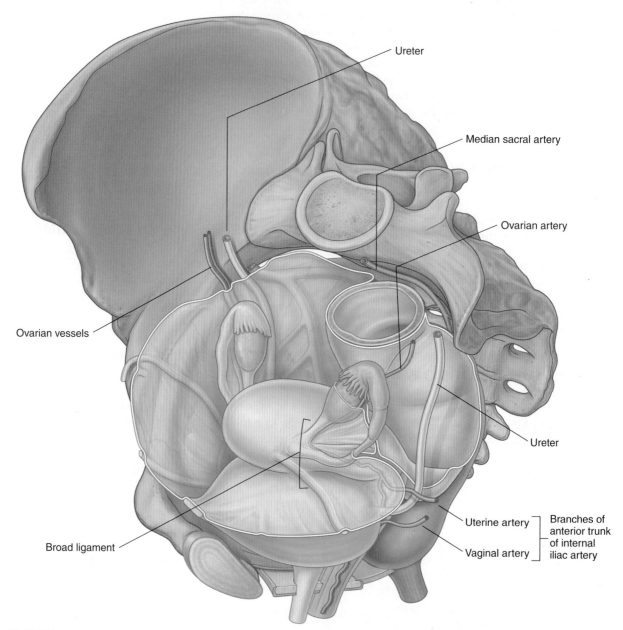

FIGURE 4-15 Blood supply to the female internal reproductive organs. (Drake R, Vogl W and Mitchell A: *Gray's Anatomy for Students.* Churchill Livingstone, 2004. Fig. 5-65.)

WHAT ARE THE MORPHOLOGIC CHARACTERISTICS OF A SEROUS CYSTADENOCARCINOMA OF THE OVARY?

Serous cystadenocarcinoma of the ovary has the following morphologic characteristics:

- Bilateral involvement of the ovaries occurs 66% of the time.

- Tumor is derived from or involves the surface of the ovary.
- Tumor mass exhibits papillary growths (Fig. 4-14).
- Epithelial stratification of the papillary growths
- Infiltration of cancer into the underlying stroma
- Cancer cells display atypia and may become undifferentiated.

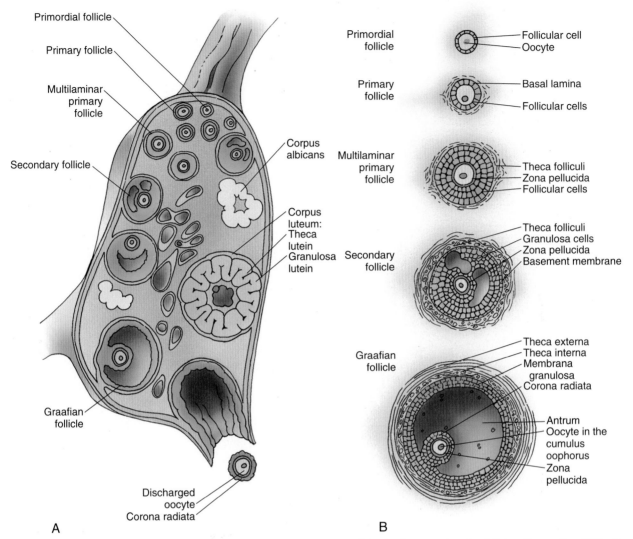

FIGURE 4-16 **A,** Illustration of the structure of an ovary. **B,** Illustration of the development of ovarian follicles. (Gartner L and Hiatt J: *Color Textbook of Histology, 2e.* WB Saunders, 2001. Fig. 20-2.)

A 54-year-old African-American man presented to his physician with complaints of frequent urination and a decreased force of urination. The physician detected a dense nodular region of the prostate gland during a digital rectal examination. Furthermore, a blood test indicated that the patient's prostate-specific antigen (PSA) was high (8 ng/mL). Based on these observations, a biopsy was obtained from the prostate gland and submitted to pathology for analysis. The pathology report confirmed the physician's suspicion that his patient had prostate adenocarcinoma, a common form of prostate cancer.

WHAT STRUCTURES CAN BE PALPATED DURING A DIGITAL RECTAL EXAMINATION?

The structures that can be palpated during a digital rectal examination in males and females are identified in Table 4-2.

WHAT IS THE ARTERIAL SUPPLY TO THE PROSTATE GLAND?

The prostate gland is principally fed by distal branches of the inferior vesical artery, a branch of the internal iliac. Branches from the internal pudendal and the middle rectal arteries, both branches of the internal iliac, also contribute rami that supply the gland.

WHAT IS THE VENOUS DRAINAGE OF THE PROSTATE GLAND?

Venous blood from the prostate gland drains into the prostatic venous plexus located along its lateral walls and base. Blood from the plexus then drains into internal iliac veins. The prostatic venous plexus communicates with the vesical venous plexus and vertebral venous plexuses.

WHAT IS THE LYMPHATIC DRAINAGE OF THE PROSTATE GLAND?

Principal lymphatic drainage of the prostate is to the internal iliac, obturator, and sacral nodes.

HOW IS THE PROSTATE GLAND DESCRIBED HISTOLOGICALLY?

The prostate gland has an average mass of 20 g and is divided into fibromuscular and glandular regions. The fibromuscular region is located along the anterior border of the gland. The glandular component, which comprises two-thirds of the prostate, contains 30 to 50 compound tubuloalveolar glands that reside in three distinct histologic zones (Fig. 4-17):

TABLE 4-2 Palpable Structures During A Digital Rectal Examination	
Male	**Female**
Penile bulb	Uterine cervix
Prostate gland	Pathological changes in the:
Seminal vesicles, if enlarged	Ovaries
Base of bladder, if distended	Uterine tubes
Inferior sacrum and coccyx	Broad ligaments
Ischial spines and tuberosities	Recto-uterine pouch
Internal iliac lymph nodes, if enlarged	

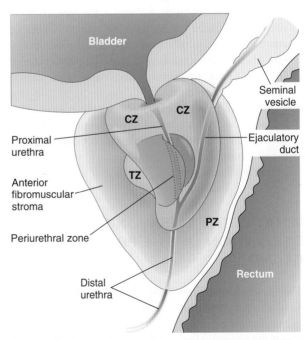

FIGURE 4-17 Prostate gland and its zones. (Kumar V, Abbas A and Fausto N: *Robbins & Cotran Pathologic Basis of Disease*, 7e. WB Saunders, 2004. Fig. 21-30.)

- The tissue that surrounds the urethra proximal to the ejaculatory ducts is referred to as the *transition zone*.
- A larger *central zone* surrounds the ejaculatory ducts and portions of the urethra located proximal and distal to the transitional zone.
- The outer region, which is the largest zone, is called the *peripheral zone*.

The peripheral zone, which houses the main glands of the prostate, is the chief site of adenocarcinoma of the prostate. Because prostatic adenocarcinoma frequently occurs in a posterior location, it is usually detected upon digital rectal examination. The transition zone is also clinically relevant as it contributes to the development of benign prostatic hypertrophy in most cases. In a severe case of benign prostatic hypertrophy, the gland attains a mass in excess of 300 g.

The signature characteristics of the prostate gland histologically are:

- The stroma contains the usual complement of connective elements as well as smooth muscle cells.
- The secretory units of the prostate gland are lined by simple columnar to pseudostratified columnar epithelium.
- The epithelium and the underlying lamina propria are arranged as folds or infoldings. The infoldings project into the lumina of the glands.
- The most conspicuous feature is the presence of corpora amylacea (prostatic concretions). Corpora amylacea are typically observed in the older prostate gland and increase with age. The concretions are calcified glycoproteins and their significance remains to be elucidated.
- The cells of the epithelium possess the typical constellation of organelles of protein-secreting cells: well-developed rough endoplasmic reticulum, large Golgi complex, abundant secretory vesicles, and numerous lysosomes.

WHAT IS THE EMBRYONIC DERIVATION OF THE PROSTATE GLAND?

The prostate gland is derived from endoderm and mesenchyme (mesoderm). The endoderm, which develops into the prostatic glandular tissue, lines the future site of the prostatic urethra within the urogenital sinus (Fig. 4-18). Several outgrowths of this endoderm then extend into the neighboring mesenchyme to form the

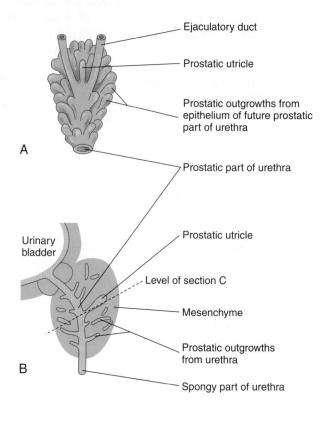

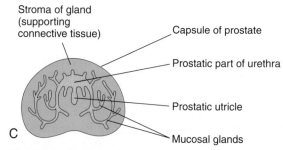

FIGURE 4-18 **A**, Dorsal view of the developing prostate at 11 weeks. **B**, Illustration of the developing prostate showing the endodermal prostatic outgrowths from the urethra. **C**, Section of prostate at 16 weeks obtained from the level shown in B. (Moore K and Persaud TVN: *The Developing Human*, 7e. WB Saunders, 2003. Fig. 13-34.)

compound tubuloalveolar glands. The surrounding mesenchyme differentiates into the fibrous stroma and smooth muscle of the prostate gland.

WHAT HORMONE IS REQUIRED FOR THE NORMAL DEVELOPMENT OF THE PROSTATE GLAND?

Development and growth of the prostate gland is dependent on dihydrotestosterone. Prostatic stromal cells contain the enzyme, 5α-reductase, which converts testosterone to its active form, dihydrotestosterone. In response to dihydrotestosterone, stromal cells synthesize and secrete growth factors that stimulate growth and proliferation of the stromal and secretory (epithelial) cells. The mitogenic effect of dihydrotestosterone can be reduced by administering finasteride, a 5α-reductase inhibitor. As a result, this therapy is effective in regressing benign hypertrophy of the prostate gland.

WHAT IS THE CYTOLOGIC ORIGIN OF PSA AND WHAT IS THE FUNCTION OF PSA?

PSA is a proteolytic enzyme synthesized and secreted by the prostatic glandular (epithelial) cells. The function of PSA is to liquefy the seminal coagulum to increase sperm motility. Prostate serum acid phosphatase (PSAP) is another protease secreted by the glandular cells. PSA and PSAP are widely used tumor markers, although PSA also is elevated in noncancerous conditions, such as benign prostatic hypertrophy and prostatitis. Elevated PSAP levels indicate a more advanced disease state.

WHAT IS THE MORPHOLOGY OF THE PROSTATE ADENOCARCINOMA?

The morphologic characteristics of prostate adenocarcinoma are:

- Cancerous glands are smaller and more crowded than benign glands.
- The epithelium lining the cancerous glands is simple cuboidal to low simple columnar.
- Cancerous glands are characteristically devoid of branching and folds of epithelium and lamina propria.
- Prostatic cancer cells typically show a loss of E-cadherins, which are transmembrane linker proteins that anchor cells to one another. Loss of these proteins allows cancer cells to dissociate from one another, facilitating their metastases.

BASED ON ANATOMIC RELATIONSHIPS, PROSTATIC CANCER MAY SPREAD LOCALLY INTO WHAT STRUCTURES?

The structures most commonly invaded by the local spread of prostate cancer are the seminal vesicles and the base of the urinary bladder. Invasion of the urinary bladder may lead to obstruction of one or both ureters.

WHAT ARE THE SITES OF PROSTATE CANCER METASTASES?

Prostate cancer has a proclivity to metastasize to the axial skeleton (Fig. 4-19). The bones of the axial

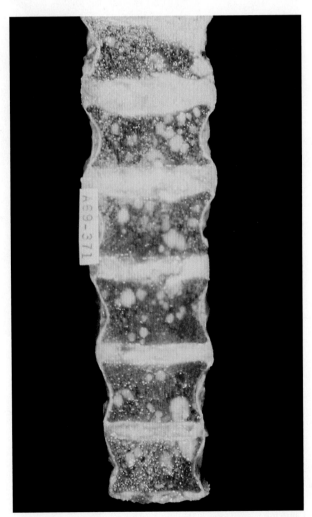

FIGURE 4-19 Prostatic metastases to the vertebral bodies. (Kumar V, Abbas A and Fausto N: *Robbins & Cotran Pathologic Basis of Disease*, 7e. WB Saunders, 2004. Fig. 21-35.)

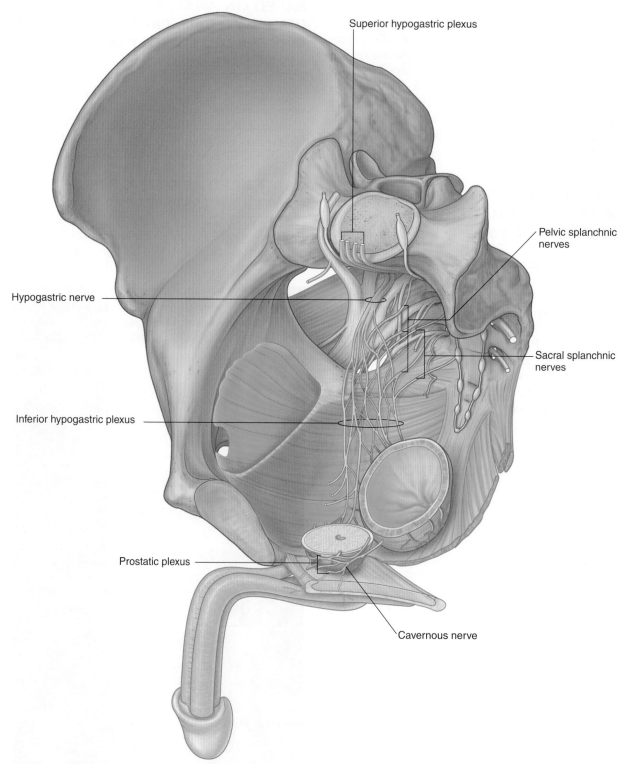

FIGURE 4-20 Innervation of urinary bladder, prostate, and penis. (Drake R, Vogl W and Mitchell A: *Gray's Anatomy for Students.* Churchill Livingstone, 2004. Fig. 5-62B.)

skeleton most commonly involved, in decreasing order of frequency, are:

- Lumbar vertebrae
- Proximal extremity of femur
- Os coxae (pelvis)
- Thoracic vertebrae
- Ribs

Metastases to the lumbar vertebrae are facilitated by the venous communications that exist between the prostatic venous plexus and extradural venous plexus in the vertebral canal. Another factor that tips in favor of metastases is that the venous communications lack valves.

Prostate cancer also spreads to regional lymph nodes. The cancer rarely involves the rectum and it may spread to the erectile bodies of the penis, causing priapism.

HOW DOES PROSTATE CANCER SPREAD LYMPHATICALLY?

Prostate cancer spreads to lymph nodes in the following progression:

- Obturator nodes
- Perivesical nodes
- Hypogastric nodes
- Iliac nodes
- Para-aortic nodes

WHY IS INVASION OF THE RECTUM BY PROSTATIC CANCER LESS COMMON?

A wall of connective tissue, Denonvilliers' fascia (fascia rectoprostatica), separates the anteriorly located distal genitourinary structures from the posteriorly positioned rectum. Denonvilliers' fascia thus serves as a barrier to the invasion of the neighboring rectum by the prostatic carcinoma.

WHY ARE IMPOTENCE AND URINARY INCONTINENCE POTENTIAL COMPLICATIONS OF PROSTATE SURGERY?

The prostate gland is supplied by the prostatic plexus, an inferior continuation of the inferior hypogastric plexus. These networks are formed by a commingling of parasympathetic and sympathetic fibers.

Sympathetic fibers (axons) originate from their cell bodies located in the lateral gray horns of spinal cord segments T11-L1. The fibers enter and take a descending route through the sympathetic trunk until they synapse with postganglionic sympathetic neurons located in the first two ganglia of the pelvic part of this trunk. The postganglionic fibers then extend from these ganglia to join the inferior hypogastric plexus through which they reach the prostate gland. Preganglionic parasympathetic fibers arise from nerve cell bodies located in spinal cord segments S2-S4. The fibers then travel retroperitoneally to join the inferior hypogastric plexus. They continue their travel inferiorly, ultimately synapsing with postganglionic parasympathetic neurons near or within the prostate gland.

The fibers of the autonomic plexuses in the vicinity of the prostate also innervate the urinary bladder, the internal urinary sphincter, and the penis. The autonomic nerve fibers that innervate the penis leave the prostatic plexus as the greater and lesser cavernous nerves. The cavernous nerves enter the penis by passing underneath the pubic arch (Fig. 4-20). Because of the intimacy of the autonomic nerves to the prostate, these fibers are at risk of sacrifice during a prostatectomy. If they are damaged, the patient may suffer from erectile dysfunction and urinary incontinence.

A 28-year-old man noticed a small mass on his right testicle during self examination. Concerned, he visited an oncologic specialist. The specialist also detected a small mass on the right testicle upon palpation. Laboratory tests showed that α-fetoprotein and human chorionic gonadotrophin levels were elevated in the patient's blood. A computed tomography scan revealed involvement of lymph nodes. A radical inguinal orchiectomy was performed. Pathologic evaluation of the excised testicle led to the diagnosis of choriocarcinoma.

WHAT IS THE ARTERIAL SUPPLY AND VENOUS DRAINAGE OF THE TESTICLE?

The right and left testicular arteries spring from the abdominal aorta at the level of the second lumbar vertebra inferior to the renal arteries. They descend retroperitoneally and cross anterior to the respective psoas major muscle and external iliac artery. The artery then enters the inguinal canal to travel within the spermatic cord to reach the testis.

In addition to the testis, the artery also supplies perirenal fat, ureter, and the cremaster muscle. The testis is also partially supplied by the cremasteric branch of the inferior epigastric artery.

Veins from each testis converge to form the pampiniform plexus within the spermatic cord. The numerous small veins that comprise the pampiniform plexus ascend within the spermatic cord and prior to entering the superficial inguinal ring, the veins unite to form three to four testicular veins. The testicular veins travel through the inguinal canal to enter the abdomen through the deep inguinal ring. After passing through the deep inguinal ring, the three or four testicular veins join to form two testicular veins that accompany the testicular artery on each side. The testicular veins travel retroperitoneally anterior to the psoas major and ureter. As the paired testicular veins ascend on each side of the body, they ultimately unite to form a single testicular vein. The right testicular vein travels posterior to the distal ileum and third (horizontal) part of the duodenum before emptying into the inferior vena cava. Infrequently, the right testicular vein drains into the right renal vein. The left testicular vein passes posterior to the inferior segment of the descending colon before joining the left renal vein. The testicular veins possess valves.

Functionally, the pampiniform plexus helps to lower testicular temperature. It accomplishes its cooling effect by serving as a heat sink. Because the temperature of venous blood in the plexus is lower than that of testicular arterial blood, heat is drawn away from arterial blood being delivered to the testis. This effectively lowers the temperature of arterial blood and that of the testis.

As a clinical sidelight, the veins of the pampiniform plexus may become varicose. The varicosities are known as a *varicocele*. Varicoceles commonly form secondary to incompetent valves in the testicular veins, with the left side more frequently involved. Physicians should be suspicious of unilateral right-sided varicoceles as they may be the result of a large mass on the kidney. Or, in older men, sudden onset of a right-sided varicocele may be secondary to a retroperitoneal mass.

Varicoceles interfere with fertility by elevating testicular temperature. The congested venous blood in the varicocele soon reaches a temperature in equilibrium with arterial blood flowing in the testicular artery. This increases arterial blood temperature, which may cause infertility secondary to a raise in testicular temperature. Surgery is advised to eliminate the varicocele and has been successful in restoring fertility.

Surgical removal of the varicocele does not impede return of venous blood from the testis as one might first suspect. Instead, venous blood flow is shifted to small venous collateral channels. These collateral channels are small veins of the:

- Ductus deferens
- Cremaster
- Scrotum

WHAT IS THE LYMPHATIC DRAINAGE OF THE TESTICLE?

Testicular lymph vessels ascend in the spermatic cord and terminate in lumbar (lateral aortic) and preaortic lymph nodes. These nodes are retroperitoneal.

WHAT IS THE INNERVATION OF THE TESTES?

The testes are dually innervated by the sympathetic and parasympathetic nerves. The sympathetic fibers

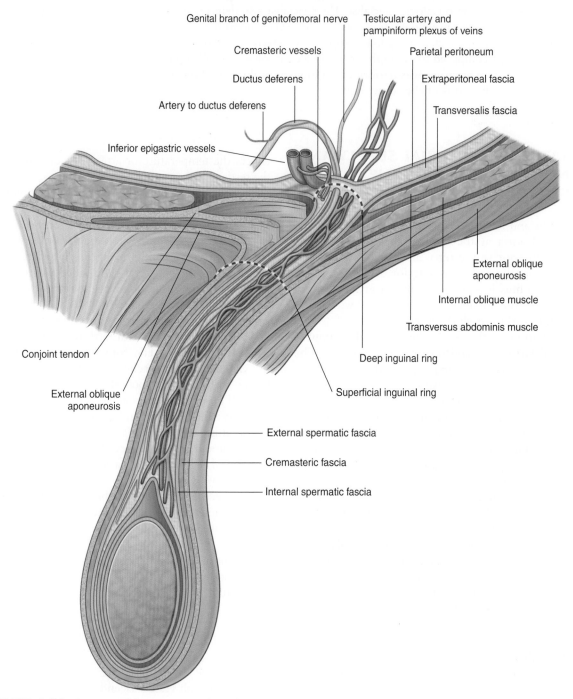

FIGURE 4-21 Coverings of the spermatic cord. (Drake R, Vogl W and Mitchell A: *Gray's Anatomy for Students*. Churchill Livingstone, 2004. Fig. 4.47.)

originate from spinal cord levels T10-T11 and the parasympathetic fibers are derived from the vagus nerves. These fibers follow the testicular artery to supply the testis.

THE SPERMATIC CORD HAS TO BE DIVIDED TO SURGICALLY EXCISE THE TESTICLE. WHAT ARE THE LAYERS OF THE SPERMATIC CORD?

The spermatic cord is composed of three layers. From external to internal, these are the (Fig. 4-21):

- External spermatic fascia. This layer formed from an extension of the aponeurosis of the external abdominal oblique muscle. It is continuous with the deep fascia of the external abdominal oblique muscle
- Cremaster muscle and cremasteric fascia. Fibers and fascia of the internal abdominal oblique muscle formed this covering
- The internal spermatic fascia is a thin covering formed from the transversalis fascia.

WHAT ARE THE HISTOLOGIC CHARACTERISTICS OF THE TESTIS?

The tunica albuginea serves as the fibrous capsule of the testis. The capsule sends septae that penetrate into the substance of the testis dividing it into lobules. Immediately deep to the tunica albuginea is the tunica vasculosa. As its name implies, it is a loose connective layer well endowed with blood vessels that follows the septa of the tunica albuginea into the testis.

Located in each lobule is a highly coiled seminiferous tubule of germinal epithelium (contains spermatogenic and Sertoli cells) with a basal lamina separating it from the tunica propria, a connective tissue coat. A seminiferous tubule may be as long as 70 cm (28 inches). Interstitial cells (of Leydig) are responsible for the synthesis and secretion of androgens. These endocrine cells are proximate to the blood vessels in the tunica vasculosa.

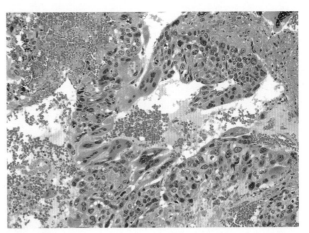

FIGURE 4-22 Choriocarcinoma of the testis. Note the clear cytotrophoblastic cells with centrally located nuclei and acidophilic syncytiotrophoblastic cells with multiple dark nuclei. Necrosis and hemorrhage are evident. (Kumar V, Abbas A and Fausto N: *Robbins & Cotran Pathologic Basis of Disease*, 7e. WB Saunders, 2004. Fig. 21-27.)

WHAT IS THE MORPHOLOGY OF A TESTICULAR CHORIOCARCINOMA?

A testicular choriocarcinoma exhibits the following morphology:

- Tumors are small in diameter, rarely exceeding 5 cm in diameter.
- Hemorrhage and necrosis are frequent.
- Two cell types are found in these cancers: syncytiotrophoblasts and cytotrophoblasts (Fig. 4-22). These cell types are described individually in the bullets below.
- Syncytiotrophoblasts are large cells with an acidophilic vacuolated cytoplasm. Nuclei are irregular in appearance, lobulated, and hyperchromatic. The cells contain human chorionic gonadotropin.
- Cytotrophoblasts are smaller cells with a clearstaining cytoplasm. The cells are described as polygonal in shape with each cell containing one nucleus that is uniform in appearance. Cytotrophoblasts grow in cords or masses.

SECTION V

Lower Limb

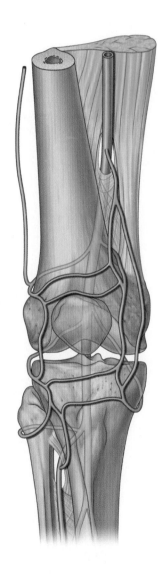

A 32-year-old man was playing a pickup basketball game at the gym. As he leaped into the air during a lay up he felt a sudden snap in the back of his right calf. One of the basketball players, who was a physician, examined the man and palpated a gap where the calcaneal tendon should be located. While standing, the doctor had the injured man attempt to stand on his toes. This action in the right foot was weak. The physician noted a positive Thompson test. The man was diagnosed with a rupture of the calcaneal tendon. The lower limb was immobilized in a cast with the foot in equinus.

WHAT MUSCLES CONTRIBUTE TO THE FORMATION OF THE CALCANEAL (ACHILLES) TENDON?

The Achilles tendon (tendocalcaneus or calcaneal tendon) is formed principally by the gastrocnemius and soleus muscles, with a minor contribution from the plantaris muscle, which are located in the superficial division of the posterior crural compartment. The gastrocnemius and soleus muscles are collectively called the *triceps surae*. The attachments, innervation, and actions of these muscles are described in Table 5-1.

WHERE DOES THE CALCANEAL TENDON TYPICALLY RUPTURE AND WHY?

Ruptures of the calcaneal tendon occur approximately 2.5 to 5 cm superior to its insertion to the calcaneal tuberosity (Fig. 5-1). Imaging studies have demonstrated a paucity of arterial vessels 2 to 6 cm superior to the tendon's insertion. The inadequate arterial supply to this area increases the tendon's vulnerability to repetitive injury, which may culminate in degeneration and eventual rupture.

WHAT IS A POSITIVE THOMPSON TEST?

With the patient in the prone position and the involved leg extended, the examiner grasps and squeezes the calf muscles. If the calcaneal tendon is intact, this test will elicit plantar flexion of the foot. A positive Thompson test is noted if plantar flexion of the foot is absent.

WHY WAS THE LOWER LIMB IMMOBILIZED WITH THE FOOT IN EQUINUS?

If left untreated, the ruptured ends of the calcaneal tendon will unite spontaneously. The downside is that the tendon will be longer than normal. Placing the foot in equinus (plantar flexion of the foot) relaxes the tendon, thus bringing the ruptured ends closer together. The net result is healing without lengthening.

Muscle	Origin	Insertion	Nerve Supply	Actions
Gastrocnemius	Lateral head: lateral condyle of femur Medial head: popliteal fossa superior to the medial femoral condyle	Posterior surface of calcaneus	Tibial nerve (S1 and S2)	Plantar flexes the foot, flexes the knee, and is active in walking, running, and jumping
Soleus	Head of fibula, superior part of fibula, soleal line of tibia, and medial border of tibia	Posterior surface of the calcaneus	Tibial nerve (S1 and S2)	Plantar flexes foot and steadies leg on foot during standing
Plantaris	Distal lateral supracondylar line of femur	Distally fuses with the medial part of the tendo calcaneus to insert on the posterior surface of the calcaneus	Tibial nerve (S1 and S2)	May act with the gastrocnemius; but is functionally insignificant

TABLE 5-1 Triceps Surae and Plantaris Muscles

Ruptured calcaneal tendon

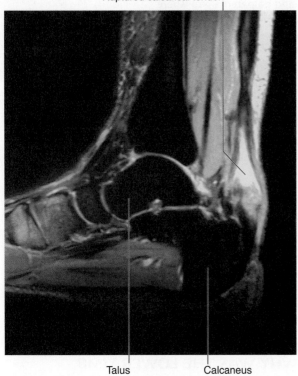

Talus

Calcaneus

FIGURE 5-1 Ruptured calcaneal tendon. (Drake R, Vogl W and Mitchell A: *Gray's Anatomy for Students*. Churchill Livingstone, 2004. Fig. 6-137.)

A 42-year-old man, a passenger in an automobile involved in a head-on collision with another vehicle, was transported to the emergency department complaining of severe pain in the right hip region and upper thigh. The patient was not wearing a seat belt and the force of the impact drove his knee into the dashboard. The physical examination revealed the following: a right limb that was shortened, medially (internally) rotated, and adducted; a contused right knee; and an unremarkable neurovascular assessment. Imaging studies showed a posterior dislocation of the hip with a small discernable fracture but no loose bodies. The dislocation was reduced and postreduction imaging studies confirmed that the maneuver was successful. The patient was prescribed ibuprofen to control the pain and inflammation, instructed to rest and ice the injury, and to perform range-of-motion exercises 1 week later to maintain normal joint flexibility.

WHAT ARE THE LIGAMENTS THAT COMPRISE THE HIP JOINT?

The hip joint is a ball-and-socket type of synovial joint (Fig. 5-2). The acetabulum, formed by the ilium, ischium, and pubis, possesses an inferior acetabular notch. This notch is bridged by the transverse acetabular ligament, which closes the defect. Other ligaments of the hip joint are the (Fig. 5-3):

- Fibrous capsule. The fibrous capsule is attached to the acetabulum proximally and to the neck of the femur distally. Some deep fibers of the capsule run circumferentially around the neck of the femur. These fibers form the zona orbicularis, which forms a fibrous belt around the neck that assists in keeping the femoral head in the acetabulum.
- Iliofemoral ligament (of Bigelow). This Y-shaped, strong ligament attaches proximally to the anterior

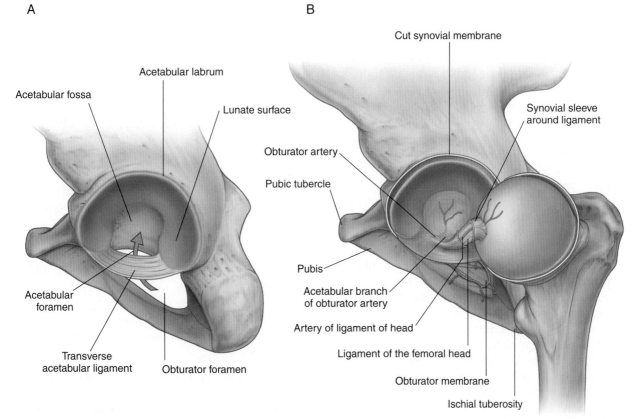

A

B

Acetabular fossa

Acetabular labrum

Lunate surface

Acetabular foramen

Transverse acetabular ligament

Obturator foramen

Cut synovial membrane

Synovial sleeve around ligament

Obturator artery

Pubic tubercle

Pubis

Acetabular branch of obturator artery

Artery of ligament of head

Ligament of the femoral head

Obturator membrane

Ischial tuberosity

FIGURE 5-2 Hip joint. **A**, Transverse acetabular ligament and acetabular labrum. **B**, Ligament of the head of the femur. (Drake R, Vogl W and Mitchell A: *Gray's Anatomy for Students.* Churchill Livingstone, 2004. Fig. 6-30.)

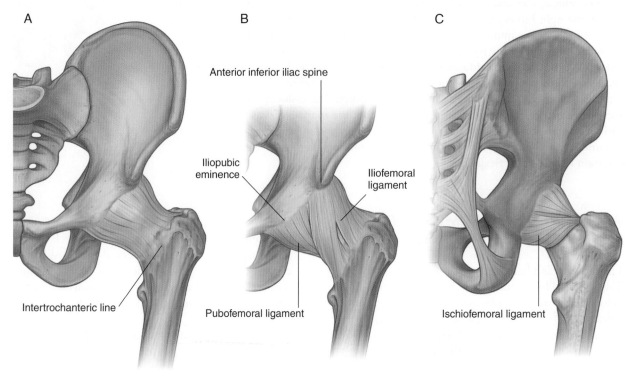

FIGURE 5-3 Joint capsule and ligaments of the hip. **A**, Joint capsule. **B**, Anterior view of iliofemoral and pubofemoral ligaments. **C**, Posterior view of ischiofemoral ligament. (Drake R, Vogl W and Mitchell A: *Gray's Anatomy for Students*. Churchill Livingstone, 2004. Fig. 6-32.)

inferior iliac spine and acetabulum and distally to the intertrochanteric line of the femur. Because of the spiral course of its fibers, the ligament becomes taut during extension. This mechanism screws the femoral head into the acetabulum. The ligament limits hyperextension and reinforces the strength of the joint.

● Pubofemoral ligament. This ligament attaches proximally to the pubic portion of the acetabular rim and the iliopectineal eminence. Distally, it attaches with the iliofemoral ligament. This ligament checks hyperabduction of the hip and becomes taut during extension.

● Ischiofemoral ligament. This ligament attaches proximally to the ischial portion of the acetabular rim and distally to the greater trochanter. The ligament screws the head of the femur into the acetabulum during extension.

● Ligamentum capitis femoris. This weak ligament is located within the capsule of the joint; thus, it is intracapsular. Medially, it attaches to the acetabular notch and the transverse acetabular ligament. Laterally, it attaches to the fovea femoris capitis. Because it is weak, it has little or no role in strengthening the joint. When present, the artery

to the head of the femur travels through the ligament to reach the femoral head.

WHAT STRUCTURE DEEPENS THE ACETABULUM?

The acetabular labrum is a fibrocartilaginous structure that attaches to the acetabular rim and the transverse acetabular ligament (Fig. 5-2). This labrum deepens the acetabulum and helps to hold the femoral head in place.

WHAT IS THE NERVE SUPPLY TO THE HIP JOINT?

The nerves that supply the hip joint are (the segmental ventral primary rami that form them are indicated in parentheses):

● Femoral nerve or its muscular branches (L2-L4)
● Obturator nerve (L2-L4)
● Accessory obturator nerve, if present (L3-L4)
● Superior gluteal nerve (L4-S1)
● Nerve to quadratus femoris (L4-S1)

WHAT IS THE ARTERIAL SUPPLY TO THE HIP JOINT?

The arteries that supply the hip joint are the (Fig. 5-2 and Fig. 5-4):

- Medial and lateral femoral circumflex arteries — branch from the profunda femoris artery (deep femoral artery), but may take origin from the femoral artery
- Superior and inferior gluteal arteries — originate from the internal iliac artery
- Acetabular artery — given off by the obturator artery
- Artery of the ligament to the head of the femur — an inconstant vessel that issues from the obturator artery, a branch of the internal iliac artery.

The circumflex femoral arteries and the gluteal arteries form a periarterial anastomosis around the proximal extremity of the femur. The medial femoral circumflex artery is the principal contributor to the anastomosis and to the femoral head. Branches from this anastomosis pierce the fibrous capsule of the hip joint and travel along the femoral neck to its head. These vessels are referred to as the retinacular arteries. These retinacular arteries are important clinically because of their vulnerability in femoral neck fractures and hip dislocations. If severely damaged, avascular necrosis of the femoral head results due to disruption of its blood supply.

Even if present, the artery to the head of the femur contributes little to the blood supply of the femoral head.

WHAT MUSCLES ACT ACROSS THE HIP JOINT?

Twenty-two muscles from the gluteal region and anterior, posterior, and medial thigh act across the hip joint to produce movements. The muscles of the gluteal region that act across the hip joint and their attachments, nerve supply, and action are described in Table 5-2.

The muscles of the anterior thigh that act across the hip joint and their attachments, nerve supply, and action are described in Table 5-3.

The muscles of the medial thigh that act across the hip joint and their attachments, nerve supply, and action are described in Table 5-4.

The muscles of the posterior thigh that act across the hip joint and their attachments, nerve supply, and action are described in Table 5-5.

WHAT WAS THE SMALL DISCERNABLE FRACTURE?

The thin, posterior rim of the acetabulum was fractured when the femoral head was forcefully driven posteriorly.

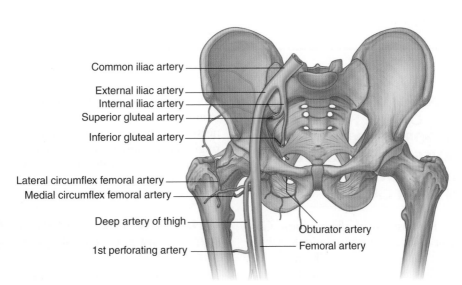

FIGURE 5-4 Arterial supply of the hip joint. (Drake R, Vogl W and Mitchell A: *Gray's Anatomy for Students.* Churchill Livingstone, 2004. Fig. 6-33.)

TABLE 5-2 Gluteal Muscles Acting Across the Hip Joint

Muscle	Origin	Insertion	Nerve Supply	Action
Gluteus maximus	Iliac crest to the superior gluteal line of ilium, posterior surface of sacrum and coccyx, and sacrotuberous ligament	Iliotibial tract and gluteal tuberosity of femur	Inferior gluteal nerve (L5, S1, and S2)	Extends and laterally rotates thigh, steadies thigh at hip, and raises trunk from a flexed position
Gluteus medius	Between the posterior and anterior gluteal lines of ilium	Lateral border of greater trochanter of femur	Superior gluteal nerve (L4, L5, and S1)	Abducts and medially rotates thigh; keeps trunk upright when contralateral foot is raised
Gluteus minimus	Between the anterior and inferior gluteal lines of ilium	Anterolateral border of greater trochanter of femur	Superior gluteal nerve (L4, L5, and S1)	Abducts and medially rotates thigh; keeps trunk upright when contralateral foot is raised
Piriformis	Anterior surface of sacrum	Superior margin of greater trochanter of femur	Ventral rami of L5, S1, and S2	Laterally rotates extended thigh and abducts flexed thigh; holds head of femur in acetabulum
Obturator internus	Bony structures surrounding the internal margin of obturator foramen and obturator membrane	Medial surface of greater trochanter of femur	Nerve to superior gemellus and obturator internus (L5 and S1)	Laterally rotates extended thigh and abducts flexed thigh; holds head of femur in acetabulum
Superior gemellus	Posterior surface of ischial spine	Medial surface of greater trochanter of femur	Nerve to superior gemellus and obturator internus (L5 and S1)	Laterally rotates extended thigh and abducts flexed thigh; holds head of femur in acetabulum
Inferior gemellus	Ischial tuberosity	Medial surface of greater trochanter of femur	Nerve to inferior gemellus and quadratus femoris (L5 and S1)	Laterally rotates extended thigh and abducts flexed thigh; holds head of femur in acetabulum
Quadratus femoris	External surface of ischial tuberosity	Quadrate tubercle on intertrochanteric crest of femur and distal to it	Nerve to inferior gemellus and quadratus femoris (L5 and S1)	Laterally rotates thigh and holds head of femur in acetabulum
Tensor fasciae latae	Anterolateral lip of iliac crest, anterior superior iliac spine, and notch below it	Iliotibial tract; a few fibers may even attach to the lateral condyle of the femur	Superior gluteal nerve (L4, L5, and S1)	Abducts, medially rotates, and flexes thigh; assists in maintaining knee in flexion; and steadies trunk on thigh

SOME PATIENTS WITH A POSTERIOR DISLOCATION OF THE HIP MAY HAVE DIFFICULTY DORSIFLEXING THEIR FOOT BECAUSE OF NEUROLOGIC COMPLICATIONS. WHAT NERVE IS INJURED IN SUCH CASES?

The sciatic nerve lies posterior to the hip joint. Consequently, posterior dislocation with posterior acetabular fracture may injure the sciatic nerve. The nerve may also be damaged when the hip is reduced. The sciatic nerve is formed by the ventral divisions of ventral primary rami L4-S3 (tibial component) and posterior divisions of the ventral primary rami from L4-S2 (common fibular component). Lesions of the sciatic nerve may produce motor deficits in the posterior thigh muscles and muscles of the leg and foot. Sensory alterations may result in the skin over the lateral surface of the leg and the skin over most of the foot.

WHAT ARE THE DORSIFLEXOR AND EVERSION MUSCLES OF THE FOOT?

The dorsiflexor and eversion muscles of the foot are located in the lateral and anterior compartments of the leg. The lateral crural compartment muscles are

TABLE 5-3 Muscles of the Anterior Thigh Acting Across the Hip Joint

Muscle	Origin	Insertion	Nerve Supply	Action
Iliacus	Superior two-thirds of iliac fossa, internal lip of iliac crest, sacroiliac and iliolumbar ligaments, and ala of sacrum	Lesser trochanter of femur	Femoral nerve (L2 and L3)	Flexes the thigh at the hip
Psoas major	Transverse processes of all five lumbar vertebrae, bodies of T12 to L5, and their intervertebral discs	Lesser trochanter of femur	Ventral primary of L1, L2, and L3	Flexes the thigh at the hip
Rectus femoris	Anterior inferior iliac spine, groove superior to acetabulum, and fibrous capsule of hip joint	Tendinous fibers converge to partially form patellar tendon; from patella to tibial tuberosity via patellar ligament	Femoral nerve (L2, L3, and L4)	Flexes thigh, extends knee, and steadies hip joint
Sartorius	Anterior superior iliac spine and superior portion of notch below it	Medial surface of tibia	Femoral nerve (L2 and L3)	Flexes knee and thigh, adducts and laterally rotates thigh

TABLE 5-4 Muscles of the Medial Thigh Acting Across the Hip Joint

Muscle	Origin	Insertion	Nerve Supply	Action
Pectineus	Pecten pubis	Pectineal line of femur	Femoral nerve (L2 and L3); occasionally receives branch from obturator nerve	Adducts and flexes thigh
Adductor magnus	Inferior pubic ramus, ischial ramus, and ischial tuberosity	Gluteal tuberosity, linea aspera, proximal part of medial supracondylar line, and adductor tubercle of femur	Obturator nerve and tibial division of the sciatic nerve (L2, L3, and L4)	Medially rotates and adducts thigh at the hip
Adductor longus	Body of pubis	Middle third of the linear aspera of femur	Anterior division of obturator nerve (L2, L3, and L4)	Medially rotates and adducts thigh at hip
Adductor brevis	External surface of pubic body and inferior ramus of pubis	Pectineal line and superior part of linea aspera of femur	Obturator nerve (L2 and L3)	Adducts thigh and minimally flexes thigh at the hip
Gracilis	Inferior half of body of pubis, inferior pubic ramus, and ischial ramus	Medial metaphyseal surface of tibia, inferior to tibial condyle	Obturator nerve (L2 and L3)	Adducts thigh at the hip, flexes leg, and medially rotates leg
Obturator externus	Bony structures surrounding and the external margin of the obturator foramen and obturator membrane	Trochanteric fossa of femur	Obturator nerve (L3 and L4)	Laterally rotates thigh holds head of femur in acetabulum

innervated by the superficial fibular nerve (L5, S1, and S2), and the muscles in the anterior (crural) compartment are innervated by the deep fibular nerve (L4, L5, and S1).

The muscles located in the lateral crural compartment, their attachments, nerve supply, and actions are described in Table 5-6.

The muscles located in the anterior crural compartment, their attachments, nerve supply, and actions are described in Table 5-7.

TABLE 5-5 Muscles of the Posterior Thigh Acting Across the Hip Joint

Muscle	Origin	Insertion	Nerve Supply	Action
Biceps femoris (long head)	Ischial tuberosity	Head of fibula, lateral collateral ligament, and lateral condyle of tibia	Long head: tibial component of sciatic nerve (L5, S1, and S2)	Flexes and laterally rotates leg; extends thigh at the hip
Semimembranosus	Ischial tuberosity	Medial condyle of tibia	Tibial component of sciatic nerve (L5, S1, and S2)	Extends thigh at the hip; flexes and medially rotates leg; extends trunk when thigh and leg are flexed
Semitendinosus	Ischial tuberosity	Medial condyle of tibia	Tibial component of sciatic nerve (L5, S1, and S2)	Extends thigh at the hip; flexes and medially rotates leg; extends trunk when thigh and leg are flexed

TABLE 5-6 Muscles of the Lateral Crural Compartment

Muscle	Origin	Insertion	Nerve Supply	Action
Fibularis (peroneus) longus	Head of fibula and the proximal two-thirds of its lateral surface, crural fascia, and anterior and posterior crural intermuscular septa	First metatarsal bone and medial (first) cuneiform bone	Superficial fibular (peroneal) nerve (L5, S1, and S2)	Everts and plantar flexes foot
Fibularis (peroneus) brevis	Distal two-thirds of fibula and anterior and posterior crural intermuscular fascia	Tuberosity of the fifth metatarsal bone	Superficial fibular (peroneal) nerve (L5, S1, and S2)	Everts foot

TABLE 5-7 Muscles of the Anterior Crural Compartment

Muscle	Origin	Insertion	Nerve Supply	Action
Tibialis anterior	Lateral condyle of tibia and proximal half of tibia and crural fascia	Medial (first) cuneiform bone and base of first metatarsal bone	Deep fibular nerve (L4 and L5)	Dorsiflexes and inverts foot
Extensor hallucis longus	Middle half of fibula and interosseous membrane	Base of distal phalanx of hallux (great toe)	Deep fibular nerve (L5 and S1)	Extends hallux and dorsiflexes foot
Extensor digitorum longus	Lateral condyle of tibia, proximal three-fourths of fibula, and interosseous membrane	Middle and distal phalanges of digits 2, 3, 4, and 5	Deep fibular nerve (L5 and S1)	Extends digits 2 to 5 and dorsiflexes foot
Fibularis (peroneus) tertius	Distal third of fibula and interosseous membrane	Dorsomedial surface of fifth metatarsal bone	Deep fibular nerve (L5 and S1)	Dorsiflexes and everts foot

Concerned about the developmental delays in motor skills of their 5-year-old boy, the parents scheduled an appointment with a pediatrician. The parents informed the physician that their son seemed uncoordinated as he had difficulty running. The results of the physical examination detected hypertrophy of the calf muscles and diminished proximal tendon reflexes. Laboratory tests revealed a deletion of the dystrophin gene and elevated serum creatine kinase levels (40 times normal). Based on this information, the boy was diagnosed with Duchenne's muscular dystrophy.

WHAT ARE THE THREE TISSUE INVESTMENTS OF MUSCLE?

Muscle is composed of millions of muscle fibers. The muscle fibers are enveloped by a thin connective tissue layer called the endomysium. Muscles fibers and their accompanying endomysium are arranged in bundles or fascicles, which are surrounded by a second connective investment, the perimysium. The entire collection of bundles forms the muscle (e.g., biceps brachii), which is ensheathed by the epimysium.

WHAT IS DYSTROPHIN AND WHAT IS ITS FUNCTION?

Dystrophin is an intracellular glycoprotein found in skeletal and cardiac muscle (Fig. 5-5) that links the microfilament actin to a group of transmembrane proteins (i.e., dystroglycans and sarcoglycans). The transmembrane proteins anchor the sarcolemma to the extracellular matrix. Functionally, dystrophin imparts structural integrity to the sarcolemma by forming a molecular interface that transmits forces from the contractile elements of the muscle cell to the extracellular matrix.

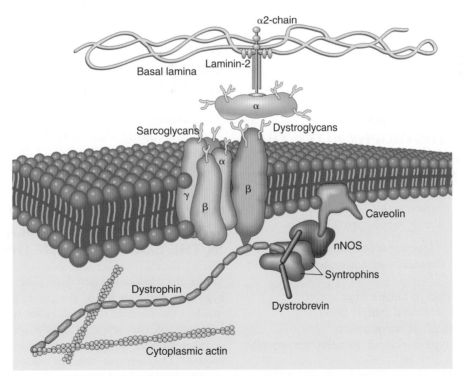

FIGURE 5-5 Illustration of the role of dystrophin in anchoring the cytoskeleton of striated muscle to the extracellular matrix *vis-à-vis* transmembrane proteins of the sarcolemma. (Kumar V, Abbas A and Fausto N: *Robbins & Cotran Pathologic Basis of Disease, 7e.* WB Saunders, 2004. Fig. 27-10.)

WHY IS CREATINE KINASE ELEVATED?

Creatine kinase (CK), formerly known as creatine phosphokinase, is an enzyme found in muscle and brain tissue that uses ATP to phosphorylate creatine to form phosphocreatine. Phosphocreatine thus represents a stored form of energy. There are three isoenzymes of CK:

- CK-BB (CK_1), found in the brain and lung, for example
- CK-MB (CK_2), found chiefly in cardiac muscle
- CK-MM (CK_3), found chiefly in skeletal muscle.

As skeletal muscle fibers degenerate, CK-MM is released into the interstitium, where it then enters the microvasculature. CK-MB also would be elevated if the heart is affected. Late in the disease, creatine kinase levels return to normal as muscle cells degenerate.

WHY ARE THE BOY'S CALF MUSCLES ENLARGED?

Initially, the enlargement of the calf muscles is the result of hypertrophy of the muscle fibers. The muscle then undergoes atrophy as muscle fibers degenerate. The lost muscle fibers are replaced by connective and adipose tissue, which gives a false impression that the calf muscles are enlarged. This phenomenon is appropriately termed *pseudohypertrophy*.

HOW DOES DUCHENNE'S MUSCULAR DYSTROPHY ALTER THE HISTOLOGIC APPEARANCE OF SKELETAL MUSCLE?

The histologic characteristics of skeletal muscle in Duchenne's muscular dystrophy are (Fig. 5-6):

- Skeletal muscle fibers that are small or hypertrophied
- Muscle fiber degeneration with phagocytosis of necrotic fibers
- Increased number of muscle fiber nuclei
- Regeneration of skeletal muscle fibers
- Increased amounts of endomysium
- Type 1 and type 2 skeletal muscles are equally affected.
- Hypercontracted muscle fibers are observed. These fibers have a hyaline (cross-striations are absent) appearance.

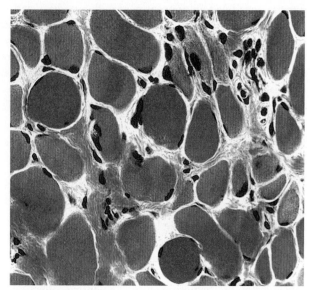

FIGURE 5-6 Duchenne muscular dystrophy. Note the variation in diameter of the skeletal muscle fibers, increase in endomysial connective tissue, and regenerating muscle fibers (blue hue). (Kumar V, Abbas A and Fausto N: *Robbins & Cotran Pathologic Basis of Disease*, 7e. WB Saunders, 2004. Fig. 27-11. Courtesy of Dr. L. Kunkel, Children's Hospital, Boston, MA.)

- Late in the disease, adipose tissue and other connective tissue elements replace most of the skeletal muscle tissue that has been lost.

WHAT ARE THE HISTOLOGIC DIFFERENCES BETWEEN TYPE 1 AND TYPE 2 SKELETAL MUSCLE FIBERS?

As mentioned above, type 1 and type 2 skeletal muscle fibers are equally affected by Duchenne's muscular dystrophy. The characteristics of these two skeletal muscle fiber types are described in Table 5-8.

WHY MIGHT A PATIENT EXHIBIT WINGING OF THE SCAPULAE LATER IN THE COURSE OF THE DISEASE?

While the reason has not been discerned, weakness begins in the muscles of the pelvic girdle and then involves the muscles of the shoulder (pectoral) girdle. Winging of the scapulae would indicate that the serratus anterior muscle has been weakened by the disease. The serratus anterior muscle originates as interdigitations from the lateral external margins of ribs 1 to 8 to insert on the anterior surface of the scapula at its vertebral (medial) border. The muscle, innervated by the long thoracic nerve (C5, C6, and C7), has three primary actions:

- Protraction of the scapula
- Fixation of the scapula against the posterior thoracic wall
- Superior rotation of the scapula's glenoid cavity

Winging of the scapula occurs because the serratus anterior muscle is too weak to hold the scapula against the posterior thoracic wall. Winging would be more pronounced when pushing an object with the upper limbs extended.

TABLE 5-8 Characteristics of the Skeletal Muscle Fiber Types

	Type I	Type IIA	Type IIB
Color	Red	Pink	White
Diameter	Small	Small to medium	Large
Mitochondria	Numerous	Intermediate	Sparse
Z-line width	Wide	Narrow	Narrow
Capillary density	High	High	Low
Myoglobin content	Rich	Intermediate	Low
Myosin ATPase activity	Slow	Fast	Fast
ATP generation	Aerobic	Aerobic	Anaerobic—glycolysis
Glycogen content	Low	Intermediate	High
Lipid content	High	Intermediate	Low
Succinate dehydrogenase	High	Intermediate to high	Low
NADH dehydrogenase	High	Intermediate to high	Low
Twitch rate	Slow	Fast	Fast
Fatigability	Slow to fatigue	Intermediate	Quickly fatigues

A 27-year-old linebacker was clipped on the posterolateral aspect of his knee during a professional football game. The player complained of severe pain in his right knee and stated that he heard his knee pop right after he was hit. The team physician immediately conducted a physical examination of the injured player's knee and observed the following: (1) the player's pain was exacerbated with medial rotation of the leg; (2) a positive anterior drawer sign was observed; and (3) abduction of the slightly flexed knee caused the medial side of the joint to separate more than normal. Several minutes later, the joint cavity of the knee swelled with blood (hemarthrosis). Imaging studies confirmed the diagnosis of the "unhappy triad" of the knee (Fig. 5-7). The player was then referred to an orthopedic surgeon for reconstructive knee surgery.

WHAT IS THE FUNCTIONAL AND ANATOMICAL CLASSIFICATION OF THE KNEE JOINT?

The knee joint is functionally classified as a diarthrosis because of it freedom of movement. Joints that are immovable or virtually immovable are designated synarthroses, whereas joints that are slightly movable are classified as amphiarthroses.

Anatomically, the articulation at the knee is classified as a type of synovial joint. Some authors classify the knee as a hinge joint but this distinction should be strictly reserved for joints that only move in one axis (uniaxial). The knee joint is more complex than a simple hinge joint as the skeletal elements (femur, tibia, and patella) permit rotation, flexion, and extension. Structurally, the femur exhibits two condyles (medial and lateral) that articulate with the corresponding plateaus of the tibial condyles. The patella possesses a saddle-shaped surface that articulates with the femur. Therefore, it is best described as having two condyloid joints and one saddle (sellar) joint.

WHAT ARE THE THREE DAMAGED STRUCTURES THAT CONSTITUTE THE "UNHAPPY TRIAD"?

The "unhappy triad" is characterized by injury to the medial (tibial) collateral ligament, the anterior cruciate ligament, and the medial meniscus (Fig. 5-7).

WHY ARE THESE STRUCTURES VULNERABLE TO INJURY?

The lateral side of the knee is more exposed than its medial surface. Therefore, as in this clinical scenario, the lateral aspect more frequently bears the force of impact. This impact causes the joint angle along the medial border of the knee to increase (valgus strain—forceful abduction of the tibia on the femur), thereby increasing the strain on the medial collateral ligament to the point of being torn. The clipping action caused a twisting motion about the knee joint. Because the deep fibers of the medial collateral ligament are attached to the medial meniscus, this abrupt rotating action tears the medial meniscus. This anatomical arrangement is not duplicated on the lateral side. Instead, the lateral meniscus and the lateral collateral ligament, which is stronger than the medial collateral ligament, are separated by the tendon of the popliteus muscle. The lateral meniscus, therefore, is less vulnerable to injury because it is not adherent to the lateral collateral ligament. The anterior cruciate ligament, which is weaker than the posterior cruciate ligament, is more vulnerable to injury during applied rotational forces that increase the tension on the ligaments. The strain on the anterior cruciate ligament was exacerbated by the anterior displacement of the tibia on the femur caused by the clipping infraction.

WHAT ARE THE FUNCTIONS OF THE COLLATERAL LIGAMENTS, THE CRUCIATE LIGAMENTS, AND THE MENISCI?

The lateral and medial collateral ligaments (Fig. 5-8) function to check extension and lateral rotation of the tibia, as well as limit side-to-side movements. Individually, the medial collateral ligament would limit abduction of the tibia, whereas its fellow would check adduction of the tibia. In the clinical scenario above, it was excessive abduction that caused the medial collateral ligament to rupture.

The anterior and posterior cruciate ligaments (Figs. 5-8 and 5-9) become taut during extension, thereby checking hyperextension. The anterior cruciate ligament also serves to limit anterior displacement of

A

Lateral meniscus   Medial meniscus

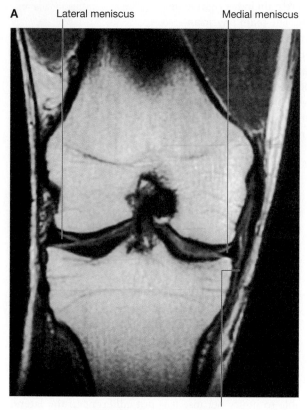

Torn tibial collateral ligament

B   Patella   Femur

Tibia   Torn anterior cruciate ligament

C

Medial femoral condyle   Torn medial meniscus

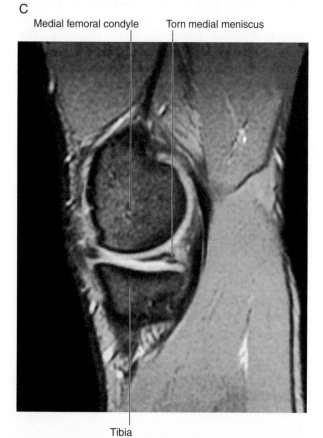

Tibia

MCL → limits TIBIAL ABDUCTN ⎫ CHECK EXTNSN,
LCL →   "   "   ADDUCTN   ⎬ Slhe-ti-sine
                          ⎭ & ROTATN

FIGURE 5-7 MRI of knee joint. **A,** Torn tibial collateral ligament. **B,** Torn anterior cruciate ligament. **C,** Torn medial meniscus. From Gray's Anatomy for Students. (Drake R, Vogl W and Mitchell A: *Gray's Anatomy for Students.* Churchill Livingstone, 2004. Fig. 6-134.)

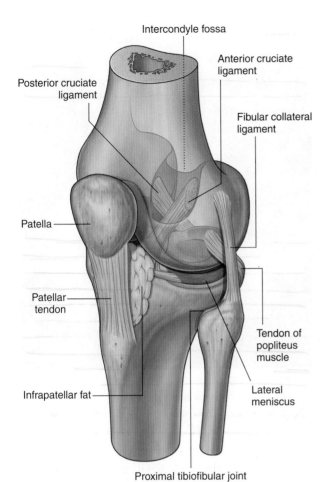

FIGURE 5-8 Knee joint with joint capsule removed. (Drake R, Vogl W and Mitchell A: *Gray's Anatomy for Students*. Churchill Livingstone, 2004. Fig. 6-68.)

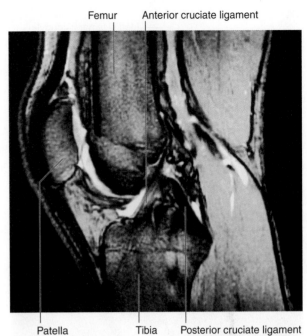

FIGURE 5-9 MRI of normal knee joint. (Drake R, Vogl W and Mitchell A: *Gray's Anatomy for Students*. Churchill Livingstone, 2004. Fig. 6-135.)

the tibia on the femur (or posterior displacement of the femur on the tibia) when the knee is flexed. Conversely, the posterior cruciate ligament checks posterior movement of the tibia on the femur (or anterior movement of the femur on the tibia) when the knee is flexed. Both cruciate ligaments serve to limit medial rotation.

The lateral and medial menisci (Figs. 5-10 and 5-11) deepen the sockets for the convex femoral condyles and in distributing the downward force of the femur laterally. This mechanism is important because it deflects the load-bearing forces away from the articular surface, thereby protecting the articular cartilage from excessive forces that would, over time, cause it to degenerate (p 392, Essential Orthopaedics and Trauma, 4th edition).

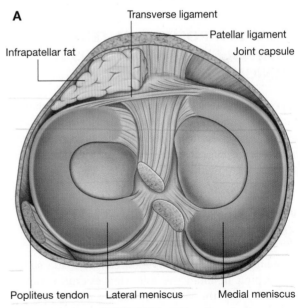

FIGURE 5-10 Superior view of the menisci of the knee joint. (Drake R, Vogl W and Mitchell A: *Gray's Anatomy for Students*. Churchill Livingstone, 2004. Fig. 6-70A.)

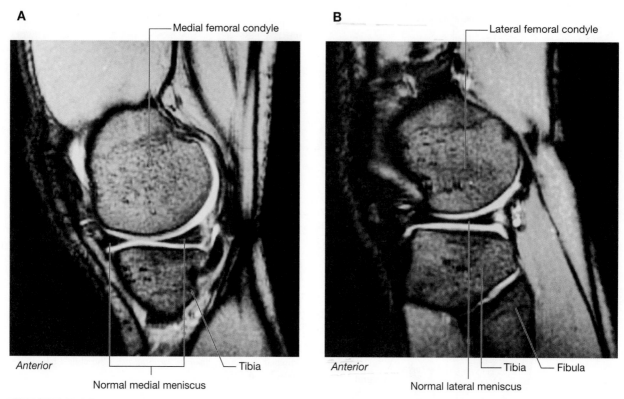

A

— Medial femoral condyle

Anterior — Tibia

Normal medial meniscus

B

— Lateral femoral condyle

Anterior — Tibia — Fibula

Normal lateral meniscus

FIGURE 5-11 MRI of normal menisci. **A**, Medial meniscus. **B**, Lateral meniscus. (Drake R, Vogl W and Mitchell A: *Gray's Anatomy for Students*. Churchill Livingstone, 2004. Fig. 6-70BC.)

WHAT IS A POSITIVE ANTERIOR DRAWER SIGN AND WHAT IS ITS CLINICAL SIGNIFICANCE?

A posterior anterior drawer sign occurs when there is excessive anterior displacement of the tibia on the femur. This indicates rupture of the anterior cruciate ligament because it is no longer intact to limit this anterior movement.

WHAT NERVES INNERVATE THE KNEE JOINT?

Remembering joint innervation can be made simple by keeping in mind the following axiom: a joint is innervated by the very same nerves that supply the muscles that move the joint and supply the skin over the joint. This axiom is known as Hilton's Law. When this law is applied to the knee joint, the innervation is the:

● Femoral nerve (supplies the quadriceps femoris muscle and overlying skin)

● Common fibular and tibial nerves (supply the hamstrings, short head of biceps femoris, and associated skin)

● Obturator nerve (supplies the skin in the popliteal fossa).

These are the nerves that are responsible for the transmission of pain to the central nervous system after injury to the joint.

WHAT IS THE PATHWAY FOR PROPRIOCEPTION?

The first-order afferent fibers from the joint receptors pass through the dorsal root to enter the spinal cord (Fig. 5-12). Upon entering the spinal cord, the fibers ascend in the ipsilateral fasciculus gracilis. The first-order fibers synapse with second-order neurons in the ipsilateral nucleus gracilis located in the caudal medulla oblongata. The second-order fibers cross the midline to ascend in the contralateral medial lemniscus of the brainstem. The fibers synapse with third-order neurons in the ventral posterolateral nucleus of the thalamus. Third-order neurons, which represent the

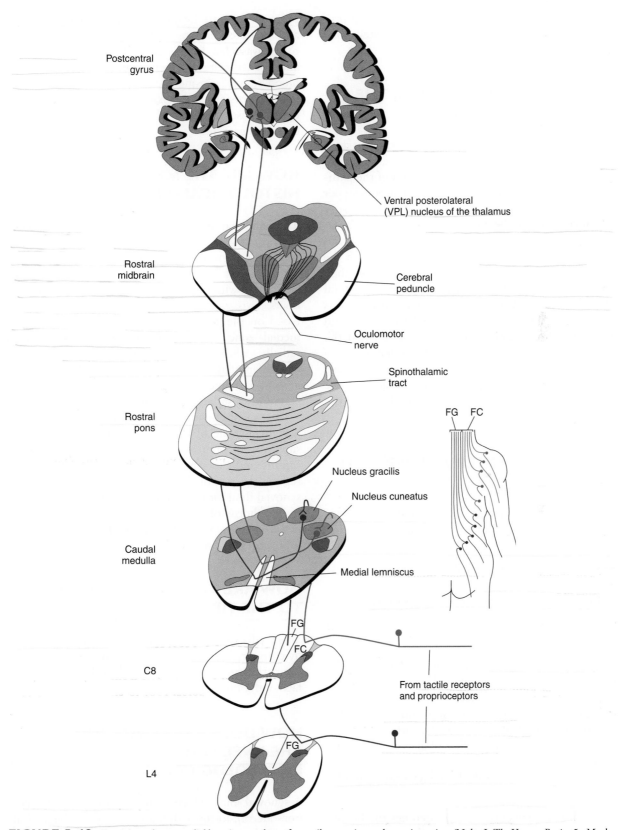

FIGURE 5-12 Posterior column-medial lemniscus pathway for tactile sensation and proprioception. (Nolte J: *The Human Brain, 5e*. Mosby, 2002. Fig. 10-17. Inset redrawn from Mettler FA: *Neuroanatomy, ed 2*, St. Louis, 1948, Mosby.)

last participant in this neuronal relay team, then project to the primary somatosensory cortex located along the medial postcentral gyrus.

WHAT IS THE PATHWAY FOR THE PERCEPTION OF PAIN?

The pathway for pain is the anterolateral spinothalamic tract. This tract also conveys temperature and some touch and pressure. The anterior portion of the pathway is responsible for the superior trunk and upper limb, whereas the lateral component conveys sensory information from the inferior trunk and lower extremity. Thus, the pathway from the knee begins with the axons from pain receptors that pass through the dorsal root to enter the spinal cord, where they then synapse with second-order neurons in the ipsilateral dorsal gray horn (Fig. 5-13). The second-order axons cross to the opposite side of the spinal cord and ascend in the lateral spinothalamic tract. In the brainstem, the second-order axons travel in the medial lemniscus to terminate in the ventral posterolateral nucleus of the thalamus. Third-order neurons then project to the primary somatosensory cortex located along the medial postcentral gyrus.

WHAT IS THE ARTERIAL SUPPLY TO THE KNEE JOINT?

The knee joint is supplied by the genicular anastomosis, which is principally formed by the following branches of the popliteal artery (Fig. 5-14):

● Superior lateral and medial genicular arteries
● Middle genicular artery
● Inferior lateral and medial genicular arteries.

Additional contributing branches to the genicular anastomosis are:

● Descending genicular. The descending genicular artery springs from the femoral artery just before it passes through the adductor hiatus
● Anterior and posterior tibial recurrent branches (both issue from the anterior tibial artery)
● Branches of the circumflex fibular artery (issues from the fibular artery)
● Descending branch of the lateral femoral circumflex artery

The medial genicular artery penetrates the fibrous capsule of the knee to supply the anterior and

posterior cruciate ligaments, the synovial membrane, and the outer margins of the menisci, which are relatively avascular. In this clinical case, rupture of the anterior cruciate ligament concomitantly tears its blood supply, causing bleeding into the joint cavity (hemarthrosis). Approximately 80% of acute hemarthroses are caused by tears of the anterior cruciate ligament.

HOW ARE THE MENISCI DESCRIBED HISTOLOGICALLY?

The semilunar menisci are composed of fibrocartilage. Fibrocartilage contains chondrocytes, type I collagen fibers, and ground substance. The chondrocytes, which occupy lacunae, are arranged in parallel rows alternating with the coarse, acidophilic type I collagen fibers. Two zones of the menisci have been identified based on the array of collagen bundles. The larger medial zone consists of collagen fibers arranged radially, whereas the smaller peripheral zone has circumferentially arrayed collagen bundles. The stiff ground substance is rich in the glycosaminoglycans chondroitin sulfate and dermatan sulfate.

The menisci are relatively avascular. Although the peripheral zone of the meniscus receives a vascular supply from branches of the arteries in the fibrous capsule and the synovial membrane that covers this region, the rest of the meniscus is dependent on the synovial fluid for its supply of nutrients and oxygen.

The horns of the menisci are well endowed with nerve endings, with the rest of the meniscus being more sparsely innervated.

HOW ARE THE MENISCI ANCHORED TO THE TIBIA?

The medial and lateral menisci are secured to the tibia by coronary ligaments. The ligaments are attached to the periphery of the menisci and to the external surface of the tibial condyles.

HOW DOES A SYNOVIAL JOINT LIKE THE KNEE FORM EMBRYOLOGICALLY?

A synovial joint, which is derived from mesenchyme (mesoderm), forms within a rod of precartilage. This means that the rod must be split into proximal and

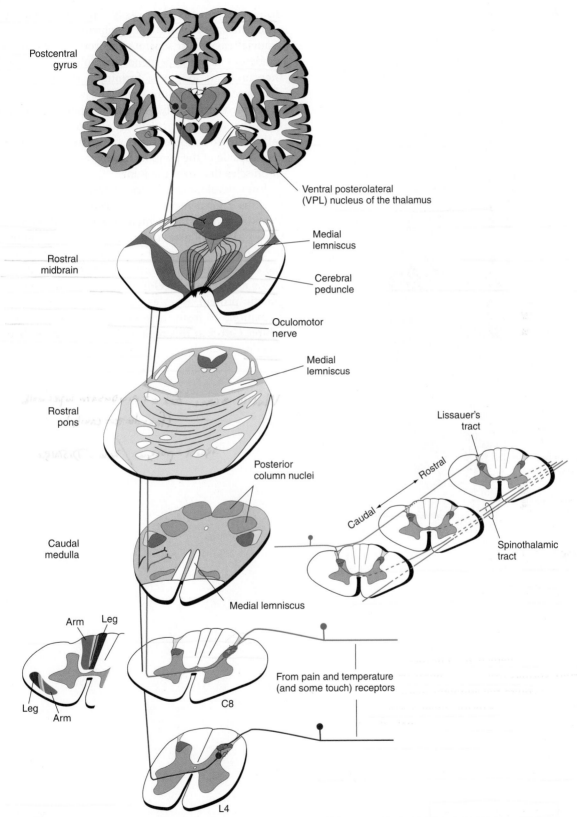

FIGURE 5-13 Spinothalamic pathway for pain, temperature, and some touch and pressure. (Nolte J: *The Human Brain*, 5e. Mosby, 2002. Fig. 10-20.)

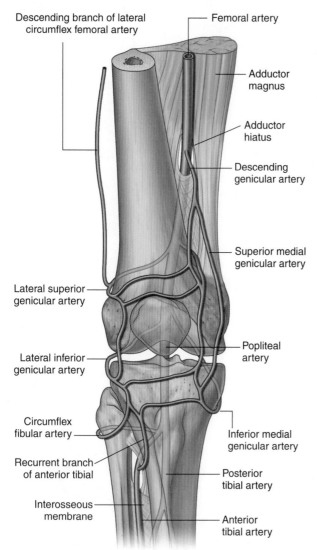

Descending branch of lateral circumflex femoral artery

Femoral artery

Adductor magnus

Adductor hiatus

Descending genicular artery

Superior medial genicular artery

Lateral superior genicular artery

Lateral inferior genicular artery

Popliteal artery

Circumflex fibular artery

Inferior medial genicular artery

Recurrent branch of anterior tibial

Posterior tibial artery

Interosseous membrane

Anterior tibial artery

FIGURE 5-14 Genicular arteries. (Drake R, Vogl W and Mitchell A: *Gray's Anatomy for Students.* Churchill Livingstone, 2004. Fig. 6-76.)

distal components that ossify into the bones that articulate at the joint. The splitting site forms the synovial cavity. To separate the rod, a zone of cells condenses along a perpendicular plane. These cells then undergo apoptosis, forming a fluid-filled space that becomes the future synovial cavity. The surfaces of the proximal and distal elements apposing the space form the articular cartilage. Additional mesenchymal cells undergo condensation to ultimately form the fibrous capsule of the joint, its ligaments, and the tendons of muscles that span the joint.

Joint development is orchestrated by an ensemble of three known regulatory molecules. These include Wnt-14, growth differentiation factor-5 (Gdf-5), and noggin. Wnt-14 plays two roles. One is to prompt the formation of the zone of cell condensation across the rod of precartilage; the other is to stimulate the synthesis and release of Gdf-5. Gdf-5, a bone morphogenetic protein, is an essential regulator of cartilage formation. To form the joint cavity, it is necessary to inhibit Gdf-5 in this region. This is accomplished by noggin.

An athletic 21-year-old man presented with a complaint of pain and weakness in his right leg when jogging. The pain and weakness intensified with continued activity but dissipated at rest. There was no history of trauma to his right lower limb and no family history of diabetes mellitus or other diseases that would lead to accelerated atherosclerosis. Lab results for cholesterol and triglycerides were normal. The dorsalis pedis arterial pulse was normal but disappeared with dorsiflexion of the right foot. Doppler measurement of blood flow velocity in the dorsalis pedis artery showed diminished velocity with dorsiflexion of the right foot and plantar flexion against resistance. Measurements in the left dorsalis pedis artery were normal. Angiography showed medial deviation of the popliteal artery with poststenotic dilatation. The patient was diagnosed with popliteal artery entrapment syndrome and it was treated surgically.

HOW DOES THE POPLITEAL ARTERY DEVELOP?

Embryologically, the popliteal artery is derived from three sources:

- The proximal segment of the popliteal artery is formed by the fusion of the femoral arterial plexus and the popliteal portion of the primitive axial (ischiadic) artery.
- The middle segment directly forms from the primitive axial artery.
- The original distal segment of the popliteal artery, which lies deep to the popliteus muscle, is a continuation of the primitive axial artery. This artery disappears at the beginning of the fetal period and is replaced by the union of two new arteries. The fusion of the vessels occurs superficial to the popliteus muscle and after the medial head of the gastrocnemius muscle has moved through the popliteal fossa.

WHAT ARE THE POSSIBLE CAUSES OF POPLITEAL ARTERY ENTRAPMENT SYNDROME?

The most frequent cause of popliteal artery entrapment is compression by a congenital abnormality of the medial head of the gastrocnemius muscle causing the popliteal artery to deviate medially. Another cause may be fibrosis of the tunica intima of the popliteal artery resulting from repetitive flexion-extension movements of the knee joint.

Six types of popliteal artery entrapment syndrome have been described. Five of these have an embryologic basis and the sixth is considered to be functional. The five embryologic types are:

- Type 1. In this type, which is the most common, development of the distal popliteal artery occurs before the medial head of the gastrocnemius muscle migrates toward its origin. As a result, the superior migration of the medial head of the gastrocnemius muscle will move the popliteal artery medially.
- Type 2. In this form, the distal popliteal artery develops ahead of schedule and prevents the medial head of the gastrocnemius muscle from completing its full ascent to its origin on the posterior surface of the medial femoral condyle. Consequently, the medial gastrocnemius muscle has a variable origin.
- Type 3. This type occurs when the popliteal artery develops within the substance of the medial head of the gastrocnemius.
- Type 4. This entrapment syndrome occurs when the primitive distal popliteal axial artery persists, rather than regresses, to form the distal popliteal artery. Because the primitive distal popliteal axial artery travels deep to the popliteus muscle, its persistence results in the entrapment of the distal part of the popliteal artery.
- Type 5. This type results when the popliteal artery and vein are both entrapped.

The sixth type of popliteal artery entrapment syndrome is considered to be functional in nature. It is postulated that exercise-induced hypertrophy of the medial head of the gastrocnemius muscle causes it to impinge on the popliteal artery.

WHAT COLLATERAL CIRCULATION IS AVAILABLE IN THE EVENT OF STENOSIS OF THE POPLITEAL ARTERY?

Collateral circulation is provided by the genicular anastomosis. This anastomosis was described with the knee joint. If the stenosis is located inferior to the superior genicular arteries, collateral blood flow is provided by the superior genicular, descending genicular, and descending branch of the lateral femoral circumflex arteries.

THE POPLITEAL ARTERY DESCENDS THROUGH THE POPLITEAL FOSSA. WHAT ARE THE BOUNDARIES OF THE POPLITEAL FOSSA?

The popliteal fossa is a diamond-shaped region located posterior to the knee. It has four borders, roof, and floor. The structures that form these demarcations are:

- The superolateral boundary is formed by the biceps femoris muscle.
- The superomedial boundary is formed by the semimembranosus and semitendinosus muscles.
- The inferolateral boundary is defined by the lateral head of the gastrocnemius muscle.
- The inferomedial boundary is defined by the medial head of the gastrocnemius muscle.
- The roof is formed by the skin and fascia (superficial and deep).
- The floor is formed by the posterior surface of the femur, popliteus fascia, and the oblique popliteal ligament, an expansion of the semimembranosus tendon.

WHAT STRUCTURES ARE FOUND IN THE POPLITEAL FOSSA?

The following structures are found in the popliteal fossa (Fig. 5-15):

- Small saphenous vein. The small saphenous vein ascends in the superficial fascia of the posterior leg, pierces the deep popliteal fascia, and empties into the popliteal vein.
- Popliteal artery and its genicular branches. The popliteal artery is a continuation of the femoral artery. When the femoral artery passes through the adductor hiatus of the adductor magnus muscle, it is called the *popliteal artery*. The popliteal artery courses along the floor of the popliteal fossa and ends at the inferior margin of the popliteus muscle by dividing into the anterior and posterior tibial arteries. The popliteal artery is the deepest structure of the popliteal fossa.
- Popliteal vein. The popliteal vein is formed by the confluence of the anterior and posterior tibial veins at the inferior border of the popliteus muscle.

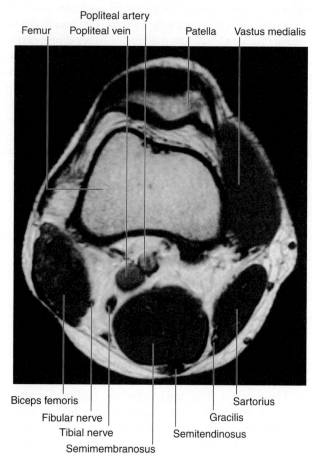

FIGURE 5-15 MRI of contents of popliteal fossa. Note that the popliteal artery is the deepest structure in the fossa. (Drake R, Vogl W and Mitchell A: *Gray's Anatomy for Students*. Churchill Livingstone, 2004. Fig. 6-133.)

- Tibial and common fibular (peroneal) nerves descend through the fossa.
- Terminal portion of the posterior femoral cutaneous nerve
- Articular branch of the obturator nerve to supply the knee joint
- Popliteal lymph nodes, popliteus fascia, lymphatic vessels, and fat

WHERE IS THE DORSALIS PEDIS ARTERY PALPABLE?

The dorsalis pedis artery is a continuation of the anterior tibial artery. It becomes the dorsalis pedis artery distal to the ankle joint. The artery is palpable between the tendon of the extensor hallucis longus and the tendon of the extensor digitorum longus to the second digit as it crosses the tarsal bones (Fig. 5-16).

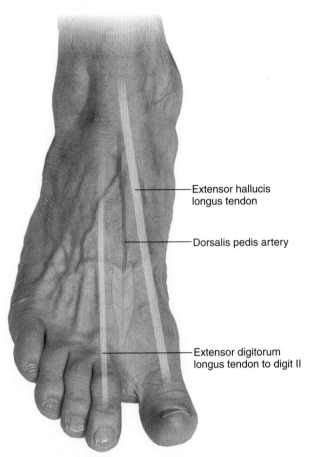

Extensor hallucis longus tendon

Dorsalis pedis artery

Extensor digitorum longus tendon to digit II

FIGURE 5-16 Locating the dorsalis pedis artery. (Drake R, Vogl W and Mitchell A: *Gray's Anatomy for Students*. Churchill Livingstone, 2004. Fig. 6-129.)

WHY DID THE DORSALIS PEDIS ARTERIAL PULSE AND BLOOD FLOW VELOCITY DIMINISH WITH DORSIFLEXION OF THE FOOT?

Popliteal artery entrapment syndrome produces a poststenotic dilatation of the popliteal artery resulting in a pressure drop distal to the obstruction. Dorsiflexion of the foot further obstructs blood flow into the dorsalis pedis artery, causing a disappearance of the pulse and diminished blood flow velocity.

A group of four men were mountain climbing when they suddenly noticed that the weather was dramatically changing for the worse. In an attempt to avoid the approaching winter blast, the climbers started to descend down a steep cliff. As the last climber was descending, he slipped and fell. After the fall, he complained of pain in his leg. One of the team members used his cell phone to call for help, but they would have to wait until the storm passed. After 4 hours, the injured man complained that his leg was tingling and burning (paresthesia). The severe weather finally passed and the man was airlifted to a nearby medical center. Lab results showed that creatine kinase was elevated, and roentgenography revealed a tibial fracture. The MRI study that followed showed increased signal intensity in the posterior compartment of the leg. The man was diagnosed with posterior compartment syndrome secondary to a tibial fracture.

WHAT ARE THE COMPARTMENTS OF THE LEG AND WHAT STRUCTURES DO THEY CONTAIN?

The leg is divided into three compartments by osseofibrous structures (Fig. 5-17). These are the anterior, lateral, and posterior compartments. The posterior compartment is further divided into superficial and deep. The contents of the crural compartments are found in Table 5-9.

WHAT ARE THE MUSCLES OF THE DEEP DIVISION OF THE POSTERIOR COMPARTMENT OF THE LEG AND WHAT ARE THEIR ATTACHMENTS, INNERVATION, AND ACTIONS?

The muscles of the deep division of the posterior compartment of the leg and their attachments, nerve supply, and actions are described in Table 5-10.

WHAT IS THE ANATOMICAL BASIS OF COMPARTMENT SYNDROME?

Compartment syndrome occurs in closed anatomical spaces, particularly the leg and the anterior forearm. In this clinical case, the closed anatomical space is the osseofibrous posterior compartment of the leg. The posterior compartment of the leg is bounded by the tibia and fibula, deep crural fascia, interosseous membrane, and the anterior intermuscular membrane (Fig. 5-17).

The number one cause of compartment syndrome is tibial fracture. Fracture of the tibia and accompanying soft tissue injury, if any, leads to an accumulation of fluid in the involved anatomical compartment.

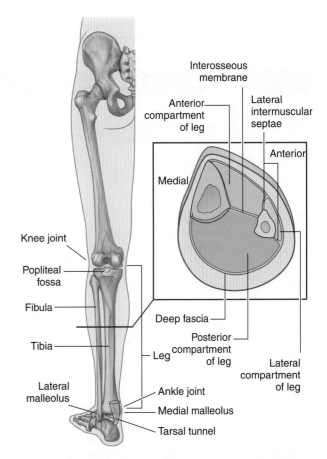

FIGURE 5-17 *Left,* Posterior view of leg. *Right,* Axial view of the left leg showing its compartments. (Drake R, Vogl W and Mitchell A: *Gray's Anatomy for Students.* Churchill Livingstone, 2004. Fig. 6-79.)

Because this occurs in a confined space, the increasing fluid causes the tissue pressure to become elevated. When tissue pressure becomes greater than perfusion (arterial) pressure, blood flow to the tissues in the compartment cannot be maintained as the elevated external tissue pressure collapses the blood vessels.

TABLE 5-9 Contents of the Crural Compartments

Structure	Anterior	Lateral	Superficial Posterior	Deep Posterior
Muscles	Tibialis anterior Extensor hallucis longus Extensor digitorum longus Fibularis tertius	Fibularis longus Fibularis brevis	Gastrocnemius Plantaris Soleus	Popliteus Flexor hallucis longus Flexor digitorum longus Tibialis posterior
Nerve	Deep fibular nerve (L4, L5, S1)	Superficial fibular (L5, S1, S2)	Tibial nerve (S1, S2)	Tibial nerve (L4, L5, S1, S2, S3)
Blood vessels	Anterior tibial artery and veins	Blood vessels do not run within this compartment. Instead branches and tributaries from the fibular artery and veins supply and drain the compartment		Posterior tibial artery and veins Fibular artery and veins

TABLE 5-10 Muscles of the Deep Division of the Posterior Crural Compartment

Muscle	Origin	Insertion	Nerve Supply	Action
Popliteus	Lateral condyle of femur and arcuate popliteal ligament	Posterior surface of tibia	Tibial nerve (L4, L5, and S1)	Rotates tibia medially or if tibia is fixed, rotates femur laterally. This action is necessary to unlock the knee joint so that flexion may occur from a fully extended state
Tibialis posterior	Interosseous membrane, posterior surface of tibia, and posterior surface of fibula	Tuberosity of navicular bone, medial, intermediate, and lateral cuneiform bones, cuboid bone, and bases of metatarsal bones 2 to 4	Tibial nerve (L4 and L5)	Plantar flexes and inverts foot
Flexor digitorum longus	Posterior surface of tibia and to fibula by an aponeurosis	Bases of the distal phalanges of digits 2 to 5	Tibial nerve (S2 and S3)	Flexes digits 2 to 5 and plantar flexes foot
Flexor hallucis longus	Distal two-thirds of posterior surface of fibula and interosseous membrane	Base of distal phalanx of first digit	Tibial nerve (S2 and S3)	Flexes first digit and plantar flexes foot

The compromised circulation leads to tissue injury and necrosis with diminished function. Injury to skeletal muscles causes release of creatine kinase, specifically CK-MM (CK_3), and myoglobin. Elevated circulating levels of myoglobin are injurious to the kidneys.

In some cases of compartment syndrome, a fasciotomy must be performed to restore perfusion to the involved limb.

AS A CAPSTONE TO THE LOWER EXTREMITY, WHAT IS THE SEGMENTAL INNERVATION OF THE MUSCLES OF THE LOWER EXTREMITY?

The segmental innervation of the muscles of the lower extremity is provided in Table 5-11.

Table 5-11 Segmental Innervation of the Lower Limb Muscles

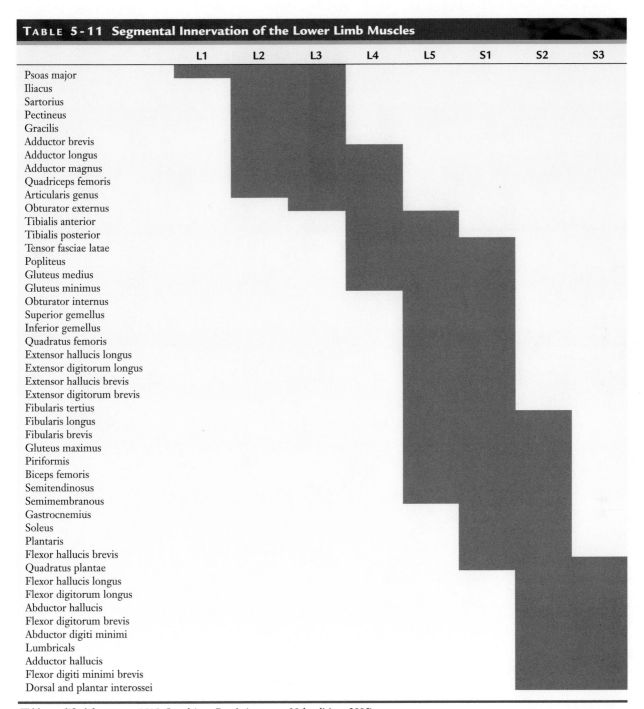

	L1	L2	L3	L4	L5	S1	S2	S3
Psoas major								
Iliacus								
Sartorius								
Pectineus								
Gracilis								
Adductor brevis								
Adductor longus								
Adductor magnus								
Quadriceps femoris								
Articularis genus								
Obturator externus								
Tibialis anterior								
Tibialis posterior								
Tensor fasciae latae								
Popliteus								
Gluteus medius								
Gluteus minimus								
Obturator internus								
Superior gemellus								
Inferior gemellus								
Quadratus femoris								
Extensor hallucis longus								
Extensor digitorum longus								
Extensor hallucis brevis								
Extensor digitorum brevis								
Fibularis tertius								
Fibularis longus								
Fibularis brevis								
Gluteus maximus								
Piriformis								
Biceps femoris								
Semitendinosus								
Semimembranous								
Gastrocnemius								
Soleus								
Plantaris								
Flexor hallucis brevis								
Quadratus plantae								
Flexor hallucis longus								
Flexor digitorum longus								
Abductor hallucis								
Flexor digitorum brevis								
Abductor digiti minimi								
Lumbricals								
Adductor hallucis								
Flexor digiti minimi brevis								
Dorsal and plantar interossei								

(Table modified from page 1415, Standring, Gray's Anatomy, 39th edition, 2005)

SECTION VI

Upper Limb

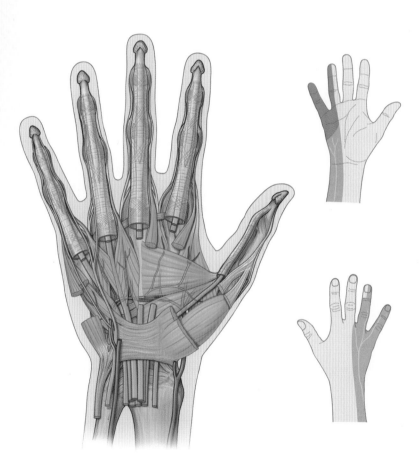

A 24-year-old woman was riding her horse in preparation for an upcoming equestrian event. At she approached one of the jumps, the horse suddenly stopped, throwing her to the ground. She landed violently on her shoulder and head causing excessive separation. The separation produced a brachial plexus injury.

WHAT IS THE ORGANIZATION OF THE BRACHIAL PLEXUS?

The brachial plexus is composed of the following elements: roots, trunks, divisions, cords, and branches (Fig. 6-1). The following mnemonic can be used to remember this basic organization: **r**ed **t**igers **d**rink **c**old **b**eer. The roots of the brachial plexus are ventral primary rami from C5, C6, C7, C8, and T1. The first pair, C5 and C6, joins to form the superior trunk, whereas C8 and T1 converge to form the inferior trunk. The middle trunk is simply a continuation of C7. Each trunk divides into an anterior division and a posterior division. The divisions then converge to form cords. The posterior cord is formed exclusively by the three posterior divisions, one from each of the three trunks. The anterior divisions form the lateral and medial cords. The anterior divisions from the superior and middle trunks unite to form the lateral cord, whereas the medial cord is simply a continuation of the anterior division from the inferior trunk. Each cord ends by dividing into two terminal branches. These are:

- Lateral cord — musculocutaneous nerve and the lateral root of the median nerve
- Medial cord — ulnar nerve and the medial root of the median nerve
- Posterior cord — axillary nerve and radial nerve

DESCRIBE THE SENSORY AND MOTOR FUNCTIONS OF THE VARIOUS ANATOMICAL LEVELS OF THE BRACHIAL PLEXUS.

The sensory and motor functions of various structural elements of the brachial plexus are described in Table 6-1.

WHAT MUSCLES ARE INNERVATED BY THE VENTRAL PRIMARY RAMI THAT CONTRIBUTE TO THE FORMATION OF THE BRACHIAL PLEXUS?

The roots (ventral primary rami) and the muscles that they innervate are found in Table 6-2.

WHAT COMPONENTS OF THE BRACHIAL PLEXUS ARE MOST LIKELY DAMAGED IN THE PATIENT?

Forceful separation of the shoulder and neck produced an upper brachial plexus injury. Upper brachial plexus injuries involve C5 and/or C6 roots, whereas lower brachial plexus injuries involve C8 and/or T1 roots. Lesions of C7 are rare.

ASSUMING AVULSIONS OF THE C5 AND C6 ROOTS IN THIS PATIENT, WHAT MOTOR AND SENSORY DEFICITS WOULD YOU EXPECT TO DETECT DURING THE PHYSICAL EXAMINATION?

The following muscles are wholly or partially innervated by ventral primary rami of C5 and C6 (based on Table 6-2):

- Serratus anterior (C5, **C6, C7**)
- Deltoid (**C5** and C6)
- Subscapularis (C5 and **C6**)
- Biceps brachii (C5 and **C6**)
- Brachialis (C5 and **C6**)
- Coracobrachialis (C5, **C6**, and C7)
- Pectoralis major (C5, **C6**, and C7 of the lateral pectoral nerve). The pectoralis major is also

[handwritten annotations: "can't abduct arm", "↓ supinatn (elbow) flexion"]

A

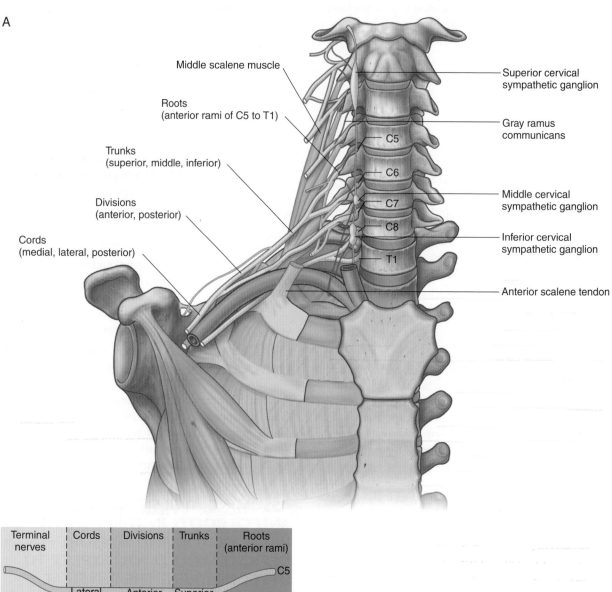

Middle scalene muscle

Roots
(anterior rami of C5 to T1)

Trunks
(superior, middle, inferior)

Divisions
(anterior, posterior)

Cords
(medial, lateral, posterior)

Superior cervical
sympathetic ganglion

Gray ramus
communicans

Middle cervical
sympathetic ganglion

Inferior cervical
sympathetic ganglion

Anterior scalene tendon

C5
C6
C7
C8
T1

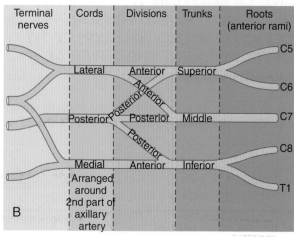

FIGURE 6-1 A, Brachial plexus structures in the neck and axilla. **B,** Schematic of the brachial plexus elements. (Drake R, Vogl W and Mitchell A: *Gray's Anatomy for Students*. Churchill Livingstone, 2004. Fig. 7-51.)

LOWER BP INJURY → Claw Hand APPEARANCE
    ↳ INTRINSIC HAND MUSCLES DEFICIT IN HANDS
        = HAND MORE DISTORTED

TABLE 6-1 Sensory and Motor Functions of the Brachial Plexus at Different Anatomical Levels

Anatomical Level	Sensory Function	Motor Function
Root of C5	Skin of lateral surface of arm and lateral surface of proximal forearm	Lateral (external) rotation and abduction of the shoulder
Root of C6	Cubital fossa, lateral side of forearm inferior to C5, and thumb	Flexion of elbow and extension and abduction of wrist (extensor carpi radialis longus muscle)
Root of C7	Digits 2,3, and 4 and dorsal-radial surface of hand	Extension of digits and wrist, flexion and abduction of wrist (flexor carpi radialis muscle), flexion of elbow (brachioradialis muscle), and pronation of forearm (pronator teres muscle)
Root of C8	Digit 5 and dorsal-ulnar surface of hand	Flexion of digits and wrist
Root of T1	Minimal	Intrinsic muscles of hand
Suprascapular nerve (branch of superior trunk)	Minimal	Lateral rotation of the shoulder (infraspinatus muscle)
Axillary nerve (branch of posterior cord)	Skin over superior surface of deltoid muscle	Abduction of shoulder (deltoid muscle)
C7 contribution to lateral cord	Digits 1, 2, and 3	Pronation of forearm (pronator teres muscle) and flexion and abduction of wrist (flexor carpi radialis muscle)
Lateral cord	Cubital fossa, radial side of forearm, and digits 1, 2, and 3. This does not include dorsal surface of digit 1.	Flexion of elbow, pronation of forearm, and flexion and abduction of wrist (flexor carpi radialis muscle)
Musculocutaneous nerve	Cubital fossa and radial side of forearm	Flexion of elbow
Middle trunk	Digits 1, 2, and 3, radial side of forearm, and radial-dorsal hand	Extension of elbow, flexion of elbow (brachioradialis muscle), and extension of wrist and digits
Posterior cord	Skin over superior surface of deltoid muscle	Abduction of shoulder, extension of elbow, flexion of elbow (brachioradialis muscle), and extension of wrist and digits
Inferior trunk and medial cord	Digits 4 and 5 and medial arm and forearm	Flexion of wrist and fingers and intrinsic hand muscles innervated by the median and ulnar nerves

(Table adapted from p. 10, Boone, the Brachial Plexus, 1997)

innervated by the medial pectoral nerve. This nerve is formed by C8 and T1 and is not involved in an upper brachial plexus injury.

- Latissimus dorsi (**C6**, **C7**, and C8)
- Triceps brachii (C6, **C7**, and **C8**)
- Teres major (**C6** and C7)
- Teres minor (**C5** and C6)
- Supraspinatus (C4, **C5**, and C6)
- Infraspinatus (**C5** and C6)
- Brachioradialis (C5, **C6**, and C7)
- Pronator teres (C6 and **C7**)
- Flexor carpi radialis (C6 and **C7**)
- Extensor carpi radialis longus (C6 and C7)
- Rhomboid major and minor (C4 and **C5**).

Motor deficits of an upper brachial plexus injury involve the C5 and C6 myotomes. Clinically, a patient would have motor deficits in abducting and laterally rotating his or her arm, flexing a forearm, and extending a wrist (Fig. 6-2 and Table 6-1). Sensory alterations would involve the C5 and C6 dermatomes. Consequently, the skin over the lateral arm, lateral forearm, and thumb would be involved (Fig. 6-2 and Table 6-1).

WITH SOME LESIONS OF THE BRACHIAL PLEXUS, A NERVE TRANSFER MAY SUCCESSFULLY RESTORE SOME FUNCTION TO THE UPPER EXTREMITY. WHICH NERVES ARE SUITABLE CANDIDATES FOR SURGICAL NERVE TRANSFERS?

Some of the common nerve transfer procedures are:

- Transfer the accessory nerve (CN XI) to the suprascapular nerve. This improves the function of the

Table 6-2 Ventral Primary Rami of C3-T1 and Their Muscular Distribution

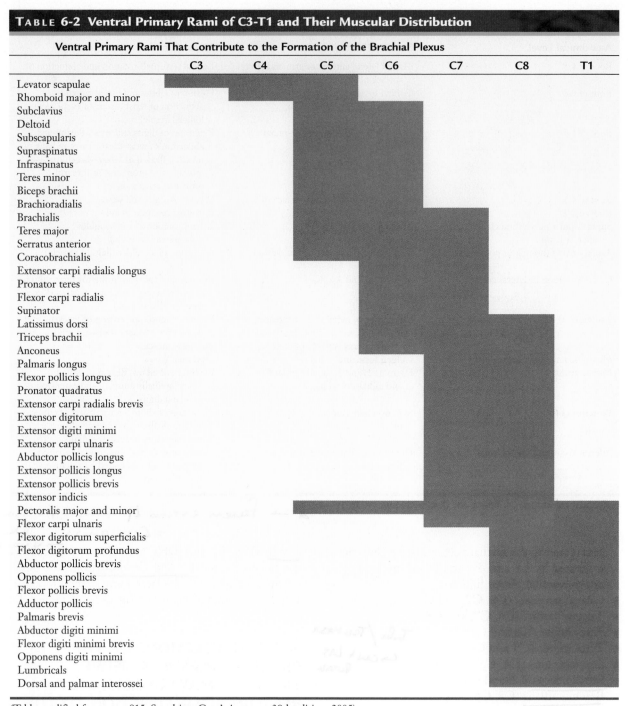

Ventral Primary Rami That Contribute to the Formation of the Brachial Plexus							
	C3	C4	C5	C6	C7	C8	T1
Levator scapulae	▓	▓	▓				
Rhomboid major and minor		▓	▓				
Subclavius			▓	▓			
Deltoid			▓	▓			
Subscapularis			▓	▓			
Supraspinatus			▓	▓			
Infraspinatus			▓	▓			
Teres minor			▓	▓			
Biceps brachii			▓	▓			
Brachioradialis			▓	▓			
Brachialis			▓	▓			
Teres major			▓	▓	▓		
Serratus anterior			▓	▓	▓		
Coracobrachialis			▓	▓	▓		
Extensor carpi radialis longus				▓	▓		
Pronator teres				▓	▓		
Flexor carpi radialis				▓	▓		
Supinator				▓	▓		
Latissimus dorsi				▓	▓	▓	
Triceps brachii				▓	▓	▓	
Anconeus				▓	▓	▓	
Palmaris longus					▓	▓	
Flexor pollicis longus					▓	▓	
Pronator quadratus					▓	▓	
Extensor carpi radialis brevis					▓	▓	
Extensor digitorum					▓	▓	
Extensor digiti minimi					▓	▓	
Extensor carpi ulnaris					▓	▓	
Abductor pollicis longus					▓	▓	
Extensor pollicis longus					▓	▓	
Extensor pollicis brevis					▓	▓	
Extensor indicis					▓	▓	
Pectoralis major and minor			▓	▓	▓	▓	▓
Flexor carpi ulnaris					▓	▓	▓
Flexor digitorum superficialis					▓	▓	▓
Flexor digitorum profundus					▓	▓	▓
Abductor pollicis brevis						▓	▓
Opponens pollicis						▓	▓
Flexor pollicis brevis						▓	▓
Adductor pollicis						▓	▓
Palmaris brevis						▓	▓
Abductor digiti minimi						▓	▓
Flexor digiti minimi brevis						▓	▓
Opponens digiti minimi						▓	▓
Lumbricals						▓	▓
Dorsal and palmar interossei						▓	▓

(Table modified from page 815, Standring, Gray's Anatomy, 39th edition, 2005)

supraspinatus and infraspinatus muscles. The accessory nerve also may be transferred to the axillary nerve.

● Transfer the third or fourth intercostal nerve to the musculocutaneous nerve. This improves the function of the biceps brachii, brachialis, and coracobrachialis muscles.

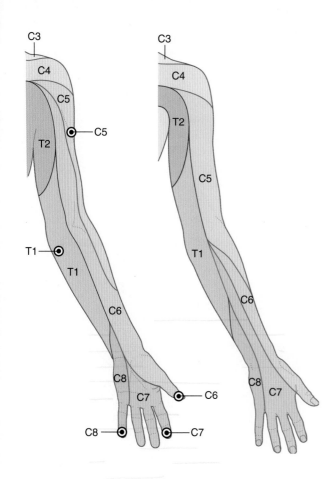

FIGURE 6–2 Dermatomes of the upper limb. (Drake R, Vogl W and Mitchell A: *Gray's Anatomy for Students*. Churchill Livingstone, 2004. Fig. 7-15.)

A 28-year-old woman presented to her physician with the chief complaint of altered sensibility of her lateral three and one-half digits. The patient was 7 months pregnant and worked as a data entry clerk. The patient stated that the symptoms began 4 days ago and become worse at night. Tinel's sign was noted on examination and nerve conduction studies showed prolonged conduction over the carpal tunnel. The patient was diagnosed with carpal tunnel syndrome. She was treated with an injection of corticosteroids into the carpal tunnel and was instructed to splint her wrist during sleep.

WHAT STRUCTURES FORM THE BOUNDARIES OF THE CARPAL TUNNEL?

The carpal tunnel (Fig. 6-3), an osseofibrous opening, is formed as follows: the proximal and distal rows of the carpal bones constitute the lateral and medial walls and the floor of the tunnel. The lateral wall is composed proximally of the triquetrum and pisiform and distally by the hamate. The hook of the hamate (hamulus) makes a minor contribution to the lateral roof of the carpal tunnel. The medial wall is formed proximally by the tubercle of the scaphoid and distally by the trapezium. The roof of the tunnel is principally formed by the fibrous flexor retinaculum. The retinaculum is attached laterally to the pisiform and hamulus and medially to the tubercle of the scaphoid and the trapezium.

WHAT STRUCTURES ARE TRANSMITTED THROUGH THE CARPAL TUNNEL?

The osseofibrous carpal tunnel transmits the tendons of the flexor digitorum superficialis, flexor digitorum profundus, and flexor pollicis longus muscles and the median nerve (Fig. 6-3).

WHAT ARE THE ATTACHMENTS, INNERVATION, AND ACTIONS OF THE MUSCLES THAT TRANSMIT THEIR TENDONS THROUGH THE CARPAL TUNNEL?

The muscles that transmit their tendons through the carpal tunnel are the long flexors of the digits. The muscles are described in Table 6-3.

BASED ON THE SENSORY AND MOTOR DISTRIBUTION OF THE MEDIAN NERVE, WHAT ARE THE EXPECTED NEUROLOGIC DEFICITS?

Since the lesion of the median nerve is located in the carpal tunnel, the sensory and motor deficits are observed in the hand. The sensory distribution is to the first three digits and the radial half of the fourth anteriorly and the dorsal skin over the proximal and distal phalanges of the same digits (Fig. 6-4). It also innervates the palm of the hand that corresponds to its digital distribution. Compression of the median nerve leads to a loss of sensation from the first three and one-half digits. The palmar skin is spared because it is innervated by a small nerve twig from the median nerve that courses outside of the carpal tunnel, anterior to the flexor retinaculum, to reach its destination.

The median nerve innervates five muscles in the hand. The muscles are described in Table 6-4.

WHAT IS TINEL'S SIGN?

Tinel's sign is observed when:

- Tapping the roof of the carpal tunnel causes paresthesias along the distribution of the median nerve.
- Prolonged flexion of the wrist elicits paresthesias.

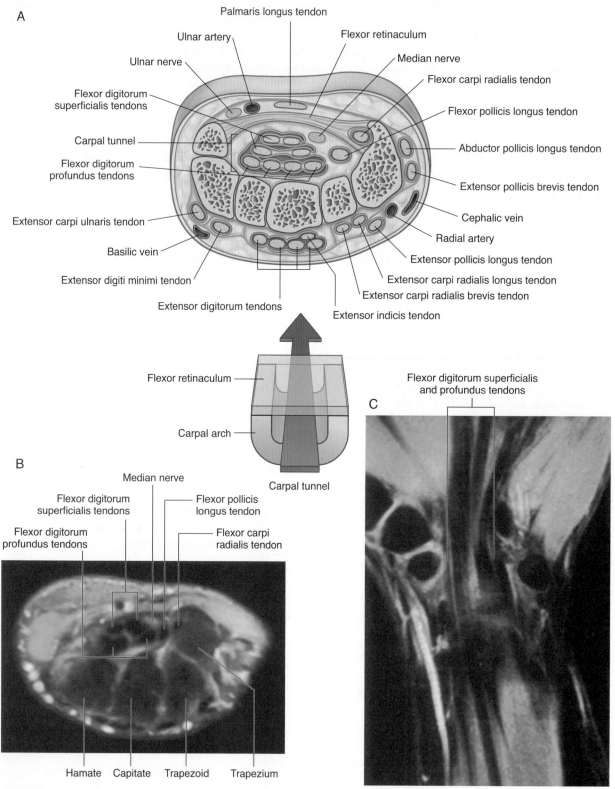

FIGURE 6–3 Carpal tunnel. **A,** Structures traversing the carpal tunnel. **B,** MRI of a normal wrist in the axial plane. (Drake R, Vogl W and Mitchell A: *Gray's Anatomy for Students.* Churchill Livingstone, 2004. Fig. 7-94.)

TABLE 6-3 Muscles That Transmit Their Tendons Through the Carpal Tunnel

Muscle	Origin	Insertion	Nerve Supply	Action
Flexor digitorum superficialis	Humeroulnar head: medial epicondyle of humerus, ulnar collateral ligament, and coronoid process of ulna. Radial head: proximal half of radius.	The tendons to digits 2 to 5 split and attach to the medial and lateral sides of the shafts of the corresponding middle phalanges	Median nerve (C8 and T1)	Flexes digits at the proximal interphalangeal joints and the metacarpo-phalangeal joints. Also flexes the hand.
Flexor digitorum profundus	Superior three-fourths of the ulna and interosseous membrane	Base of the distal phalanx of digits 2 to 5	Ulnar nerve (C8 and T1) to the medial part to digits 4 and 5 Median nerve (C8 and T1) to the lateral part to digits 2 and 3	Flexes distal interphalangeal joints
Flexor pollicis longus	Radius and interosseous membrane	Base of distal phalanx of pollex (thumb)	Anterior interosseous nerve (C7 and C8), a branch of the median nerve	Flexes thumb at interphalangeal and metacarpophalangeal joints

TABLE 6-4 Hand Muscles Innervated by the Median Nerve

Muscle	Origin	Insertion	Nerve Supply	Action
Abductor pollicis brevis	Flexor retinaculum, tubercle of scaphoid, and tubercle of trapezium	Radial side of the base of the proximal phalanx of thumb	Recurrent branch of median nerve (C8 and T1)	Abducts thumb at carpometacarpal joint and assists in opposition
Flexor pollicis brevis	Flexor retinaculum and tubercle of scaphoid	Radial side of the base of the proximal phalanx of thumb	Recurrent branch of median nerve (C8 and T1)	Flexes thumb at the carpometacarpal and metacarpophalangeal joints
Opponens pollicis	Flexor retinaculum and tubercle of scaphoid	Radial side of the first metacarpal bone	Recurrent branch of median nerve (C8 and T1)	Opposes thumb and medially rotates thumb
Lumbricals 1 and 2	Radial tendons of the flexor digitorum profundus	Radial sides of the extensor expansion of digits 2 and 3	Median nerve (C8 and T1)	Flexes digits 2 and 3 at the metacarpophalangeal joints and extends the interphalangeal joints of digits 2 and 3

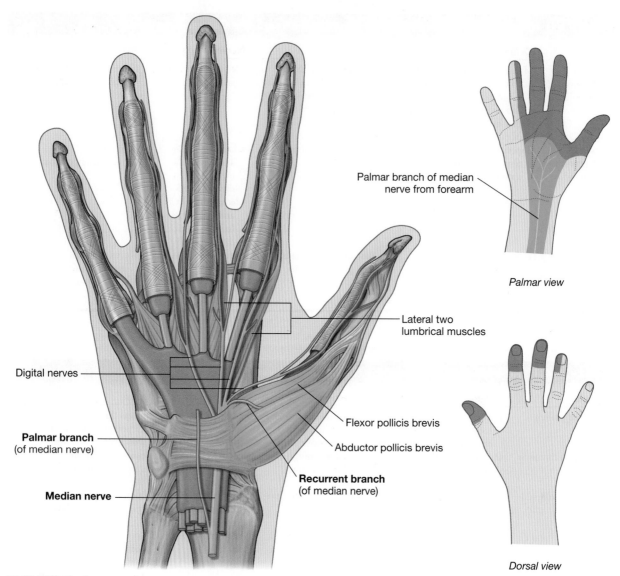

Palmar branch of median nerve from forearm

Palmar view

Lateral two lumbrical muscles

Digital nerves

Flexor pollicis brevis

Palmar branch (of median nerve)

Abductor pollicis brevis

Recurrent branch (of median nerve)

Median nerve

Dorsal view

FIGURE 6–4 Distribution of median nerve in the hand. (Drake R, Vogl W and Mitchell A: *Gray's Anatomy for Students*. Churchill Livingstone, 2004. Fig. 7-109.)

A 55-year-old man with diabetes mellitus presented with a complaint of contracture of his left fourth digit. He informs you that his father had the same condition many years ago. A nodule was discovered in the patient's palm during examination. The patient was diagnosed with Dupuytren's disease (contracture) and the deformity was surgically corrected.

WHAT STRUCTURE WAS THICKENED, RESULTING IN THE NODULE IN THE PATIENT'S PALM?

Dupuytren's contracture is the result of an abnormal fibrotic thickening of the palmar aponeurosis. The aponeurosis contracts as it thickens, causing flexion of the metacarpophalangeal joint and the proximal interphalangeal joint (Fig. 6-5).

The palmar aponeurosis is the deep fascia of the hand (Fig. 6-6). It is strong and triangular in appearance. Proximally, the apex of the aponeurosis attaches to the flexor retinaculum, and the tendon of the palmaris longus muscle splays into it. The distal base of the aponeurosis gives rise to four longitudinal bands that extend into the digits to attach to the bases of the proximal phalanges of digits two to five. The longitudinal bands also attach to the fibrous flexor tendinous sheaths and to the deep transverse metacarpal ligaments.

WHICH DIGITS ARE MORE SERIOUSLY FLEXED IN DUPUYTREN'S DISEASE?

Serious flexion deformities are usually limited to the fourth and fifth digits.

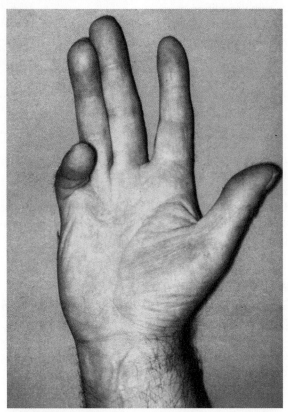

FIGURE 6–5   Dupuytren's contracture involving the fifth digit. A thickened band of the palmar aponeurosis is visible proximal to the flexed digit. (Dandy D and Edwards D: *Essential Orthopaedics and Trauma, 4e.* Churchill Livingstone, 2003. Fig. 23.19A.)

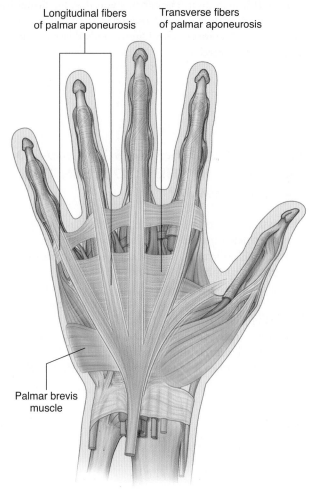

Longitudinal fibers of palmar aponeurosis

Transverse fibers of palmar aponeurosis

Palmar brevis muscle

FIGURE 6–6   Palmar aponeurosis. (Drake R, Vogl W and Mitchell A: *Gray's Anatomy for Students.* Churchill Livingstone, 2004. Fig. 7-95.)

A 55-year-old woman fell on an icy sidewalk. As she fell she caught herself with her outstretched right hand. As bystanders approached to assist, she complained of pain around her elbow joint. An ambulance was summoned to transport her to the emergency room where she was examined. Upon examination, there was swelling around the right elbow joint, and the forearm appeared shortened with a prominent olecranon. Neural assessment revealed a reduction in the strength of opposition of the right thumb and a reduction in sensation to the palmar surfaces of the lateral three and a half digits. Radiographs confirmed that the patient had suffered a dislocation of the elbow joint (Fig. 6-7). The dislocation was successfully reduced and the patient regained normal sensation and motor control of opposition.

WHAT LIGAMENTS ARE ASSOCIATED WITH THE ELBOW JOINT?

The elbow joint is classified as a hinge type of synovial joint. The joint is formed by two articulations (Fig. 6-8):

- Humeroulnar articulation occurs between the trochlea of the humerus and the trochlear notch of the ulna.
- Humeroradial articulation occurs between the capitulum of the humerus and the head of the radius.

The elbow joint is complicated by the presence of the proximal radioulnar articulation. This articulation occurs between the head of the radius and the radial notch of the ulna.

The elbow articulation is composed of three ligaments (Fig. 6-9):

- Articular capsule. The articular capsule is attached anteriorly to the humerus superior to the coronoid and radial fossae. Posteriorly, the capsule is attached just inferior to the olecranon fossa. Its distal attachments are to the lateral border of the trochlear notch, margin of the coronoid process, and anular ligament. The weakest parts of the capsule are its anterior and posterior parts, and it is strengthened laterally and medially by radial and ulnar collateral ligaments, respectively.
- Radial (lateral) collateral ligament. This strong, triangular-shaped ligament is proximally attached to the lateral epicondyle of the humerus and distally to the annular ligament, with some of its fibers blending with the attachments of the supinator and extensor carpi radialis brevis muscles.
- Ulnar (medial) collateral ligament. This triangle-shaped ligament is composed of three parts or bands:

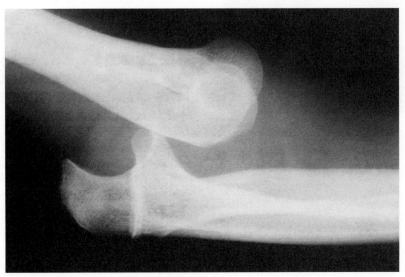

FIGURE 6–7 Posterior dislocation of the elbow. (Dandy D and Edwards D: *Essential Orthopaedics and Trauma, 4e*. Churchill Livingstone, 2003. Fig. 6.7B.)

A

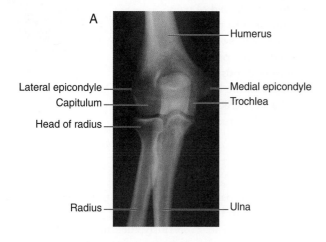

- Humerus
- Lateral epicondyle
- Capitulum
- Head of radius
- Medial epicondyle
- Trochlea
- Radius
- Ulna

B

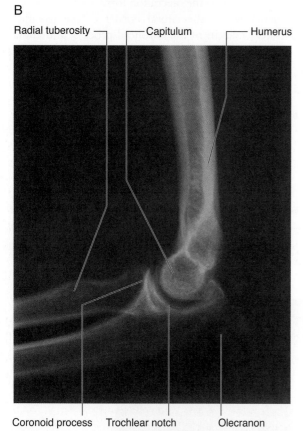

Radial tuberosity — Capitulum — Humerus

Coronoid process — Trochlear notch — Olecranon

FIGURE 6–8 **A**, Anteroposterior radiograph of the elbow. **B**, Lateral radiograph of the elbow. (Drake R, Vogl W and Mitchell A: *Gray's Anatomy for Students*. Churchill Livingstone, 2004. Fig. 7-61B & 7.62B.)

anterior, posterior, and oblique. Proximally, the anterior and posterior bands are attached to the medial epicondyle of the humerus. The anterior band has a distal attachment to the tubercle on the coronoid process of the ulna, whereas the posterior band fans out to attach to the medial margin of the

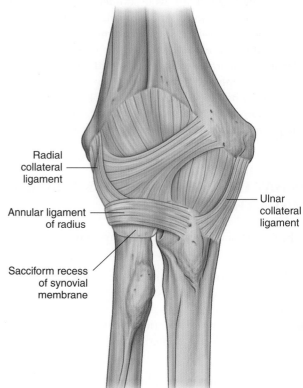

- Radial collateral ligament
- Annular ligament of radius
- Sacciform recess of synovial membrane
- Ulnar collateral ligament

FIGURE 6–9 Joint capsule and ligaments of the elbow joint (anterior view). (Drake R, Vogl W and Mitchell A: *Gray's Anatomy for Students*. Churchill Livingstone, 2004. Fig. 7-72.)

olecranon. The oblique band connects the anterior and posterior bands. The ulnar collateral ligament checks abduction at the elbow (i.e., limits valgus stress) and is commonly damaged in elbow injuries.

THE SYNOVIAL MEMBRANE LINES THE ARTICULAR CAPSULE. HOW IS THIS MEMBRANE DESCRIBED HISTOLOGICALLY?

The synovial membrane (Fig. 6-10) is composed of cellular and connective tissue elements. Because the membrane lacks a continuous epithelium, in contrast to membranes that line body cavities, some authorities prefer synovial layer. Two primary cell types are found in the synovial layer:

- Type A cells. These cells are macrophages and are responsible for phagocytosing tissue debris that results from the normal wear-and-tear of joint movements.

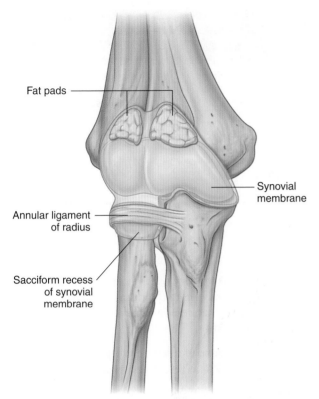

Fat pads

Synovial
membrane

Annular ligament
of radius

Sacciform recess
of synovial
membrane

FIGURE 6–10 Synovial membrane of the elbow joint and annular ligament of the radioulnar joint. (Drake R, Vogl W and Mitchell A: *Gray's Anatomy for Students*. Churchill Livingstone, 2004. Fig. 7-71.)

- Type B cells. These cells are similar to fibroblasts and synthesize and secrete the collagen and proteoglycans found in the synovial layer.

In addition to these two primary cell types, a few lymphocytes are present in the deeper layer of the synovium.

The synovial layer is highly vascular with a network of fenestrated capillaries. The fenestrated capillaries provide a functional filter to form the synovial fluid from plasma. This fluid is modified by type B cells that contribute hyaluronic acid and lubrican, substances with lubricating properties. The synovial fluid, which is constantly being produced, is drained by lymphatic capillaries.

HOW ARE DISLOCATIONS OF THE ELBOW JOINT CLASSIFIED?

Clinically, elbow dislocations are classified on the basis of movement of the ulna and radius relative to the humerus. Most frequently (more than 90%), elbow dislocations are classified as posterior. These dislocations occur when someone, such as an athlete, falls on his or her outstretched hand. The force is transmitted to the radius and ulna, driving the forearm bones posteriorly through the weak posterior portion of the fibrous capsule (Fig. 6-7).

BASED ON ANATOMICAL RELATIONSHIPS, WHAT ARE THE POTENTIAL COMPLICATIONS OF ELBOW DISLOCATIONS?

Possible complications of elbow dislocations are fractures and neurovascular compromise. Fractures may include the radial head or neck, coronoid process, and the medial or lateral epicondyles of the humerus. Neurovascular structures that may be injured are the brachial artery, median nerve, and the ulnar nerve. The median nerve also may be injured during a reduction.

BASED ON THE NEURAL ASSESSMENT IN THIS PATIENT, WHICH NERVE WAS INVOLVED?

The patient had difficulty opposing her right thumb and she had diminished sensation on the skin of the palmar surfaces of the lateral three and a half digits. Based on this assessment, the median nerve was entrapped.

WHAT IS THE ARTERIAL SUPPLY TO THE ELBOW JOINT?

An arterial anastomosis supplies the elbow joint. The anastomosis is formed by the:

- Superior ulnar collateral artery, a branch of the brachial artery
- Inferior ulnar collateral artery, which also springs from the brachial artery
- Radial collateral artery, a branch of the profunda brachii artery
- Anterior ulnar recurrent, a branch of the ulnar, joins the inferior ulnar collateral artery
- Posterior ulnar recurrent, a branch of the ulnar, joins the superior ulnar collateral artery
- Radial recurrent artery, issues from the radial artery, joins the radial collateral artery

WHAT IS THE NERVE SUPPLY TO THE ELBOW JOINT?

The following nerves supply articular branches to the elbow joint:

- Musculocutaneous nerve
- Radial nerve
- Median nerve
- Ulnar nerve
- Anterior interosseous nerve, a branch of the median nerve

Of the above nerves, the principal supply to the elbow joint is from the musculocutaneous and radial nerves.

WHAT SHOULD THE PHYSICIAN BE WARY OF IN ASSESSING RADIOGRAPHS FROM PEDIATRIC PATIENTS WITH ELBOW DISLOCATIONS?

In children, the physician must not confuse ossification centers with fractures. The elbow joint in children has six ossification centers. These ossification centers are the:

- Capitulum
- Radial head
- Internal (medial) epicondyle
- Trochlea
- Olecranon
- External (lateral) epicondyle

These six ossification centers can be remembered by the mnemonic CRITOE. The age of appearance of the secondary ossification centers is found in Table 6-5.

LONG BONES, SUCH AS THE HUMERUS, UNDERGO ENDOCHONDRAL OSSIFICATION. WHAT ARE THE STAGES OF ENDOCHONDRAL OSSIFICATION?

Endochondral bone formation occurs within a template of hyaline cartilage that is destined to develop into a bone. Ossification of the cartilaginous model of a long bone is initiated in a single primary center of ossification in the middle of the diaphysis followed by

TABLE 6-5 Age of Appearance of the Secondary Ossification Centers of the Elbow Joint

Ossification Center	Age (year) When Ossification Center Appears
Capitulum	1
Radial head	5
Internal (medial) epicondyle	5
Trochlea	11
Olecranon	12
External (lateral) epicondyle	13

two centers of secondary ossification; one in the proximal epiphysis and one in the distal epiphysis.

Five distinctive zones are observed in the secondary center of ossification. These are the:

- Zone of rest (zone of reserve cartilage). Chondrocytes in this zone, which resembles hyaline cartilage, are mitotically active.
- Zone of proliferation. Proliferating chondrocytes align themselves along the parallel axis of bone growth. The chondrocytes are found in isogenous groups.
- Zone of hypertrophy. Chondrocytes mature and hypertrophy. Hypertrophy of the chondrocytes leads to enlargement of their lacunae, which erodes the matrix that separates them.
- Zone of calcification. Death of hypertrophied chondrocytes causes the thin matrix separating the lacunae to degrade. As a result, two or more smaller lacunae merge to form one larger lacuna. The cartilaginous matrix that remains is calcified.
- Zone of ossification. Osteoprogenitor cells migrate into the region and morph into osteoblasts. The osteoblasts deposit organic matrix on the calcified remnants of cartilage. The organic matrix then becomes calcified, forming bone tissue.

WHAT STRUCTURE WAS MOST LIKELY FRACTURED?

Forceful anterior displacement of the humerus causes it to slide over the coronoid process of the ulna (Fig. 6-7). This forceful displacement may result in a fracture of the coronoid process.

A 12-year-old girl fell off her bicycle and landed on her right arm. She ran into the house in obvious pain and found her mother, who drove her to the nearby medical clinic. The physician noticed that the right arm was shortened and swollen. Neurovascular function remained intact. Radiographs revealed a fracture of the midshaft of the humerus. The patient was treated by immobilizing her arm in a cast.

WHAT NEUROVASCULAR STRUCTURES ARE VULNERABLE TO INJURY IN A MIDSHAFT FRACTURE OF THE HUMERUS?

Fractures of the humerus produce bony spike fragments that may be injurious to surrounding tissue. In the midshaft region, these fragments may involve the radial nerve and/or vessels of the profunda brachii as they travel in the radial groove located on the posterior surface of the humerus (Fig. 6-11). The incidence of radial nerve injury secondary to a humeral shaft fracture is 16%.

WHAT MUSCLES ARE INNERVATED BY THE RADIAL NERVE AND WHAT ARE THEIR ATTACHMENTS AND ACTIONS?

The muscles innervated by the radial nerve are located in the posterior (extensor) compartments of the arm and forearm. The muscles of the posterior compartment of the arm and their attachments, innervation, and actions are described in Table 6-6.

The superficial muscles of the posterior compartment of the forearm and their attachments, innervation, and actions are described in Table 6-7.

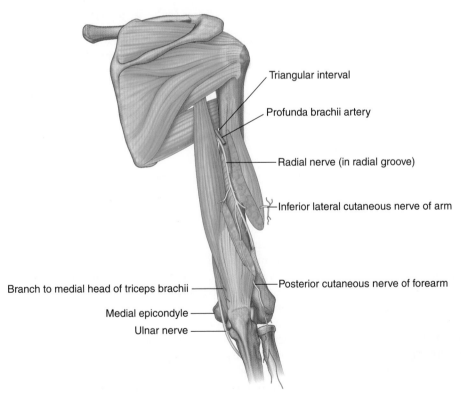

Triangular interval

Profunda brachii artery

Radial nerve (in radial groove)

Inferior lateral cutaneous nerve of arm

Branch to medial head of triceps brachii

Posterior cutaneous nerve of forearm

Medial epicondyle

Ulnar nerve

FIGURE 6–11 Radial nerve in the arm. (Drake R, Vogl W and Mitchell A: *Gray's Anatomy for Students.* Churchill Livingstone, 2004. Fig. 7-68.)

TABLE 6-6 Muscles of the Posterior Compartment of the Arm

Muscle	Origin	Insertion	Nerve Supply	Action
Triceps brachii	Long head: infraglenoid tubercle of scapula Lateral head: proximal to radial groove of humerus Medial head: distal to radial groove of humeral shaft	Upper surface of olecranon	Radial nerve (C6, C7, and C8)	Medial head is active in all forms of extension of forearm. Lateral and long heads are active in extension against resistance.
Articularis cubiti	Distal to radial groove. Fibers blend with deep fibers of medial head of triceps	Cubital capsule	Radial nerve (C6, C7, and C8)	Pulls cubital capsule superior during extension of the elbow

TABLE 6-7 Superficial Muscles of the Posterior Forearm

Muscle	Origin	Insertion	Nerve Supply	Action
Brachioradialis	Proximal two-thirds of supracondylar ridge of humerus	Distal end of radius proximal to its styloid process	Radial nerve (C5 and C6)	Flexes elbow
Extensor carpi radialis longus	Distal third of lateral supracondylar ridge of humerus	Base of second metacarpal bone	Radial nerve (C6 and C7)	Extends and abducts hand at wrist
Extensor carpi radialis brevis	Lateral epicondyle of humerus	Base of third metacarpal bone	Deep branch of radial nerve (C7 and C8)	Extends and abducts hand at wrist
Extensor digitorum	Lateral epicondyle of humerus	Dorsal expansions of digits 2 to 5	Posterior interosseous branch of radial nerve (C7 and C8)	Extends digits 2 to 5 at interphalangeal and metacarpophalangeal joints
Extensor digiti minimi	Lateral epicondyle of humerus	Extensor expansion of digit 5	Posterior interosseous branch of radial nerve (C7 and C8)	Extends digit 5 at interphalangeal and metacarpophalangeal joints
Extensor carpi ulnaris	Lateral epicondyle of humerus and ulna	Base of fifth metacarpal bone	Posterior interosseous branch of radial nerve (C7 and C8)	Extends and adducts hand at the wrist
Anconeus	Lateral epicondyle of humerus	Lateral surface of olecranon and ulna	Radial nerve (C6, C7, and C8)	Extends and stabilizes elbow joint; abducts ulna during pronation

The deep muscles of the posterior compartment of the forearm and their attachments, innervation, and actions are described in Table 6-8.

WHAT EVENTS ACCOMPANY HEALING OF BONE FRACTURES?

There are four stages of bone healing after a fracture: inflammation, soft callus formation, hard callus formation, and remodeling.

● Inflammation is characterized by hemorrhage, thrombus formation, edema, and pain. The inflammatory response involves mast cells, neutrophils, and macrophages, which secrete cytokines that regulate the reparative process. Macrophages and osteoclasts are activated to cleanse necrotic bone and debris from the site of injury and to prepare the bone tissue for healing.

● Soft callus formation overlaps inflammation and is nearly a month-long process. The soft callus is composed of collagen, glycoproteins, fibroblasts, and preosteoblasts. The soft callus is well vascularized.

TABLE 6-8 Deep Muscles of the Posterior Forearm

Muscle	Origin	Insertion	Nerve Supply	Action
Supinator	Lateral epicondyle of humerus, radial collateral ligament, annular ligament, supinator crest and fossa of ulna	Lateral surface of proximal third of radius	Deep branch of the radial nerve (C6 and C7)	Supinates forearm
Abductor pollicis longus	Posterior ulnar surface and interosseous membrane	Base of first metacarpal bone	Posterior interosseous nerve, the terminal branch of the deep radial nerve (C7 and C8)	Abducts thumb and extends it at metacarpophalangeal joint
Extensor pollicis brevis	Posterior surface of radius and interosseous membrane	Base of proximal phalanx of thumb	Posterior interosseous nerve, the terminal branch of the deep radial nerve (C7 and C8)	Extends thumb at proximal phalanx and first metacarpal bone
Extensor pollicis longus	Middle third of posterior ulnar surface and interosseous membrane	Base of distal phalanx of thumb	Posterior interosseous nerve, the terminal branch of the deep radial nerve (C7 and C8)	Extends thumb at interphalangeal and metacarpophalangeal joints
Extensor indicis	Posterior surface of ulna	Extensor expansion of second digit	Posterior interosseous nerve, the terminal branch of the deep radial nerve (C7 and C8)	Extension of index finger and wrist

Chondroblasts and cartilage contribute to callus formation. The soft callus begins to stabilize the bone fracture.

● A hard callus is formed when the soft callus is replaced with woven bone. Endochondral and intramembranous ossification processes are involved in forming a hard callus.

● Remodeling involves the degradation of the woven bone followed by the formation of lamellar bone. The thickened periosteal bone collar is gradually thinned to normal by osteoclastic activity and the medullary cavity is restored. Remodeling is a lengthy process and until it is complete, the bone has not been restored to its full functional state.

A 34-year-old man who was painting ceilings with a brush for 3 days presented to his physician with the chief complaint of shoulder pain. The pain started 2 days ago and is worse at night and when he lifts his arm over his head. The examination showed that the patient's pain was greater with active abduction of the arm against resistance. An impingement sign was noted with passive flexion of the humerus. The patient's passive range of motion was normal. The patient was diagnosed with tendinitis of the supraspinatus tendon and was instructed to rest and take nonsteroidal anti-inflammatory drugs for the pain.

WHAT MUSCLES CONSTITUTE THE ROTATOR CUFF MUSCLE GROUP?

Four muscles form the rotator muscle group. The muscles and their attachments, nerve supply, and actions are described in Table 6-9 and are shown in Figure 6-12.

In addition to the actions described in the table above, the rotator cuff muscles also function to hold the head of the humerus in the glenoid cavity.

WHAT ARE THE OTHER TWO MUSCLES OF THE SCAPULAR REGION?

The deltoid and the teres major are the other two muscles of the scapular region. Their attachments, nerve supply, and actions are described in Table 6-10.

WHICH TENDON OF THE ROTATOR CUFF GROUP MOST COMMONLY RUPTURES?

The supraspinatus tendon is most commonly ruptured proximate to its insertion. It is postulated that the tendon has an inadequate blood supply and, as a result, degenerates over time. Because the tendon blends with the fibrous articular capsule, the capsule is frequently involved.

TABLE 6-9 Muscles of the Rotator Cuff				
Muscle	Origin	Insertion	Nerve Supply	Action
Supraspinatus	Supraspinous fossa of scapula	Superior facet of greater tubercle of humerus	Suprascapular nerve (C5 and C6)	Initiate abduction of humerus and prevent inferior displacement of the adducted humerus when carrying a heavy weight
Infraspinatus	Infraspinous fossa of scapula	Middle facet of greater tubercle of humerus	Suprascapular nerve (C5 and C6)	Lateral rotation of humerus
Teres minor	Superior portion of lateral border of scapula	Inferior facet of greater tubercle of humerus	Axillary nerve (C5 and C6)	Lateral rotation of humerus and assists in its adduction
Subscapularis	Subscapular fossa of scapula	Lesser tubercle of humerus	Upper and lower subscapular nerves (C5 and C6)	Medial rotation and adduction of humerus

TABLE 6-10 Deltoid and Teres Major Muscles

Muscle	Origin	Insertion	Nerve Supply	Action
Deltoid	Anterior fibers: lateral third of clavicle Middle fibers: acromion Posterior fibers: spine of scapula	Deltoid tuberosity of humerus	Axillary nerve (C5 and C6)	Anterior fibers: flex and medially rotate humerus Middle fibers: abduct humerus Posterior fibers: extend and laterally rotate arm
Teres major	Posterior surface of inferior angle of scapula	Medial crest of intertubercular sulcus of humerus	Lower subscapular nerve (C5, C6, and C7)	Adduct and medially rotate humerus

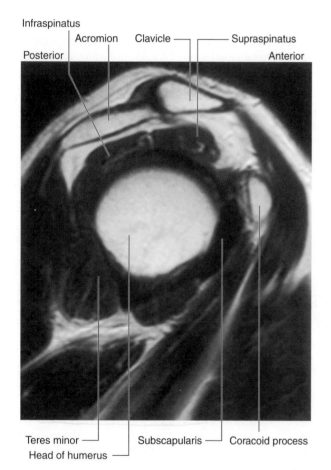

FIGURE 6–12 MRI of a normal shoulder joint. (Drake R, Vogl W and Mitchell A: *Gray's Anatomy for Students.* Churchill Livingstone, 2004. Fig. 7-29.)

During a college football game, the 21-year-old right-handed quarterback preparing to pass the football was tackled from behind by the opposing linebacker. As he was tackled, the quarterback's abducted left arm was driven into the turf. After the tackle, the quarterback was in excruciating pain and was unable to move his left arm at the shoulder joint. He was transported to the affiliated University Medical Center for medical care. During his physical examination, the physician noted that the patient's left arm was slightly abducted and was laterally (externally) rotated and the range of motion was limited. The doctor also was able to palpate the left humeral head. A neurologic examination revealed paralysis of the deltoid muscle and a loss of skin sensation over the central area of the deltoid. A series of radiographs confirmed the diagnosis of dislocation of the glenohumeral joint (Fig. 6-13) and a MRI study showed a Bankart's lesion. The dislocation was reduced and the Bankart's lesion was surgically repaired.

BESIDES THE DELTOID, TERES MAJOR, AND ROTATOR CUFF MUSCLES, WHAT OTHER MUSCLES ACT ACROSS THE SHOULDER JOINT?

The additional muscles and their attachments, innervation, and actions that act across the shoulder joint are described in Table 6-11.

WHAT ARE THE FUNCTIONAL AND ANATOMICAL CLASSIFICATIONS OF THE GLENOHUMERAL JOINT?

The glenohumeral joint permits a wide range of movement so it is functionally classified as a diarthrosis. Anatomically, it is a ball-and-socket type of synovial joint. The shallow socket of the joint is deepened by the presence of a ring of fibrocartilage called the *glenoid labrum*.

A
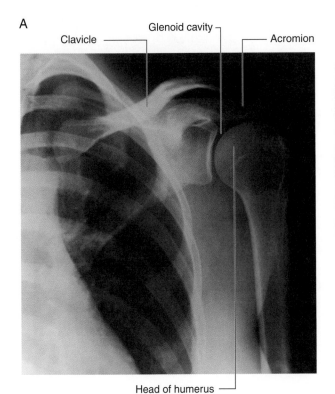
Clavicle — Glenoid cavity — Acromion

Head of humerus —

B
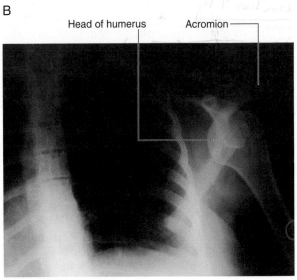
Head of humerus — Acromion —

FIGURE 6–13 A, Radiograph of a normal shoulder joint. **B**, Radiograph showing an anterior dislocation of the shoulder joint. (Drake R, Vogl W and Mitchell A: *Gray's Anatomy for Students.* Churchill Livingstone, 2004. Fig. 7-52B & 7.31.)

Table 6-11 Muscles Acting Across the Shoulder Joint

Muscle	Origin	Insertion	Nerve Supply	Action
Pectoralis major	Clavicular head: medial half of clavicle Sternocostal head: sternum, first six costal cartilages, and aponeurosis of external abdominal oblique	Lateral crest of intertubercular groove of humerus	Lateral and medial pectoral nerves: clavicular head is C5 and C6 and sternocostal head is C6, C7, C8, and T1.	Adducts and medially rotates humerus, clavicular head flexes humerus, sternocostal head extends humerus, protracts scapula and pulls it inferiorly
Biceps brachii	Long head: supraglenoid tubercle of scapula Short head: coracoid process of scapula	Radial tuberosity of radius and bicipital aponeurosis	Musculocutaneous nerve (C5 and C6)	Supinates forearm, flexes forearm, and flexes humerus
Coracobrachialis	Coracoid process of scapula	Middle third of humerus	Musculocutaneous (C5, C6, and C7)	Flexes and adducts arm
Triceps brachii	Previously described in Table 6-6			
Latissimus dorsi	Spinous processes of thoracic vertebrae 7-12, inferior 3 or 4 ribs, iliac crest, and thoracolumbar fascia	Floor of intertubercular groove of humerus	Thoracodorsal (C6, C7, and C8)	Adducts, extends, and medially rotates humerus; pulls body towards humerus when humerus is fixed

The fibrous capsule of the joint extends from the margin of the glenoid cavity to the anatomical neck of the humerus. The joint is reinforced anteriorly and superiorly by intrinsic ligaments and anteriorly, superiorly, and posteriorly by the rotator cuff muscles. Because the inferior portion of the fibrous capsule is not strengthened, this represents its weakest point.

The intrinsic ligaments of the joint are the (Fig. 6-14):

- Three glenohumeral ligaments
- Coracohumeral ligament. This ligament attaches to the base of the coracoid process of the scapula and to the anatomical neck of the humerus near the greater tubercle. The ligament reinforces the superior part of the fibrous articular capsule.
- Transverse humeral ligament. This ligament attaches to the lesser tubercle of the humerus, bridges the intertubercular groove, and attaches to the greater tubercle. The ligament secures the tendon of the long head of the biceps brachii muscle as it travels in the intertubercular groove to attach to the supraglenoid tubercle of the scapula.

HOW CAN LIGAMENTS BE DESCRIBED HISTOLOGICALLY?

Ligaments are examples of dense regular collagenous connective tissue (Fig. 6-15). Ligaments are composed

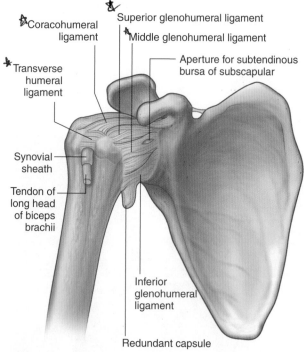

FIGURE 6–14 Capsule of the shoulder joint. (Drake R, Vogl W and Mitchell A: *Gray's Anatomy for Students*. Churchill Livingstone, 2004. Fig. 7-27.)

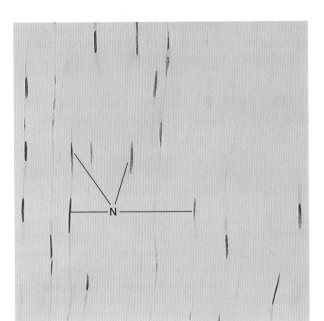

FIGURE 6–15 Micrograph of dense collagenous connective tissue that typifies ligaments. (Gartner L and Hiatt J: *Color Textbook of Histology*, 2e. WB Saunders, 2001. Fig. 6-18.)

of closely packed, acidophilic, type I collagen fibers arrayed parallel to one another. Located between the collagen fibers are fibroblasts and extracellular matrix. The extracellular matrix contains proteoglycans, glycoproteins, water, and a few elastic fibers.

WHAT ARE THE CYTOLOGIC FEATURES OF AN ACTIVE FIBROBLAST?

The active fibroblast possesses the following cytologic attributes:

- Branched cytoplasmic processes
- Oval, euchromatic nucleus with a prominent nucleolus
- Well endowed with rough endoplasmic reticulum. This imparts a basophilic characteristic to the cytoplasm with staining.
- Well-developed Golgi apparatus
- Most of the mitochondria are located around the nucleus.
- Actin microfilaments are numerous in the cytoplasm next to the plasmalemma. Alpha-actinin accompanies the actin microfilaments.

- Microtubules extend out from the pair of centrioles in the centrosome to maintain cell shape.
- Myosin is found throughout the cytoplasm.

WHAT ARE THE STEPS INVOLVED IN THE SYNTHESIS OF TYPE I COLLAGEN?

There are eight steps involved in the synthesis of type I collagen. These steps are:

- Transcription of mRNA in the nucleus
- Translation of mRNA to preprocollagen in the rough endoplasmic reticulum
- Hydroxylation of preprocollagen in the rough endoplasmic reticulum
- Glycosylation of preprocollagen in the rough endoplasmic reticulum
- Three preprocollagen molecules form a triple helix of procollagen in the rough endoplasmic reticulum.
- Procollagen is transported to the Golgi complex, packaged into secretory vesicles, and secreted.
- In the extracellular milieu, the procollagen molecules are cleaved by collagen peptidases to form tropocollagen molecules.
- Tropocollagen molecules self-assemble to from collagen fibrils.

WHAT NERVES INNERVATE THE GLENOHUMERAL JOINT?

Innervation of the glenohumeral (shoulder) joint complies with the Law of Hilton, which states that a joint is innervated by the same nerves that supply the muscles that move the joint and the skin covering the joint. Thus, the nerve supply to the shoulder joint is from the: → Getsinjued nhotrimus Drpsinkeere

- Axillary nerve—deltoid and teres major muscles
- Suprascapular nerve—supraspinatus and infraspinatus muscles
- Lateral pectoral nerve—pectoralis major muscle
- Independent branches from the posterior cord of the brachial plexus—the posterior cord also issues separate branches (i.e., thoracodorsal, upper and lower subscapular, and radial nerves) that innervate muscles (latissimus dorsi, subscapularis, teres minor, and triceps brachii) that move the shoulder joint.

Of these nerves, the axillary and suprascapular nerves are the principal supply to the joint.

→ RADIAL N. CAN ALSO BE STRETCHED

WHAT ARTERIES SUPPLY THE SHOULDER JOINT?

The arteries that supply the joint have *circumflex* and/or *scapular* as part of their name. These vessels are the:

- Anterior and posterior humeral circumflex arteries, branches of the axillary artery
- Suprascapular artery, a branch of the thyrocervical trunk that springs from the subclavian artery
- Circumflex scapular artery, a branch of the subscapular artery that issues from the axillary artery

DISLOCATIONS OF THE GLENOHUMERAL JOINT MOST COMMONLY OCCUR IN WHAT DIRECTION?

Clinically, most glenohumeral dislocations occur anteriorly. An anterior dislocation results when the arm is forcefully abducted and laterally (externally) rotated. The forced abduction drives the humeral head through the inferior capsule, its weakest part. Lateral rotation of the humerus causes its head to move ante-riorly. These movements result in the head of the humerus lying anterior to the infraglenoid tubercle and inferior to the glenoid cavity.

WHAT NERVES ARE VULNERABLE TO INJURY WITH A DISLOCATION OF THE SHOULDER JOINT?

The axillary and radial nerves may be injured with a dislocated shoulder joint. The axillary nerve is transmitted through the quadrangular space inferior to the articular capsule. Consequently, anteroinferior displacement of the humeral head may injure the axillary nerve. The radial nerve is vulnerable for a different reason. Inferior movement of the humerus lengthens the distance from the point of the shoulder to the elbow. This lengthening results in stretching of the radial nerve.

WHAT IS A BANKART'S LESION?

A Bankart's lesion is a tear of the fibrocartilaginous glenoid labrum. The torn labrum can be surgically reattached.

[handwritten note in box] ANT. DISLOCATION of the shoulder Jun

[handwritten notes at bottom left]

Factors that ↑ lig. strength

1. Diameter (↑D = ↑strength)
2. Collagen Cross links (All normal lys have stable crosslinks)
3. Elastic fibers
   ↳ all injured lys have unstable cross-links

A 17-year-old high school hockey player was violently checked into the boards during a game. The force of the impact was borne by the player's right acromion. The player was in severe pain from the impact and complained of restricted movement at the right shoulder. He was transported to the local medical center and the physical examination showed a prominent right clavicle and inferior displacement of the right acromion. The inferior displacement of the acromion was more pronounced when the patient held a 15-lb weight in his right hand. Subsequent imaging studies confirmed the diagnosis of separation of the right acromioclavicular (AC) joint (Fig. 6-16). The separation was surgically repaired.

ANATOMICALLY DESCRIBE THE AC JOINT.

The AC joint is a plane type of synovial joint formed by the acromial end of the clavicle and the medial surface of the acromion (Fig. 6-17). Fibrocartilage covers the articular surfaces, which are separated by a small articular disc that is cuneiform in appearance. The joint is enclosed by a fibrous capsule and strengthened by a superior band of fibrous connective tissue, the AC ligament. Because these ligaments are relatively weak, the joint is stabilized by stronger extrinsic ligaments known as *conoid* and *trapezoid* ligaments. Collectively, these ligaments form the coracoclavicular ligament (Fig. 6-17).

WHAT LIGAMENTS WERE TORN IN THIS SEPARATION OF THE AC JOINT?

The fibrous capsule and the conoid and trapezoid components of the coracoclavicular ligament were torn. Tearing of these ligaments frees the acromion and coracoid process from the clavicle, allowing for the inferior displacement of the upper extremity (Fig. 6-16).

WHAT IS THE NERVE SUPPLY TO THE AC JOINT?

The nerve supply to the AC joint is from the:

- Suprascapular nerve (C5-C6)
- Lateral pectoral nerve (C5-C7), a branch of the medial cord of the brachial plexus

WHAT IS THE ARTERIAL SUPPLY TO THE AC JOINT?

Branches of the suprascapular and thoracoacromial arteries supply the AC joint. The suprascapular artery takes its origin from the thyrocervical trunk, a branch of the subclavian artery. The thoracoacromial trunk is the first branch from the second part of the axillary artery.

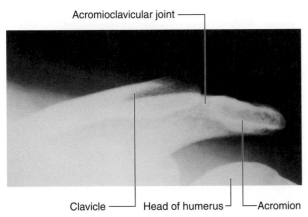

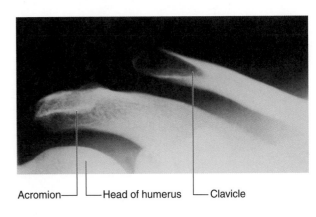

FIGURE 6–16 Radiographs of the acromioclavicular joints. **A**, Normal joint. **B**, Dislocated joint. (Drake R, Vogl W and Mitchell A: *Gray's Anatomy for Students*. Churchill Livingstone, 2004. Fig. 7-30.)

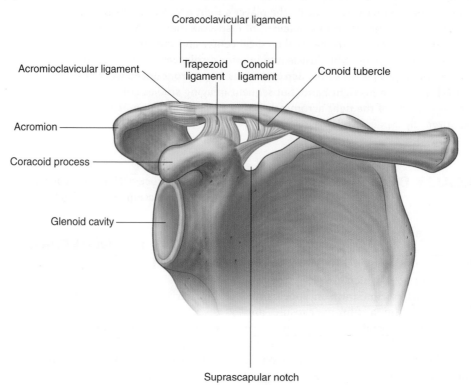

FIGURE 6–17 Ligaments of the acromioclavicular joint. (Drake R, Vogl W and Mitchell A: *Gray's Anatomy for Students.* Churchill Livingstone, 2004. Fig. 7-24.)

A 55-year-old man presented to his physician with complaints of numbness in his right dominant hand and clumsiness of finger movements. As a child, he had suffered a supracondylar fracture of his right humerus. Healing of the fracture resulted in cubitus valgus. The physical examination detected a modest degree of wasting of the intrinsic hand muscles and a sensory deficit of the skin supplied by the ulnar nerve. The diagnosis was ulnar nerve compression at the elbow. Surgery was performed to move the ulnar nerve to a safer location anterior to the medial epicondyle.

WHAT IS CUBITUS VALGUS AND HOW DOES IT CONTRIBUTE TO ULNAR NERVE COMPRESSION?

Valgus means *bent outwards* or *away from the body*. When the normal elbow is fully extended, the forearm is not in a straight line with the humerus, but is slightly abducted away from the midline. Therefore, the forearm normally exhibits a minimal amount of valgus. In men, this deviation is approximately 10 degrees and, in women, it is about 15 degrees. When this angulation becomes excessive, the condition is known as *cubitus valgus*.

Healing of supracondylar fractures of the humerus can lead to cubitus valgus. Because of the exaggerated angulation of the forearm, the ulnar nerve is pulled more sharply as it travels in the osseofibrous tunnel between the olecranon and the medial epicondyle (Fig. 6-18). This subjects the ulnar nerve to greater frictional forces, which can lead to friction neuritis of the nerve. In turn, the inflammation causes fibrosis and nerve thickening within the confined osseofibrous tunnel.

WHERE ELSE CAN THE ULNAR NERVE BECOME COMPRESSED?

The ulnar nerve also can be compressed, albeit less frequently, as it passes between the two heads of the flexor carpi ulnaris as it enters the forearm and in Guyon's canal. Guyon's canal is an osseofibrous canal formed by three carpal bones: triquetrum, pisiform, and hamate. The fibrous component is a ligament that attaches to the pisiform and the hamulus of the hamate. Because of its attachments, the ligament is called the pisohamate ligament. Compression of the ulnar nerve in Guyon's canal results in a motor neuropathy as sensory innervation is preserved. Sensory innervation remains intact because the sensory branch of the ulnar nerve to the hand passes outside of Guyon's canal.

WHAT IS THE MOTOR DISTRIBUTION OF THE ULNAR NERVE?

The principal motor distribution of the ulnar nerve is to the hand with additional distribution to the anterior compartment of the forearm. The muscles of the anterior compartment of the forearm innervated by the ulnar nerve, their attachments, and actions are summarized in Table 6-12.

The muscles of the hand innervated by the ulnar nerve, their attachments, and actions are summarized in Table 6-13.

WHAT HAPPENS TO THE HAND IF THE ULNAR NERVE IS SEVERELY DAMAGED?

The intrinsic muscles of the hand undergo wasting due to the loss of their nerve supply. As the muscles waste, they shorten, which can cause digits four and five, and sometimes digit three to assume a clawhand (main-en-griffe; French for *clawhand*) position.

WHAT IS THE SENSORY DISTRIBUTION OF THE ULNAR NERVE?

The sensory distribution of the ulnar nerve is to the wrist and hand (Fig. 6-19). Specifically, it supplies the ulnar one and one-half digits (anterior and dorsal surfaces) and the corresponding palm and anterior wrist and the corresponding dorsum of the hand and wrist.

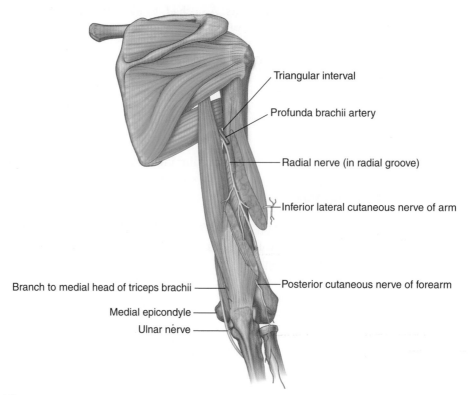

FIGURE 6–18   Ulnar nerve and its relationship to the elbow. (Drake R, Vogl W and Mitchell A: *Gray's Anatomy for Students*. Churchill Livingstone, 2004. Fig. 7-68.)

TABLE 6-12 Muscles of the Anterior Forearm Innervated by the Ulnar Nerve				
Muscle	**Origin**	**Insertion**	**Nerve Supply**	**Action**
Flexor carpi ulnaris	Humeral head: medial epicondyle of humerus Ulnar head: olecranon and posterior surface of ulna	Pisiform bone, hamulus of hamate bone, and 5th metacarpal bone	Ulnar nerve (C7, C8 and T1)	Flexes the hand and adducts the hand
Flexor digitorum profundus	Medial and anterior surfaces of ulna and interosseous membrane	Bases of distal phalanges of digits 2, 3, 4, and 5.	Ulnar nerve (C8 and T1) innervates portion of profundus that inserts on digits 4 and 5	Flexes digits at the distal interphalangeal joint and assists in flexing the wrist

TABLE 6-13 Muscles of the Hand Innervated by the Ulnar Nerve

Muscle	Origin	Insertion	Nerve Supply	Action
Adductor pollicis	Oblique head: capitate bone and 2nd and 3rd metacarpal bones Transverse head: anterior surface of the 3rd metacarpal bone	Base of proximal phalanx	Deep branch of ulnar nerve (C8 and T1)	Adducts thumb
Abductor digiti minimi (quinti)	Pisiform bone and pisohamate ligament	Ulnar side of base of proximal phalanx of 5th digit	Deep branch of ulnar nerve (C8 and T1)	Abducts the little finger
Flexor digiti minimi brevis	Hamulus of hamate bone and flexor retinaculum	Ulnar side of base of proximal phalanx of 5th digit	Deep branch of ulnar nerve (C8 and T1)	Flexes proximal phalanx of 5th digit
Opponens digiti minimi	Hamulus of hamate bone and flexor retinaculum	Ulnar and anterior surfaces of the 5th metacarpal bone	Deep branch of ulnar nerve (C8 and T1)	Flexes and laterally rotates 5th digit, opposing it to the thumb
Lumbricals 3 and 4	Ulnar three tendons of the flexor digitorum profundus muscles	Radial sides of the extensor expansions of digits 4 and 5	Deep branch of ulnar nerve (C8 and T1)	Flexes digits at the metacarpophalangeal joints and extends the digits at the interphalangeal joints
Dorsal interossei (4 in number)	Adjacent sides of metacarpal bones	Extensor expansions and bases of proximal phalanges of digits 2, 3, and 4	Deep branch of ulnar nerve (C8 and T1)	Abduct digits 2-4, flexes digits 2-4 at metacarpophalangeal joints, and extends digits 2-4
Palmar interossei (3 in number)	1st palmar interosseous arises from ulnar side of 2nd metacarpal, 2nd and 3rd palmar interossei arise from radial sides of metacarpal bones 4 and 5, respectively	Extensor expansions and bases of proximal phalanges of digits 2, 4, and 5	Deep branch of ulnar nerve (C8 and T1)	Adducts digits 2, 4, and 5, flexes same digits at metacarpophalangeal joints, and extends same digits
Palmaris brevis	Flexor retinaculum	Dermis of ulnar aspect of anterior hand	Superficial branch of ulnar nerve (C8 and T1)	Wrinkles skin and may contribute to grip

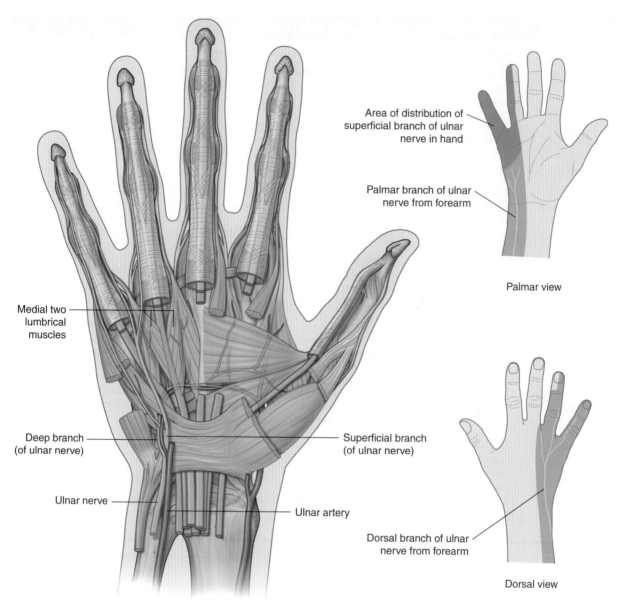

Area of distribution of
superficial branch of ulnar
nerve in hand

Palmar branch of ulnar
nerve from forearm

Palmar view

Medial two
lumbrical
muscles

Deep branch
(of ulnar nerve)

Superficial branch
(of ulnar nerve)

Ulnar nerve

Ulnar artery

Dorsal branch of ulnar
nerve from forearm

Dorsal view

FIGURE 6–19 Distribution of ulnar nerve in the hand. (Drake R, Vogl W and Mitchell A: *Gray's Anatomy for Students*. Churchill Livingstone, 2004. Fig. 7-108)

SECTION VII

Head and Neck

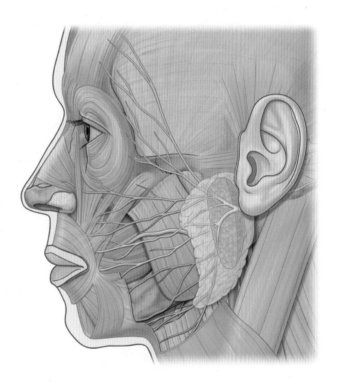

A 68-year-old woman accompanied by her 40-year-old daughter appeared in your office. The daughter was concerned about her mother's mental condition. She said her mother was experiencing difficulty learning new information and was forgetting recent events. The daughter also said her mother had recently gotten lost driving to her house. When the physician asked if anyone else in the family ever had these symptoms, the mother responded with verbal hesitancy that her father had Alzheimer's disease. An MRI study of the brain supported the diagnosis of Alzheimer's disease. The patient was treated with the acetylcholinesterase inhibitor, donepezil.

ALZHEIMER'S DISEASE IS ASSOCIATED WITH A DECREASE IN CHOLINERGIC INPUT TO THE CEREBRAL CORTEX. WHAT NUCLEUS OF THE BRAIN CONTAINS THESE CEREBRAL CORTEX-PROTECTING, CHOLINERGIC NEURONS THAT DEGENERATE IN ALZHEIMER'S?

The large, basophilic cell bodies of these cholinergic neurons reside in the basal nucleus (of Meynert) located in the substantia innominata (substance with no name). The substantia innominata occupies the basal forebrain under the anterior commissure. The therapeutic purpose of an acetylcholinesterase inhibitor is to prolong the action of a limited number of acetylcholine molecules by hindering their enzymatic degradation.

ALZHEIMER'S DISEASE IS ALSO ASSOCIATED WITH A LOSS OF NEURONS IN TWO REGIONS OF THE BRAIN INVOLVED IN THE FORMATION OF NEW MEMORIES AND LEARNING. WHAT ARE THESE REGIONS AND WHAT ARE THE CLASSIC MICROSCOPIC ABNORMALITIES THAT ARE OBSERVED IN THESE AREAS?

Neuronal loss is evident in two regions of the temporal lobe of the cerebral cortex involved in the formation of new memories and learning:

- Hippocampal formation
- Parahippocampal gyrus

As the disease progresses, neuronal loss becomes evident in other areas of the cerebral cortex. Cortical atrophy is pronounced in the:

- Frontal lobes
- Temporal lobe
- Parietal lobes.

This global decrease in neurons results in gross pathologic changes, such as cerebral atrophy, widening of the sulci, and dilatation of the ventricles (Fig. 7-1).

Several derangements in microscopic structure are observed in Alzheimer brains:

- Neuritic plaques
- Neurofibrillary tangles
- Amyloid angiopathy
- Granulovacuolar degeneration.

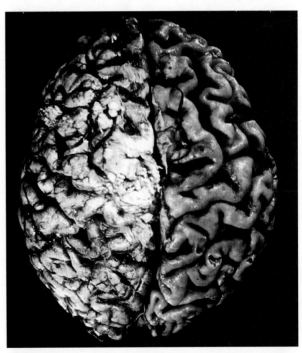

FIGURE 7-1 Alzheimer brain demonstrating cortical atrophy with widening of the sulci. This is best seen on the right where the meninges have been removed. (Kumar V, Abbas A and Fausto N: *Robbins & Cotran Pathologic Basis of Disease*, 7e. WB Saunders, 2004. Fig. 28-34. Courtesy of Dr. E.P. Richardson, Jr., Massachusetts General Hospital, Boston, MA.)

The two pathologically classic abnormalities are neuritic plaques and neurofibrillary tangles. Neuritic plaques are focal aggregations of argyrophilic (silver-loving) dystrophic neurites (dystrophic neurites are thickened or irregular processes of neurons) surrounding a central core of amyloid (Fig. 7-2A, B). Microglia and astrocytes are found at the periphery of the neuritic plaques. At the ultrastructural level, dystrophic neurites contain abnormal mitochondria and paired filaments arrayed as a helix. These helical filaments are principally constituted of the microtubule-associated protein, tau, which is hyperphosphorylated. Other moieties of these filaments are ubiquitin and MAP2, another microtubule-associated protein.

Neurofibrillary tangles are aggregates of these same helical filaments in the cytoplasm of neurons (Fig. 7-2C, D). These filaments, which are best demonstrated with silver stains, displace or surround the nucleus of the neuron. Another characteristic feature of these filaments is their resistance to proteolysis. Consequently, these tangles remain even after the death of the nerve cell.

Amyloid deposition in the walls of cerebral blood vessels is another microscopic abnormality seen in Alzheimer's disease (Fig. 7-2B). This deposition causes a condition known as *cerebral amyloid angiopathy*. Because of the amyloid accumulation, the walls of these vessels may deteriorate, thereby increasing the risk for cerebral hemorrhage.

Two forms of granulovacuolar degeneration are observed in Alzheimer's disease. First, neurons in the hippocampus and olfactory bulbs form clear vacuoles in their cytoplasm. Each of these granules contains a silver-staining (argyrophilic) granule. The other form of granulovacuolar degeneration is the accumulation of eosinophilic vacuoles, called *Hirano bodies*, in pyramidal cells of the hippocampus. The principal molecular moiety found in Hirano bodies is actin.

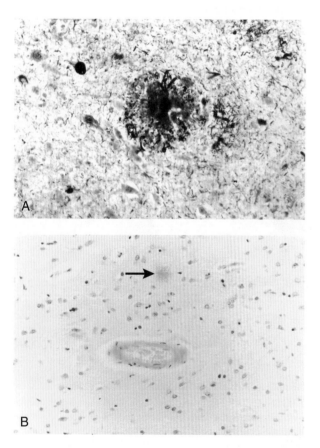
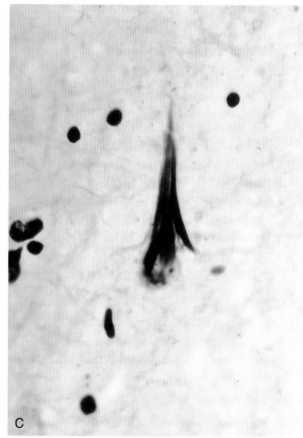

FIGURE 7-2 Histologic changes associated with Alzheimer disease. **A,** Neuritic plaque. **B,** Congo red stain demonstrating amyloid deposition in a neuritic plaque (*arrow*) and in a blood vessel of the cerebral cortex. **C,** Silver stain highlighting a neurofibrillary tangle in a neuron. (Kumar V, Abbas A and Fausto N: *Robbins & Cotran Pathologic Basis of Disease,* 7e. WB Saunders, 2004. Fig. 28-35.)

APOPTOSIS HAS BEEN IMPLICATED AS A MECHANISM OF NEURONAL DEATH IN ALZHEIMER'S DISEASE. WHAT ARE THE REGULATORS OF APOPTOSIS AND WHAT ROLE DOES IT PLAY IN ALZHEIMER'S DISEASE?

Programmed cell death (apoptosis) involves the activation of a family of proteolytic enzymes called caspases. Activation of caspase occurs through the extrinsic or intrinsic pathway. The extrinsic and intrinsic pathways are also known as the *death receptor-initiated* and the *mitochondrial pathways*, respectively.

The extrinsic pathway is activated by ligands that bind to death receptors on the surface of the cell that is to undergo apoptosis. The array of death receptors all belong to the tumor necrosis factor family of death receptors. The two best characterized death receptors are the type 1 tumor necrosis factor receptor and another protein called *Fas*. Activation of the death receptors activates a caspase cascade.

The intrinsic pathway is triggered by an injurious event (e.g., radiation, toxins, and free radicals) that damages the genetic apparatus of a cell. The damaged DNA overexpresses p53, which promotes the release of cytochrome C from mitochondria. The release of cytochrome C activates a caspase cascade.

The caspase cascade, triggered by either apoptotic pathway, results in a breakdown of intracellular structures. The degradation products are pinched off from the cell as apoptotic bodies, which are earmarked for destruction by professional phagocytic cells.

WHAT IS THE ROLE OF AMYLOID PRECURSOR PROTEIN IN THE PATHOGENESIS OF ALZHEIMER'S DISEASE?

Amyloid precursor protein (APP) is a ubiquitous transmembrane protein whose function is becoming elucidated. Experimental evidence suggests that a normal, cytoplasmic cleavage fragment of APP has a signaling role in the nucleus to regulate transcription involved in the growth of neurites. However, abnormal proteolytic cleavage of APP has been implicated in the etiology of Alzheimer's disease (Fig. 7-3). When APP is improperly cleaved at its extracellular domain, Aß peptide fragments in the neural interstitium are produced. The Aß fragments readily aggregate forming amyloid fibrils. The amyloid fibrils, which are resistant to proteolysis, have a direct neurotoxic effect and attract astrocytes and microglia.

HOW IS AXONAL TRANSPORT ACCOMPLISHED IN NEURONS AND HOW IS THIS TRANSPORT SYSTEM DISRUPTED IN ALZHEIMER'S DISEASE?

Axons exhibit bidirectional transport of macromolecules and organelles. The transport of substances from the cell body to the axon terminal is termed *anterograde transport*, whereas the movement of material from the axon terminal to the cell body is called *retrograde transport*. This transport occurs at three distinct velocities:

- Slow velocity moves proteins and actin microfilaments.
- Intermediate velocity transports mitochondria.
- Fast velocity moves vesicles containing neurotransmitters.

Important to the transport of mitochondria and neurotransmitter-containing vesicles are microtubules and microtubule-associated proteins. The microtubules function as molecular highways along which transport occurs. They also direct the flow of traffic because of their polarity. The plus-ends of the microtubules are directed toward the axon terminal, and their minus-ends are directed toward the nucleus.

The microtubule-associated proteins are motors fueled by ATP. The motors drive along microtubules, the molecular highways. Dynein is the motor responsible for retrograde transport, movement toward the cell body (minus-ends of the microtubules). Another motor is kinesin, which is responsible for anterograde transport to the axon terminal (plus-ends of the microtubules). By hitching cargo to these motors, transport will occur. For example, peptide neurotransmitters synthesized in the cell body of the neuron are packaged into synaptic vesicles by the Golgi apparatus. The vesicles are then molecularly hitched to kinesin, which shuttles the cargo to the axon terminal so that the vesicles can release their neurotransmitters.

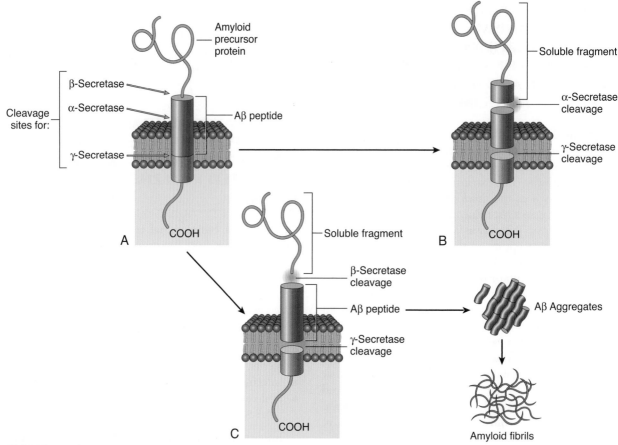

FIGURE 7-3   Mechanism of amyloid deposition in Alzheimer's disease. Amyloid precursor protein (APP) possesses three potential cleavage sites (**A**). Note the Aß domain. If APP is cleaved by α-secretase and γ-secretase, Aß is not formed (**B**). When APP is cleaved by ß-secretase and γ -secretase, Aß is produced (**C**). Aß aggregates into amyloid fibrils. (Kumar V, Abbas A and Fausto N: *Robbins & Cotran Pathologic Basis of Disease*, 7e. WB Saunders, 2004. Fig. 28-36.)

Neurons affected in Alzheimer's disease demonstrate impaired anterograde axonal transport. This reduction in transport begins with mutations of presenilin 1, an integral membrane protein. Mutated presenilin 1 increases the activity of glycogen synthase kinase 3ß (GSK3ß). The more active GSK3ß increases the phosphorylation of an isoform of kinesin. The phosphorylation of kinesin causes it to release its cargo, thereby disrupting the transport system. This reduction in transport makes the neurons more vulnerable to injury and cell death.

A 52-year-old white man presented to his family physician complaining of a bleeding growth on his nose. The patient states that his job requires him to frequently work outside and that he seldom uses protection against the sun even though he is of fair complexion. Visual examination of the growth showed that it was shiny and pink-colored with dilated blood vessels and a white rolled margin (Fig. 7-4A). The center of the papule was ulcerated and bleeding and measured 2 cm in diameter. Microscopic examination of a biopsy of the papule confirmed a diagnosis of basal cell carcinoma. The lesion was surgically excised.

HOW DOES SKIN FORM EMBRYOLOGICALLY?

The skin is formed from two germ layers. The epidermis is derived from ectoderm, whereas the underlying dermis develops from mesoderm-derived mesenchyme. The basic events of development of the epidermis are (Fig. 7-5):

- The primordium of the epidermis is represented by simple cuboidal ectoderm.

- At 4 weeks post-fertilization, a second epithelial layer has been formed by the mitotic activity of the basal layer. This superficial layer, the periderm, is composed of squamous cells that undergo keratinization and desquamation. Because of their mitotic capacity, the basal layer of cells is called the *stratum germinativum*.

- Continued mitotic activity of the stratum germinativum forms an intermediate layer of cells between it and the periderm. The intermediate layer forms at about 11 weeks.

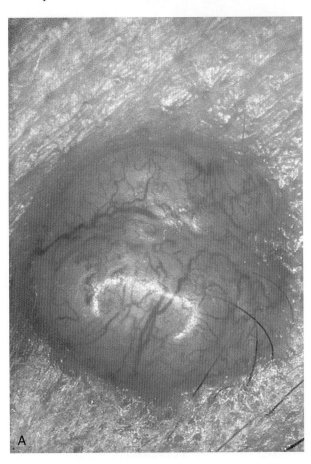

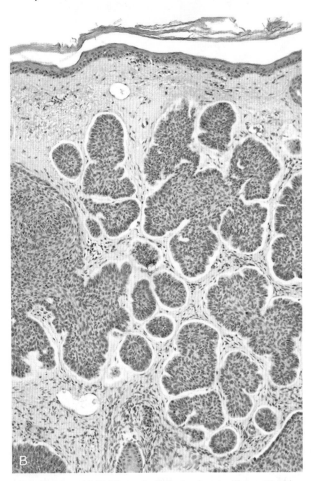

FIGURE 7-4 Basal cell carcinoma. **A**, Pearly nodule with blood vessels (telangiectatic). **B**, Nests of cells in the dermis. (Kumar V, Abbas A and Fausto N: *Robbins & Cotran Pathologic Basis of Disease*, 7e. WB Saunders, 2004. Fig. 25-15.)

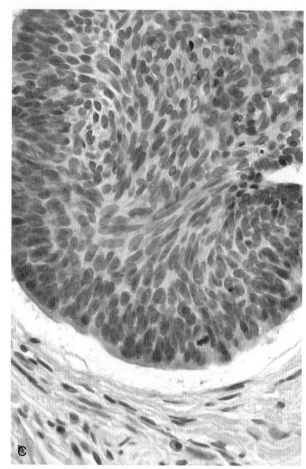

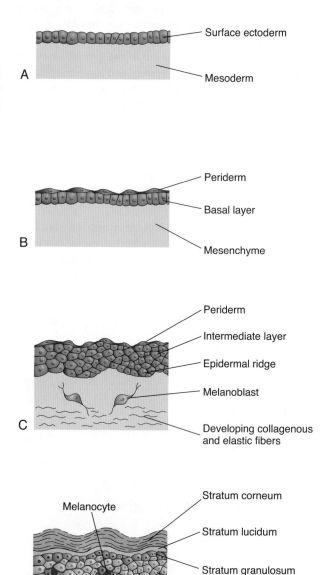

FIGURE 7-4, cont'd C, Cleft separating cell nest from stroma. (Kumar V, Abbas A and Fausto N: *Robbins & Cotran Pathologic Basis of Disease*, 7e. WB Saunders, 2004. Fig. 25-15.)

FIGURE 7-5 Stages of skin development. **A**, 4 weeks. **B**, 7 weeks. **C**, 11 weeks. **D**, Newborn. (Moore K and Persaud TVN: *The Developing Human*, 7e. WB Saunders, 2003. Fig. 20-1.)

● The stratum corneum replaces the cells of the periderm at approximately 21 weeks.

The dermis of the skin is primarily formed from the primitive mesenchyme. The mesenchyme that ultimately forms the dermis is derived from two mesodermal sources:

● Lateral somatic mesoderm
● Dermatomes of the somites

Most of the dermis differentiates from the lateral somatic mesoderm.

HOW IS SKIN ON THE NOSE DESCRIBED HISTOLOGICALLY?

Based on the thickness of the epidermis, skin can be classified as thin or thick. In this case, the skin on the nose is categorized as thin skin. Microscopically, four layers can be observed in the epidermis of thin skin. From deep to superficial, these layers are (Fig. 7-6):

- Stratum basale (also known as the stratum germinativum)
- Stratum spinosum
- Stratum granulosum
- Stratum corneum

Thick skin has the same four layers as thin skin, plus an additional layer called the *stratum lucidum*. The stratus lucidum is located between the stratum granulosum and the stratum corneum and its keratinocytes, which are devoid of organelles and contain keratin filaments and eleidin.

In the stratum basale, a single row of cuboidal to short columnar cells, termed *keratinocytes*, rests on a basal lamina. The mitotically active cells of the stratum basale are joined to one another and to the cells in the stratum spinosum by intercellular junctions.

The stratum spinosum contains a few layers (more layers are found in thick skin) of keratinocytes that are connected by numerous desmosomes. The cells are beginning to accumulate tonofilaments, a type of intermediate filament constituted of cytokeratin. As the keratinocytes migrate toward the skin surface through the stratum spinosum, the tonofilaments, whose synthesis is maintained, aggregate to form larger bundles termed *tonofibrils*. The presence of tonofibrils imparts an eosinophilic appearance to the cells. Keratinocytes in the stratum spinosum are also mitotically active. The two mitotically active layers (basale and spinosum) are collectively referred to as the *Malpighian layer*.

Two to three layers of basophilic keratinocytes form the stratum granulosum. The basophilia of these cells is due to the presence of keratohyalin granules. In contrast, thick skin possesses three to five layers of cells in this stratum.

The stratum corneum is the outermost layer of thin skin. It is composed of several layers of squamous cells. The cells, which are nonviable and devoid of organelles, are filled with the keratin intermediate filaments ensconced in an amorphous matrix. As the cells migrate to the external surface, they lose their desmosomes before being sloughed off.

WHAT IS THE MOLECULAR CONFIGURATION OF DESMOSOMES THAT JOIN KERATINOCYTES AND HEMIDESMOSOMES THAT ANCHOR THE BASAL LAYER OF KERATINOCYTES TO THE BASAL LAMINA?

Desmosomes and hemidesmosomes are junctional complexes constituted of three basic structural elements:

- Cytoskeleton
- Intracellular attachment (anchor) proteins
- Transmembrane adhesion proteins

These three basic structural components are described below.

As a clinical aside, pemphigus is a blistering skin disease that disrupts the integrity of desmosomes and hemidesmosomes. It is an autoimmune disease, as patients have antibodies that are directed against selected molecules that form either desmosomes or hemidesmosomes.

MALIGNANT TUMOR CELLS HAVE DEVELOPED MECHANISMS THAT ENABLE THEM TO METASTASIZE. WHAT ARE THESE MECHANISMS?

The mechanisms of metastasis involve:

- Disruption of adhesion complexes
- Remodeling of cytoskeleton
- Proteolysis of the basal lamina and extracellular matrix
- Migration into blood vessels or lymphatic vessels

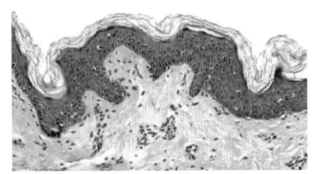

FIGURE 7-6 Histologic features of thin skin. Note the presence of melanin in the basal layer of the epidermis. (Kerr J: *Atlas of Functional Histology*. Mosby, 1999. Fig. 8-3b.)

● Migration out of blood vessels or lymphatic vessels into the tissue of a distant site

Normal epithelial cells are connected to one another and to the basal lamina by an array of adhesion complexes. For a cancer to become metastatic, its cells must orchestrate the disassembly of their molecular interconnections. The molecular constituents include cytoskeletal elements (actin microfilaments and keratin intermediate filaments), transmembrane adhesion proteins (E-cadherins and integrins), and intracellular anchor proteins (catenins, pectin, and BP230). Intracellular anchor proteins link the cytoskeletal elements of the cells to the transmembrane adhesion (linker) protein. The transmembrane adhesion protein molecularly links to a transmembrane adhesion protein from a neighboring cell or to extracellular matrix proteins (e.g., basal lamina).

To break these adhesion complexes, cancer cells decrease the expression of E-cadherin, resulting in decreased numbers on the plasma membrane. They also underexpress catenins or express dysfunctional catenin molecules.

Integrin synthesis is additionally altered by cancer cells. Integrin synthesis is reduced but does not completely cease. Instead, the cancer cells express altered integrin molecules. The modified integrin molecules allow the cell to migrate through the extracellular environment and the walls of blood or lymphatic vessels.

Disruption of the adhesion complexes causes a disarray of the cytoskeleton. This allows the cell to remodel its cytoskeletal network. This reorganization endows the cell with ambulation. Motility of the cell is accomplished by cytoplasmic extensions.

Although the cancer cell has now acquired the characteristics of a motile cell, a barrier still remains. The barrier is a wall of extracellular matrix, which includes the basal lamina. Cancer cells can digest this connective tissue wall by secreting proteases, by prompting other cells to release proteases, or both. Participating proteases are matrix metalloproteinases, urokinase-type plasminogen, and cathepsin-B.

Once cancer cells have broken through the connective tissue barrier, they migrate toward vascular or lymphatic vessels. They enter the vessels by passing through narrow channels between the endothelial cells. To protect themselves from the harsh physical environment and from immunosurveillance, the cancer cells may travel in a mass or they may shield themselves with platelets to escape detection by immune cells. The cancer cells that survive this vascular or lymphatic journey use carbohydrate receptors to snag selectin. Selectin is a carbohydrate receptor on the surface of endothelial cells. This ligand-receptor interaction slows the cancer cell down as the cell rolls along the surface of the endothelium. The rolling comes to a standstill by the braking action of stronger integrin interactions. Once stopped, the cancer cell migrates across the vascular wall into the extracellular space, thereby seeding a distant site with cancer cells.

WHAT ARE THE PATHOLOGIC CHARACTERISTICS OF BASAL CELL CARCINOMA?

The pathologic characteristics of basal cell carcinoma are (Fig. 7-4):

● Appear as pearly papules
● Prominent dilated blood vessels are often found in the superficial layer of the dermis. These are referred to as *telangiectasias*.
● These neoplasms may contain melanin; thus, they may appear similar to melanomas.
● Ulceration may occur in advanced lesions.
● With long-term neglect, the tumor may invade bone and paranasal sinuses.
● Tumor cells appear similar to the normal cells of the stratum basale.
● One growth pattern is multifocal, where tumor cells extend over several centimeters of skin surface but do not penetrate deeply into the skin.
● The other growth pattern forms nodular lesions. These lesions penetrate deeply into the dermis with tumor cells arranged as cords or nests. The cells are basophilic with hyperchromatic nuclei. The cell cords or nests are usually surrounded by many fibroblasts and lymphocytes.

GRANULATION TISSUE IS FORMED DURING WOUND HEALING. WHAT IS GRANULATION TISSUE?

Granulation tissue is formed as a part of the body's normal healing process. The tissue has three signature attributes (Fig. 7-7):

● Numerous blood vessels. Angiogenesis is responsible for the numerous blood vessels that are observed in granulation tissue. Vascular endothelial-derived growth factor and angiopoietins serve as important

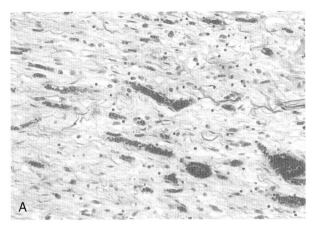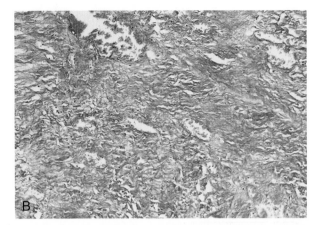

FIGURE 7-7 **A**, Characteristic appearance of granulation tissue: numerous blood vessels, edema, and loose extracellular matrix. **B**, Dense collagenous connective tissue of a mature scar (trichrome stain). (Kumar V, Abbas A and Fausto N: *Robbins & Cotran Pathologic Basis of Disease*, 7e. WB Saunders, 2004. Fig. 3-17.)

molecular conductors in the development and sta-bilization of new blood vessels.

● Edematous. Newly formed blood vessels are leakier than normal. The increased permeability leads to edema.

● Loose extracellular matrix. An orchestra of growth factors causes migration of fibroblasts to the tissue. This is followed by their proliferation. Fibroblasts elaborate the components of the extracellular matrix.

WHAT ARE THE EVENTS OF CUTANEOUS WOUND HEALING AFTER REMOVAL OF THE LESION?

Cutaneous wound healing involves three phases:

● Inflammation (early and late)
● Formation of granulation tissue and generation of new epithelial cells
● Wound contraction, deposition of extracellular matrix, and remodeling

Since the lesion was surgically excised and the clean edges of the skin were approximated by sutures, the wound will undergo healing by first intention. Wounds that are infected, gaping, and/or jagged undergo healing by second intention. The sequences of events in healing by first intention are (Fig. 7-8):

● Neutrophils migrate toward the margins of the fibrin clot. Epithelial cells deposit basal lamina elements at the interface between the dermis and epidermis. The epithelial cells eventually form a thin epidermal layer that covers the dermis. This occurs underneath the scab surface.

● Macrophages replace the neutrophils and granulation tissue forms. Granulation tissue is characterized by angiogenesis, edema, and loose extracellular matrix. The epithelial cells become mitotically active causing the thin epidermal layer to thicken.

● Granulation tissue becomes more abundant, angio-genesis peaks, and collagen fibrils become more numerous, filling in the incision. The epidermis assumes a normal architecture.

● Granulation tissue becomes almost completely re-placed by collagen and a proliferation of fibroblasts.

● Inflammatory cells have disappeared and a scar re-presents the site of wound healing. The scar tissue is remodeled over the next several months to in-crease its tensile strength.

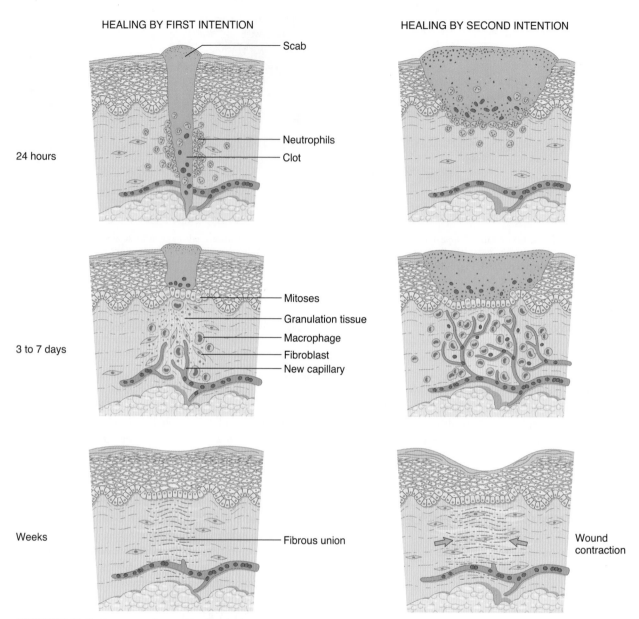

HEALING BY FIRST INTENTION

HEALING BY SECOND INTENTION

24 hours

- Scab
- Neutrophils
- Clot

3 to 7 days

- Mitoses
- Granulation tissue
- Macrophage
- Fibroblast
- New capillary

Weeks

- Fibrous union

Wound contraction

FIGURE 7-8 Processes of wound healing by first intention (left). Note on the right that healing by second intention is characterized by greater amounts of granulation tissue and contraction of the wound. (Kumar V, Abbas A and Fausto N: *Robbins & Cotran Pathologic Basis of Disease*, 7e. WB Saunders, 2004. Fig. 3-21.)

A 71-year-old woman woke up in the morning with weakness and numbness on the right side of her face. Fearful that she had suffered a stroke, she called 911 and paramedics responded to transport her to the emergency department of a nearby medical center. During the history, the physician learned that the patient had just recently recovered from an upper respiratory tract infection and that she was drooling from the right corner of her mouth. The physical examination showed that the patient was unable on the right side of her face to wrinkle the skin of her forehead, close the eye, flare her nostril, or raise the corner of her mouth. Tear flow was also noted on the right side of her face. All other cranial nerves were normal. Imaging studies ruled out any abnormalities. The patient was diagnosed with Bell's palsy, treated with corticosteroids, and instructed on eye care.

WHAT CRANIAL NERVE IS INVOLVED AND WHAT IS ITS COURSE?

Bell's palsy involves the facial nerve. The two divisions of the facial nerve (large motor root and a small intermediate nerve) exit the brainstem at the pontomedullary junction. The motor root is responsible for the innervation of the muscles of facial expression, and the intermediate nerve conveys gustatory, parasympathetic, and somatosensory fibers. The facial nerve leaves the cranial cavity by entering the internal acoustic meatus, traversing the facial canal in the petrous portion of the temporal bone, and exiting at the stylomastoid foramen (Fig. 7-9). Because of its long intraosseous journey, the facial nerve is vulnerable to compression within the facial canal.

Once it exits the stylomastoid foramen, the facial nerve branches into the posterior auricular nerve and a main trunk (Fig. 7-10). The main trunk and the parotid plexus that it forms are embedded in the parotid gland. The plexus gives rise to the five ter-

minal branches of the facial nerve: temporal, zygomatic, buccal, marginal mandibular, and cervical (Fig. 7-10). The distribution of the five terminal branches and the posterior auricular nerve are purely motor. Table 7-1 describes the muscular distribution of the facial nerve. In addition to the many muscles listed in the table, the facial nerve also innervates the stapedius, a small muscle in the middle ear.

DESCRIBE THE THREE CONNECTIVE TISSUE INVESTMENTS OF A NERVE.

The three connective tissue investments of a nerve are (Fig. 7-11):

- Endoneurium (*Among fascicles*)
- Perineurium (*Around Bundles/axons*)
- Epineurium (*outer*)

A nerve is composed of many axons, myelinated and unmyelinated. Single axons (fibers) and their associated Schwann cells are enveloped by a thin, delicate connective layer called the *endoneurium*. Aggregations of axons and their accompanying investments are called *bundles* or *fascicles*. Fascicles are enveloped by another connective tissue element, the perineurium. The entire nerve, formed by the fascicles, is ensheathed by the outermost connective tissue layer, the epineurium. These connective tissue investments maintain the structural array of the nerve and transmit blood vessels to nourish the fibers and cells.

Noxious stimuli (e.g., cold and infections) evoke an inflammatory response. The resultant increase in permeability of the microvasculature causes tissue swelling of the connective tissue investments leading to nerve compression within the facial canal. This explains the constellation of symptoms in a patient with Bell's palsy. Corticosteroids are prescribed to reduce the inflammatory response thereby decompressing the nerve.

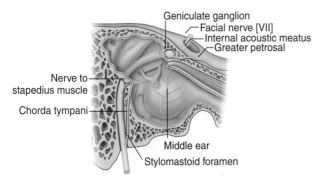

FIGURE 7-9 Facial nerve traversing facial canal of temporal bone. (Drake R, Vogl W and Mitchell A: *Gray's Anatomy for Students.* Churchill Livingstone, 2004. Fig. 8-124)

Geniculate ganglion
Facial nerve [VII]
Internal acoustic meatus
Greater petrosal
Nerve to stapedius muscle
Chorda tympani
Middle ear
Stylomastoid foramen

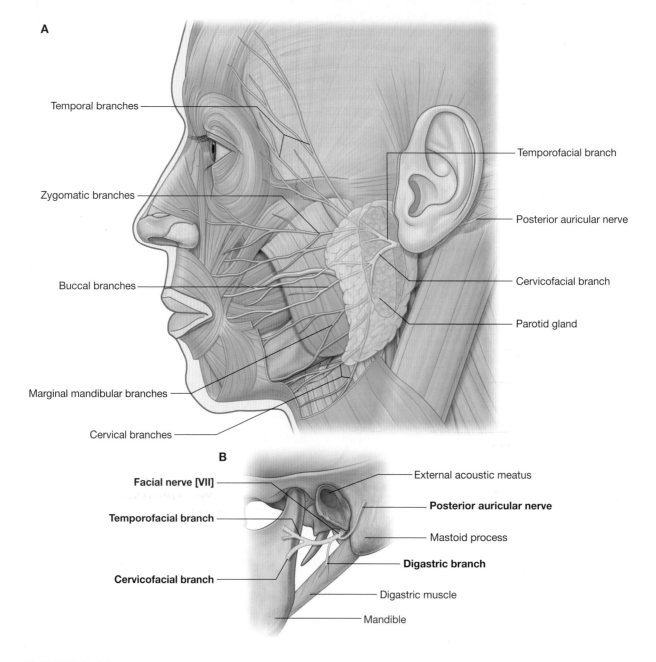

FIGURE 7-10 **A**, Terminal branches of facial nerve on the face. **B**, Branches of facial nerve before penetrating the parotid gland. (Drake R, Vogl W and Mitchell A: *Gray's Anatomy for Students.* Churchill Livingstone, 2004. Fig. 8-60)

WHAT IS THE EMBRYOLOGIC BASIS OF THE STRUCTURES INNERVATED BY THE FACIAL NERVE?

Embryologically, the second pharyngeal arch is supplied by the facial nerve. The derivatives of the second pharyngeal arch are:

- Muscles of facial expression
- Stapedius
- Posterior belly of digastric
- Stylohyoid

Thus, in the adult form, the muscles retain their embryologic innervation.

TABLE 7-1 Muscular Distribution of Facial Nerve Branches

Facial Nerve Branch	Muscular Distribution
Posterior auricular	Auricularis posterior (auricular branch)
	Occipital belly of occipitofrontalis (occipital branch)
	Posterior belly of digastric (digastric branch)
	Stylohyoid (stylohyoid branch)
Temporal	Auricularis superior
	Auricularis inferior
	Frontal belly of occipitofrontalis
	Corrugator supercilii
	Superior portion of orbicularis oculi
Zygomatic	Inferior part of orbicularis oculi
Buccal	Procerus
	Nasalis
	Depressor septi
	Buccinator
	Levator labii superioris alaeque nasi
	Levator labii superioris
	Zygomaticus major
	Zygomaticus minor
	Levator anguli oris
	Superior parts of orbicularis oris
Marginal mandibular	Mentalis
	Depressor labii inferioris
	Depressor anguli oris
	Inferior parts of orbicularis oris
	Risorius
Cervical	Platysma

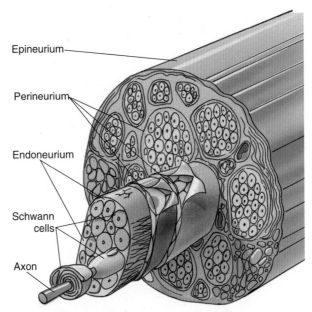

FIGURE 7-11 Diagram of the connective tissue investments of a nerve. (Gartner L and Hiatt J: *Color Textbook of Histology, 2e.* WB Saunders, 2001. Fig. 9-22.)

WHY WAS THE PATIENT INSTRUCTED ON EYE CARE?

Paralysis of the orbicularis oculi muscle causes the lower eyelid to droop and bend away from the surface of the eye. Consequently, lacrimal fluid spills down the side of the face. This diversion of lacrimal fluid away from the eye accompanied by the inability of the orbicularis oculi to close and wipe lacrimal fluid across the corneal surface and conjunctiva lead to dehydration.

Anatomically, the facial nerve conveys parasympathetic fibers to the lacrimal gland that stimulate lacrimal secretion. This innervation remains intact because the lesion producing Bell's palsy in this patient is distal to the course of these parasympathetic fibers that are conveyed in the intermediate branch of the facial nerve.

After the birth of their son, the parents were informed that their child was born with a bilateral posterior cleft defect. The concerns of the parents were assuaged when the physician informed them that the congenital defect could be surgically corrected.

C A S E

53

HOW DOES THE PALATE DEVELOP?

Development of the palate is a 7-week process that begins at the end of the fifth week and culminates during the twelfth week. The adult palate is formed from the embryonic primary and secondary palates (Fig. 7-12).

The primary palate, or median palatine process, develops from the intermaxillary segment of the maxilla. The median palatine process is an outgrowth of mesenchyme from the maxillary prominences. The primary palate, which eventually undergoes ossification, is anterior to the incisive fossa. Consequently, it represents a minor part of the adult palate.

The secondary palate develops from two lateral palatine processes. The lateral palatine processes, like the median palatine process, are mesenchymal outgrowths of the maxillary prominences. The lateral palatine processes grow toward the midline and ultimately fuse. The ventral parts of the lateral palatine processes ossify, forming the hard palate posterior to the incisive fossa. The dorsal parts of the lateral palatine processes, which do not ossify, form the soft palate, including its uvula. The median palatine raphe is a visible landmark representing the line of fusion of the lateral palatine processes.

WHAT IS THE EMBRYOLOGIC BASIS OF A POSTERIOR CLEFT DEFECT?

Posterior cleft anomalies develop posterior to the incisive fossa (Fig. 7-13). With a bilateral posterior cleft defect, the migration of both lateral palatine processes abates. This migration failure causes clefts to appear lateral to the nasal septum. In the case of a unilateral posterior defect, only one lateral palatine process fails to migrate, causing only one cleft to form lateral to the nasal septum.

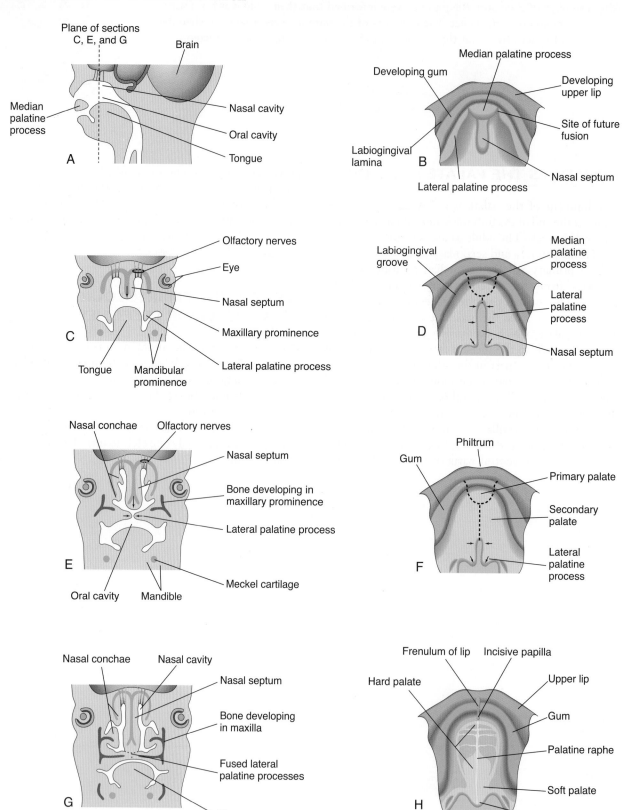

FIGURE 7-12 **A**, Sagittal section of head at end of sixth week showing median palatine process. **B**, **D**, **F**, and **H**, Roof of mouth showing development of the palate between weeks 6 and 12. **C**, **E**, and **G**, Coronal sections of head showing the fusion of the lateral palatine processes and nasal septum. This divides the nasal and oral cavities. (Moore K and Persaud TVN: *The Developing Human*, 7e. WB Saunders, 2003. Fig. 10-37.)

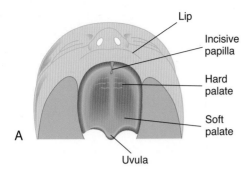

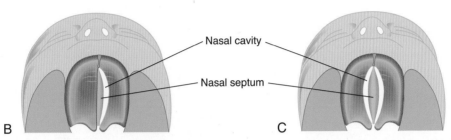

FIGURE 7-13 **A**, Normal lip and palate. **B**, Unilateral posterior cleft palate. **C**, Bilateral posterior cleft palate. (Moore K and Persaud TVN: *The Developing Human*, 7e. WB Saunders, 2003. Fig. 10-40.)

A 36-year-old woman presented to her family practitioner with complaints of weight gain, muscle weakness, ruddy complexion (plethora), a rounded face ("moon" face), and streaks on her skin (striae). She also informed her physician that she was concerned about her elevated blood pressure after a recent self-administered measurement at the local drugstore. Dexamethasone suppression tests indicated a pituitary cause of excess ACTH and a MRI study demonstrated an adenoma of the pituitary gland. The patient was diagnosed with an ACTH-secreting pituitary gland tumor (Cushing's disease).

WHAT IS THE ARTERIAL SUPPLY TO THE PITUITARY GLAND?

The pituitary gland is supplied by the following arteries (Fig. 7-14):

- Pair of inferior hypophyseal arteries
- Several pairs of superior hypophyseal arteries

Each inferior hypophyseal artery arises from each internal carotid within the cavernous sinus. The superior hypophyseal arteries issue from multiple parent vessels. These are the supraclinoid segments of the internal carotid arteries and the anterior and posterior cerebral arteries.

WHERE ARE ACTH-SECRETING CELLS LOCATED IN THE PITUITARY GLAND AND HOW ARE THEY DESCRIBED HISTOLOGICALLY?

The cells responsible for secreting ACTH are called *corticotrophs*. Corticotrophs are observed in the pars distalis of the anterior pituitary (also known as the *adenohypophysis*).

Histologically, the cells of the adenohypophysis are classified on the basis of their staining characteristics. The resident cells of the adenohypophysis are:

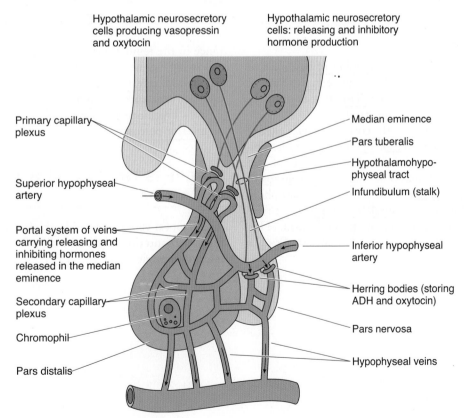

Hypothalamic neurosecretory cells producing vasopressin and oxytocin

Hypothalamic neurosecretory cells: releasing and inhibitory hormone production

Primary capillary plexus

Superior hypophyseal artery

Portal system of veins carrying releasing and inhibiting hormones released in the median eminence

Secondary capillary plexus

Chromophil

Pars distalis

Median eminence

Pars tuberalis

Hypothalamohypophyseal tract

Infundibulum (stalk)

Inferior hypophyseal artery

Herring bodies (storing ADH and oxytocin)

Pars nervosa

Hypophyseal veins

FIGURE 7-14 Illustration of the circulation of the pituitary gland. (Gartner L and Hiatt J: *Color Textbook of Histology, 2e*. WB Saunders, 2001. Fig. 13-2.)

- Acidophils, which have an affinity for acid dyes
- Basophils, which react with basic dyes
- Chromophobes, which are cells that fail to react with dyes

Corticotrophs are a type of basophil. Typically, basophils are located at the periphery of the pars distalis. At the ultrastructural level, corticotrophs exhibit an eccentric nucleus in a cell that is round to oval in shape. The organelles are not well developed and the cytoplasm contains secretory vesicles (250–400 nm in diameter). The secretory vesicles are known to contain several hormones:

- ACTH
- Pro-opiomelanocortin
- Melanocyte-stimulating hormone
- Endorphins
- Lipotropin

WHAT ARE THE PATHOLOGIC CHARACTERISTICS OF THE PITUITARY GLAND IN CUSHING'S DISEASE?

The pathologic characteristics of the pituitary gland in Cushing's disease are:

- There is an increase in the number of basophils in the pars distalis. This increase can be in the form of a discrete adenoma or hyperplasia that is diffusely distributed throughout the gland.
- The basophilic nature of the corticotrophs is altered by the excessive stimulation of glucocorticoids. The normal basophilic granulated appearance of the corticotroph's cytoplasm is replaced by a uniform, lightly basophilic substance. This lightly basophilic feature is due to an accumulation of keratin, a type of intermediate filament, in the cytoplasm. This alteration in the cytoplasm is termed *Crooke's hyaline change*.

IN THIS CASE SCENARIO, THE CORTICOTROPH CELL ADENOMA IS LARGE ENOUGH TO BE DETECTED BY MRI. THIS IS NOT ALWAYS THE CASE, AS SOME ADENOMAS ARE TOO SMALL OR THERE IS DIFFUSE HYPERPLASIA OF CORTICOTROPHS. WHEN IMAGING STUDIES ARE UNREMARKABLE, ANOTHER CLINICAL PROCEDURE MUST BE PERFORMED TO DISTINGUISH CUSHING'S DISEASE FROM OTHER CAUSES OF CUSHING SYNDROME. THIS PROCEDURE, WHICH MEASURES ACTH-INDUCED SECRETION FROM THE ADENOHYPOPHYSIS, IS INFERIOR PETROSAL SINUS SAMPLING. STARTING FROM THE FEMORAL VEIN, WHAT IS THE ROUTE THAT A CATHETER WILL TAKE TO REACH THE INFERIOR PETROSAL SINUS?

Once in the femoral vein the catheter would take the following sequential course through the venous circulation: external iliac vein → common iliac vein → inferior vena cava → right atrium → superior vena cava → brachiocephalic vein → internal jugular vein → inferior petrosal sinus.

WHERE IS THE FEMORAL VEIN LOCATED?

The femoral vein is located in the femoral triangle of the superoanterior thigh. The three boundaries of the femoral triangle are (Fig. 7-15):

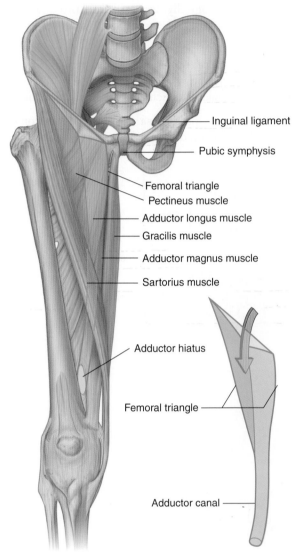

FIGURE 7-15 Boundaries of the femoral triangle. (Drake R, Vogl W and Mitchell A: *Gray's Anatomy for Students*. Churchill Livingstone, 2004. Fig. 6-41)

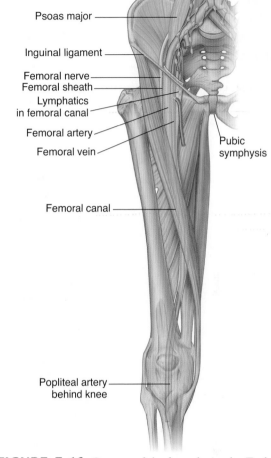

FIGURE 7-16 Contents of the femoral triangle. (Drake R, Vogl W and Mitchell A: *Gray's Anatomy for Students*. Churchill Livingstone, 2004. Fig. 6-42)

- The superior boundary or base is formed by the inguinal ligament.
- The lateral boundary is formed by the medial border of the sartorius muscle.
- The medial boundary is formed by the medial margin of the adductor longus muscle.

The femoral triangle contains neurovascular structures and lymphatic vessels. These structures are arranged in a specific order. From lateral to medial, the structures are (Fig. 7-16):

- Femoral nerve
- Femoral artery
- Femoral vein
- Lymphatic vessels

The mnemonic NAVeL is useful in remembering the lateral to medial sequence of these structures. The femoral vein is found by first locating the femoral artery. The pulse of the femoral artery is located inferior to the midpoint of the inguinal ligament. The femoral vein is just medial to the artery.

WHERE ARE THE TARGET CELLS FOR ACTH CHIEFLY LOCATED IN THE SUPRARENAL GLAND AND WHAT HORMONES ARE SECRETED BY THE TARGET CELLS?

The target cells for ACTH (corticotropin) are located in the cortex of the suprarenal glands. These cortical cells are histologically arranged into three layers or zonae. From external to internal, these layers are (Fig. 7-17):

- Zona glomerulosa
- Zona fasciculata
- Zona reticularis, which abuts the inner medulla

The zona glomerulosa secretes aldosterone, a mineralocorticoid, the zona fasciculata chiefly secretes

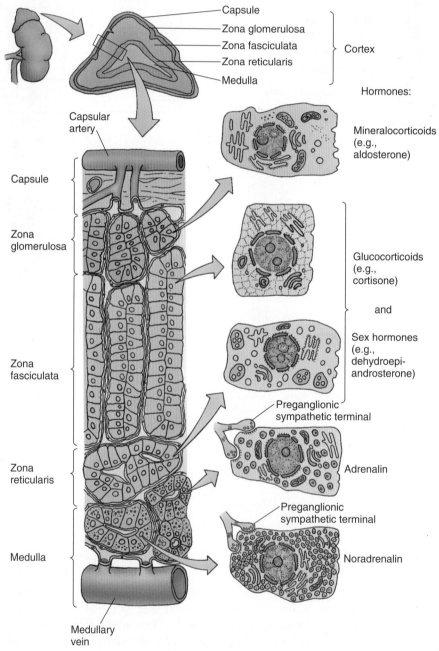

FIGURE 7-17 Illustration of the suprarenal gland and its cell types. (Gartner L and Hiatt J: *Color Textbook of Histology, 2e.* WB Saunders, 2001. Fig. 13-10.)

cortisol, a glucocorticoid, and small quantities of androgens, and the zona reticularis secretes principally androgens and small amounts of cortisol.

The zona fasciculata, which comprises 75% of the adrenal cortex, contains cells arrayed in columns, one to two cell layers thick, like spokes in a wheel. The lightly acidophilic cells are joined by gap junctions and exhibit the typical ultrastructural attributes of steroid-secreting cells. The cells are:

- Well endowed with smooth endoplasmic reticulum that contains enzymes bound to its membranous network necessary for the synthesis of steroids. Because steroids are freely diffusable across cell membranes, they are not sorted and packaged into membrane-limited secretory vesicles. Instead, the hormones are produced on demand and readily leave the cell by diffusion across its plasmalemma.

- Mitochondria possessing tubular cristae are also numerous. The tubular cristae are unique to mitochondria contained in steroid-secreting cells. Their significance, however, is an enigma. In tandem with the endoplasmic reticulum, mitochondria participate in steroid synthesis by housing some of the requisite enzymes on its inner mitochondrial membrane.

- The last characteristic to highlight is the presence of several lipid droplets that provide the precursor lipids for the steroid synthetic pathway. During tissue preparation for light microscopy, the lipid droplets are dissolved and removed. Because the lipid extraction imparts a vacuolated appearance to these cells, they are termed *spongiocytes*.

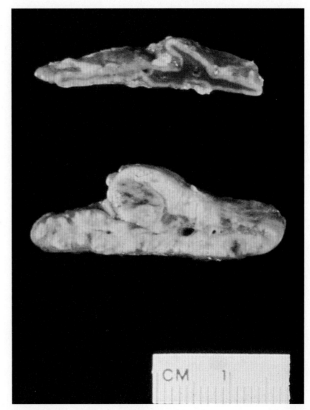

FIGURE 7-18 Normal suprarenal gland on top contrasted with the enlarged suprarenal gland below. Note that the cortex of the suprarenal gland below is yellow and wider because of hyperplasia and hypertrophy of the lipid-laden zonae fasciculata and reticularis. (Kumar V, Abbas A and Fausto N: *Robbins & Cotran Pathologic Basis of Disease*, 7e. WB Saunders, 2004. Fig. 24-47.)

HOW DO REGIONS OF THE ADRENAL GLAND RESPOND TO AN EXCESSIVE LEVEL OF CIRCULATING ACTH?

An excessive level of ACTH has an enhanced stimulatory effect on the cortical cells principally located in the zona glomerulosa and the zona reticularis. This increased stimulation causes significant cortical hypertrophy. The normal adrenal gland has a mass of 4 g, whereas an adrenal gland may have a mass of 25 to 40 g in Cushing's disease (Fig. 7-18). In most cases, the hypertrophy is the result of diffuse hyperplasia of the cortical cells of the inner two zones. Though the cells of the zona glomerulosa require the presence of ACTH for aldosterone secretion, ACTH exerts little effect on their rate of secretion.

THE ADRENAL GLAND HAS A RICH ARTERIAL BLOOD SUPPLY FROM THE SUPERIOR, MIDDLE, AND INFERIOR SUPRARENAL ARTERIES. WHAT ARE THE PARENT VESSELS OF THE SUPRARENAL ARTERIES?

The acronym "IPAR" is helpful in remembering that the inferior phrenic (IP), aorta (A), and renal (R) arteries give rise to the superior, middle, and inferior suprarenal arteries, respectively. There is dominance in which arteries supply the adrenal gland. In the right gland, the superior and inferior suprarenal arteries are the principal supply, whereas the left gland is primarily supplied by the middle and inferior suprarenal arteries.

WHAT LETTER OF THE ALPHABET BEST REPRESENTS THE APPEARANCE OF THE SUPRARENAL GLANDS ON CT IMAGING?

Because of its triangular shape, an axial CT image of the suprarenal gland appears as the letter Y (Fig. 7-19). It has also been described as the "Mercedes-Benz" sign due to its resemblance to this luxury automaker's emblem.

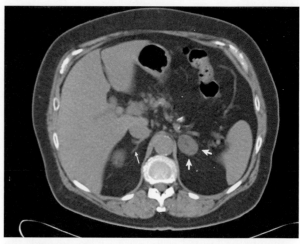

FIGURE 7-19 Normal right suprarenal gland is shown at the small *arrow*. Note its Y-shaped appearance. (Towsend C et al.: *Sabiston Textbook of Surgery, 17e*. WB Saunders, 2004. Fig. 37-24.)

A 62-year-old woman visited her ophthalmologist for her annual examination. The examination showed some peripheral visual field defects, and morphologic changes of the optic disc and retina were detected by visual inspection and optical coherence tomography, respectively. Intraocular pressure measured 20 mm Hg, which was four points higher than last year's value. The patient was diagnosed with primary open angle glaucoma.

WHAT STRUCTURE PRODUCES AQUEOUS HUMOR AND HOW IS THIS HUMOR DRAINED?

Located between the ora serrata and the margin of the lens is a wedge-shaped extension of choroid called the *ciliary body* (Fig. 7-20, *upper left*). Extending from the anterior part of the ciliary body toward the lens are numerous (approximately 70) ciliary processes. Attached to the ends of these processes and to the lens are the suspensory ligaments of the lens. Most of the ciliary body, except for the ciliary processes, is composed of smooth muscle forming the ciliary muscle. The ciliary muscle has three bundles of smooth

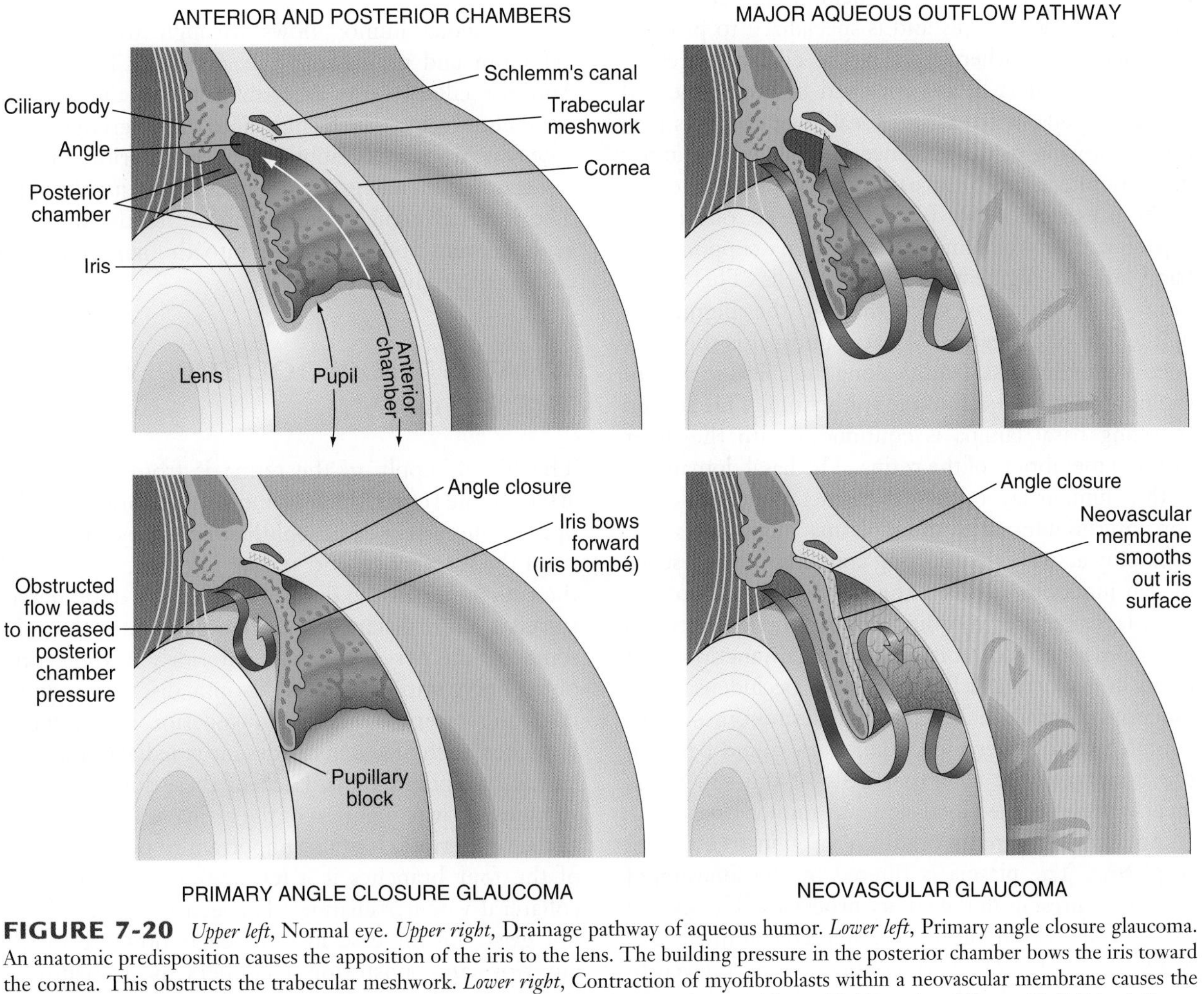

FIGURE 7-20 *Upper left*, Normal eye. *Upper right*, Drainage pathway of aqueous humor. *Lower left*, Primary angle closure glaucoma. An anatomic predisposition causes the apposition of the iris to the lens. The building pressure in the posterior chamber bows the iris toward the cornea. This obstructs the trabecular meshwork. *Lower right*, Contraction of myofibroblasts within a neovascular membrane causes the iris to appose the trabecular meshwork. This obstructs the drainage of aqueous humor. (Kumar V, Abbas A and Fausto N: *Robbins & Cotran Pathologic Basis of Disease*, 7e. WB Saunders, 2004. Fig. 29-11.)

muscle. The lateral-most muscle bundle, which abuts the sclera, stretches the choroid. This muscle, called the *tensor muscle* of the choroid and also known as the *muscle of Brücke*, facilitates drainage of aqueous humor. The other two muscle bundles are involved in accommodation for near vision. Contraction of these smooth muscle bundles paradoxically reduces the tension on the suspensory ligaments of the lens. The reduced tension increases the refractive power of the lens by increasing its thickness, thus enabling the person to view near objects. The core of the ciliary body is the vascular layer, which is composed of loose connective tissue containing elastic fibers and numerous blood vessels. The cores of the ciliary processes contain loose connective tissue supporting many fenestrated capillaries.

Lining the inner surface of the ciliary body and the ciliary processes is an epithelium, continuous with the pigmented epithelium of the retina, called the *pars ciliaris* of the retina. This epithelium consists of two layers of columnar cells and is specialized to produce aqueous humor where it lines the ciliary processes. The superficial layer is composed of nonpigmented columnar cells, whereas the basal layer contains pigmented (owing to the presence of melanin) columnar cells. An interesting feature of this stratified epithelium is the presence of two basal laminae. As one might expect with epithelium, a basal lamina supports the basal layer of pigmented columnar cells. This membrane is continuous with that of the pigmented epithelium of the retina. What is unusual is the presence of another basal lamina along the apical surface of the nonpigmented columnar epithelium. This second investing basal lamina is continuous with the inner limiting membrane of the retina. The basal domains of both columnar layers possess characteristic infoldings and interdigitations of their plasma membranes that exemplify actively transporting epithelia. The presence of gap junctions between the pigmented cells of the basal layer ensures coordination of function between the independent cell units. Intercellular junctions that typify transporting cells are zonula occludens (tight junctions), zonula adherens, and desmosomes. This complement of intercellular junctions found between the nonpigmented columnar cells of the superficial layer represents the blood-aqueous humor barrier.

Aqueous humor is a relatively protein-free filtrate of plasma. The plasma is filtered by the fenestrated capillaries present in the ciliary processes. The filtrate is then transported into the pigmented columnar cells of the basal layer of ciliary epithelium and relayed to the nonpigmented cells of the superficial layer. From this layer, aqueous humor is released in the posterior chamber of the eye, which is located between the vitreous body and the iris. Aqueous humor then flows through the pupil of the iris to enter the anterior cavity located between the iris and the cornea. To maintain normal intraocular pressure, aqueous humor, which is being constantly produced, must be drained from the anterior chamber. The biological drainage apparatus is located near the limbus. The limbus is at the junction of the cornea and sclera. The apparatus is composed of a trabecular meshwork of endothelium-lined spaces that leads to the canal of Schlemm (sinus venosus sclerae). Aqueous humor filters through this meshwork before being collected by the canal of Schlemm (Fig. 7-20, *upper right*).

HOW DOES AQUEOUS HUMOR RETURN TO THE RIGHT ATRIUM?

The aqueous humor flows through the canal of Schlemm and drains into the anterior ciliary veins. Anterior ciliary veins are tributaries of the inferior ophthalmic veins, which empty into the cavernous sinus. The cavernous sinus empties into the inferior petrosal sinus, which then empties into the internal jugular vein. The internal jugular then empties into the brachiocephalic vein and from here into the superior vena cava to the right atrium.

WHAT IS THE BLOOD SUPPLY TO THE RETINA?

The blood supply to the retina is from the central artery of the retina, the first and smallest branch of the ophthalmic artery. The ophthalmic artery originates from the internal carotid artery. The central artery of the retina pierces the dural sheath of the optic nerve, travels a short distance, and then penetrates the substance of the nerve. It travels anteriorly in the center of the nerve until it reaches the optic disc. At the optic disc, the artery divides into superior and inferior branches, each of which divides into medial (nasal) and lateral (temporal) rami. Each of these four branches supplies its own quadrant of the retina as far anteriorly as the ora serrata. It is also important to note that each of the four branches is a terminal artery; therefore, collateral vascular channels between these vessels do not exist. An increase in intraocular pressure in the anterior and posterior chambers is transmitted throughout the eye. Theoretically, if this pressure is elevated to a high enough level, it can restrict blood flow through the central artery of the retina, which may lead to blindness if the pressure is not reduced.

WHAT ARE THE LAYERS OF THE RETINA?

The retina is the third and innermost layer of the eye. It is composed of 10 layers. From external to internal, these are the (Fig. 7-21):

- Pigmented epithelium. This simple layer of cuboidal to columnar cells is supported by Bruch's membrane, which separates the pigmented epithelium from the choroid. The lateral domains of the pigment cells possess zonula occludens, zonula adherens, and desmosomes. The zonula occludens is responsible for forming the blood-retina barrier. Also present are gap junctions (nexus). A typical array of organelles is present in the cytoplasm with numerous mitochondria located along the invaginations of the basal plasmalemma abutting Bruch's membrane. The apical region of the pigment cell demonstrates many melanin granules and residual bodies containing the discarded tips of photoreceptor cells that were phagocytosed.

- Layer of photoreceptors (rods and cones). Each retina contains about 6 million cones and 100 to 120 million rods. Cones are specialized for bright light and color perception and are the exclusive photoreceptor of the fovea centralis. The number of cones decreases and the number of rods increases as you move away from the fovea. Both photoreceptors are composed of four regions or segments: outer segment, which intimately contacts the pigment cells; inner segment; nuclear regions; and the synaptic region. The shape of the outer segment is the structural feature that distinguishes rods and cones.

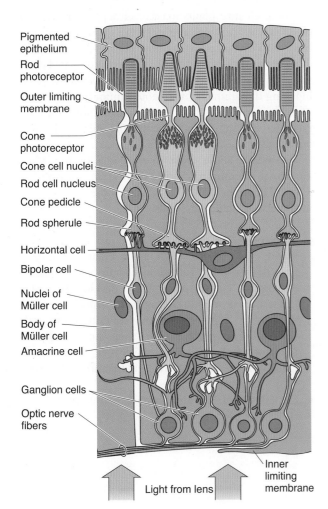

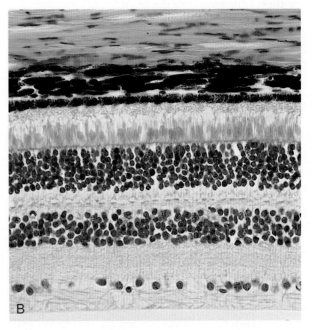

FIGURE 7-21 **A,** Illustration of the layers of the retina. **B,** Light micrograph of the layers of the retina (x270). (Gartner L and Hiatt J: *Color Textbook of Histology, 2e.* WB Saunders, 2001. Figs. 22-8 and 22.7.)

- Outer limiting membrane. This is not a true membrane. Instead it is a zone of contact, *vis-à-vis* zonulae adherens, between Müller cells and photoreceptors.
- Outer nuclear layer. This layer is represented by the nuclei of the rods and cones. The nuclei of rods are smaller, rounder, and more intensely basophilic than the cone nuclei.
- Outer plexiform layer. This layer is composed of axodendritic synapses. The axons of the rods and cones form synaptic contacts with the dendrites of bipolar and horizontal cells.
- Inner nuclear layer. This layer contains the nuclei of bipolar neurons as well as nuclei from amacrine, Müller, and horizontal cells.
- Inner plexiform layer. This layer is composed of several structural elements. Bipolar cell axons synapse with the dendrites of ganglion and amacrine cells, and processes of amacrine, ganglion, and bipolar cells form a plexus in this layer.
- Ganglion cell layer. The cell bodies of large multipolar neurons are found in this layer. The axons of these cells project to the brain.
- Optic nerve fiber layer. The unmyelinated axons of the ganglion cells pass through this layer to converge at the optic disc. When the axons pierce the sclera to exit via the optic nerve, they become myelinated.
- Inner limiting membrane. In contrast to the outer limiting membrane, this is a true membrane, which is the basal lamina of Müller cells.

HOW DOES THE RETINA DEVELOP?

An ectodermal extension of the forebrain called the optic cup develops into the retina. The optic cup is composed of two layers: an external, thin layer and an internal thick layer. The external layer differentiates into the pigmented epithelium and, under the influence of the forming lens, the internal layer develops into the neural retina. Early in development these two layers are separated by the intraretinal space. This space eventually obliterates when the two layers fuse. As is common in the nervous system of the newborn, myelination of the optic nerve fibers as they leave the eye is incomplete. Full myelination of the nerve fibers is typically complete by 10 weeks of age.

WHAT ARE THE CAUSES OF OPEN ANGLE AND ANGLE CLOSURE GLAUCOMA?

The causes of open angle and angle closure glaucoma are dependent on an understanding of the normal anatomy of the eye which is illustrated in the upper panels of Figure 7-20.

The causes of the secondary open angle glaucoma are manifold and include:

- Leakage of erythrocytes into the eye from trauma can clog the trabecular meshwork leading to the canal of Schlemm.
- Turnover (phacolysis) of lens proteins
- Pigment granules from the epithelial cells lining the iris
- Oxytalan fibers from the suspensory ligaments of the lens
- Tumors
- Elevated pressure in the episcleral veins

Angle closure glaucoma can either be primary or secondary. In primary angle closure glaucoma, the iris bows into the anterior chamber (Fig. 7-20, *lower left*). This forward displacement of the iris causes its lateral margins to abut the trabecular meshwork, thus blocking the drainage of aqueous humor into the canal of Schlemm. Production of aqueous humor continues unabated driving the intraocular pressure to dangerous levels.

Secondary angle closure glaucoma occurs when abnormal membranes with contractile capabilities develop over the anterior surface of the iris. Specific mechanisms include the following:

- In response to protracted ischemia of the retina, angiogenic factors, such as vascular endothelial growth factor, are released. It is proposed that the angiogenic factors prompt the development of a fibrovascular membrane over the anterior surface of the iris. This membrane contains contractile cells called *myofibroblasts*, and their shortening pulls the iris over the trabecular meshwork. This form of glaucoma is called neovascularization glaucoma (Fig. 7-20, *lower right*).
- Certain tumors can also promote neovascularization.

- Endothelial cells lining the cornea may rebel and migrate over the surface of the iris. Contraction of these cells also leads to obstruction of the trabecular meshwork. This type of glaucoma is called *iridocorneal syndrome*.
- Penetrating injuries to the anterior eye through surgery or trauma can cause the superficial epithelium of the cornea or conjunctiva to grow through the opening created by the injury into the anterior chamber. Contraction of these cells similarly occludes the trabecular meshwork.
- Neoplasms of the ciliary body can push the iris against the meshwork.

WHAT MORPHOLOGICAL CHANGES ACCOMPANY GLAUCOMA?

One of the hallmark morphological changes observed in patients with glaucoma is cupping of the optic disc (Fig. 7-22B). Another change is thinning of the retina due to atrophy of the optic nerve fiber layer and the ganglion cell layer (Fig. 7-22A).

WHAT GENE IS MUTATED IN A SUBSET OF PATIENTS WITH PRIMARY OPEN ANGLE GLAUCOMA?

A subgroup of patients with primary open angle glaucoma has mutations in the GLC1A gene. The gene, located on chromosome 1, is also known as the trabecular meshwork inducible glucocorticoid response gene (TIGR). TIGR encodes the protein myocilin, whose function has not been discerned. Myocilin is located in the trabecular meshwork and in other tissues of the anterior chamber. It is also found in the optic nerve. Thus, myocilin may play a role in the pathogenesis of retinal nerve damage in glaucoma.

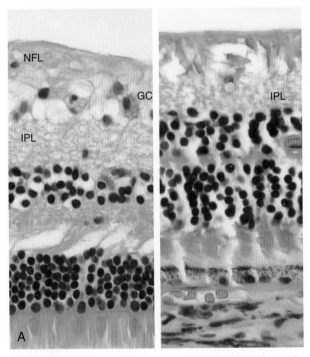

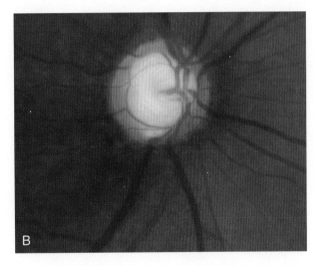

FIGURE 7-22 **A,** Normal retina is shown in the right panel and a retina in glaucoma is in the left panel. Both micrographs were taken at the same magnification. The full thickness of the glaucomatous retina is shown, whereas the normal retina only shows a portion of its overall thickness. The glaucomatous retina shows thinning. The nerve fiber layer and the ganglion cell later are noticeably atrophied in the glaucomatous retina. **B,** Nerve cupping in the glaucomatous retina. (Kumar V, Abbas A and Fausto N: *Robbins & Cotran Pathologic Basis of Disease*, 7e. WB Saunders, 2004. Fig. 29-26.)

A 27-year-old woman presented to her physician complaining of nervousness, tiredness, and difficulty sleeping. She also commented on her weight loss even though her appetite was good and she experienced little menstrual flow during her last two periods. The physical examination revealed skin that was warm and moist, thinning of the hair, tremor of outstretched hands, exophthalmos, and hyperactive tendon reflexes. The patient also had tachycardia, a widened pulse pressure, and an elevated pulse pressure. Palpation of the neck indicated that the thyroid gland was enlarged. Results from the laboratory showed that free T_3 and T_4 were elevated and thyroid-stimulating hormone (TSH) was undetectable. The patient was diagnosed with Graves' disease and was placed on propylthiouracil, an antithyroid drug.

WHAT ARE THE ANATOMICAL CHARACTERISTICS OF THE THYROID GLAND?

The salient characteristics of the thyroid gland are:

- Brownish-red and highly vascular
- Mass of approximately 25 g in adults; slightly larger in females. The gland also enlarges during menstruation and pregnancy.
- Right and left lobes are each approximately 5 cm long and are connected at their inferior poles by the isthmus.

WHAT ARE THE ANATOMICAL RELATIONSHIPS OF THE THYROID GLAND?

To truly know your anatomy is to know who the anatomical neighbors are. In the case of the thyroid gland, its anatomical relationships in the neck are:

- Deep to the sternohyoid, sternothyroid, and omohyoid muscles
- Anterior to C5 through T1 vertebrae
- Isthmus of thyroid lies anterior to the 2nd and 3rd tracheal cartilaginous rings

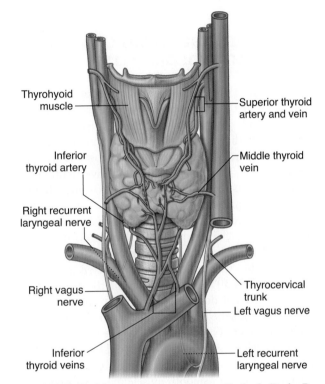

FIGURE 7-23 Vasculature of the thyroid gland. (Drake R, Vogl W and Mitchell A: *Gray's Anatomy for Students*. Churchill Livingstone, 2004. Fig. 8.169)

WHAT IS THE ARTERIAL SUPPLY TO THE THYROID GLAND?

The highly vascular thyroid gland receives its blood supply from the (Fig. 7-23):

- Superior thyroid arteries
- Inferior thyroid arteries

The superior thyroid artery is a branch of the external carotid artery, whereas the inferior thyroid artery arises from the thyrocervical trunk, which issues from the subclavian artery. Occasionally, the thyroid gland also may be supplied by the thyroid ima artery. This artery has multiple origins and has been described, for example, branching from the brachiocephalic trunk, right common carotid artery, aortic arch, and internal thoracic artery. Because of its midline ascension in the neck, the thyroid ima artery is vulnerable to injury when performing midline procedures in the neck.

HOW DO THE THYROID HORMONES REACH THE RIGHT ATRIUM?

The venous blood, which contains the thyroid hormones, is drained by the paired superior, middle, and inferior thyroid veins. The superior and middle veins are tributaries of the internal jugular vein, which then drains into the brachiocephalic vein. The inferior thyroid veins drain into the brachiocephalic veins. Blood then flows from the brachiocephalic veins to the superior vena cava before emptying in the right atrium.

HOW DOES THE THYROID GLAND FORM EMBRYOLOGICALLY?

The thyroid gland forms from the endoderm that lines the floor of the primitive pharynx between the first and second pharyngeal pouches. This endoderm thickens in the median plane and begins its descent into the ventral neck as the embryo grows. During its descent, the thyroid primordium (diverticulum) is tethered to its origin by the thyroglossal duct. Before the thyroid primordium completes its caudal migration, it bifurcates into two lobes, which are connected by an isthmus. The thyroglossal duct normally regresses, leaving behind an anatomical landmark on the base of the tongue called the *foramen cecum*. In approximately 50% of the population, the distal end of the thyroglossal duct fails to regress. This persistent segment forms the pyramidal lobe of the thyroid gland. When present, it is not unusual for the pyramidal lobe to be superiorly anchored to the hyoid bone by fibrous tissue and smooth muscle, levator of the thyroid gland, though this smooth muscle may be absent.

As a clinical aside, remnants of the thyroglossal duct may persist anywhere along its course. A remnant may then form a thyroglossal cyst. These cysts may develop in the tongue or in the anterior neck.

WHAT ARE THE HISTOLOGIC CHARACTERISTICS OF THE THYROID GLAND?

The thyroid gland is invested by a thin capsule of dense irregular collagenous tissue. Septa from the capsule extend into the substance of the gland, dividing it into lobules. The lobules contain prominent follicles, which are composed of colloid and cells (Fig. 7-24). The eosinophilic colloid represents a storage depot of thyroid hormones (triiodothyronine

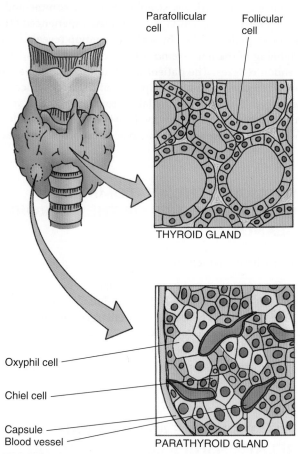

FIGURE 7-24 Illustrations of the thyroid and parathyroid glands. (Gartner L and Hiatt J: *Color Textbook of Histology, 2e.* WB Saunders, 2001. Fig. 13-6.)

and tetraiodothyronine) bound to the protein called *thyroglobulin*. The colloid is contained in the large lumen of the follicle. A ring of follicular cells surrounds the colloid, with the basal domains of these cells supported by a basal lamina. Some parafollicular (also know as clear or C) cells are found within the follicular epithelium, but they do not extend to the lumen of the follicle.

WHAT ARE THE CHARACTERISTICS OF FOLLICULAR CELLS?

The shape of the follicular cells ranges from squamous to short columnar depending on the degree of stimulation from TSH. When the follicular cells are not being stimulated by TSH, the quiescent cells assume a squamous shape. With stimulation, the cells morph into short columnar cells to accommodate the increase in volume of organelles to synthesize and release thyroid hormones.

WHAT ARE THE PATHOLOGIC CHANGES OF THE THYROID GLAND THAT ARE ASSOCIATED WITH GRAVES' DISEASE?

In Graves' disease, the thyroid gland possesses the following characteristics:

- Shows significant enlargement and may have a mass of more than 80 g (normal mass is about 25 g). The increase in size is the result of hypertrophy and hyperplasia of the follicular cells.
- In response to the sustained stimulation, the follicular cells assume a columnar profile and appear crowded in the epithelium. The colloid becomes lighter than normal and its margins appear corrugated (Fig. 7-25).
- Since this is an autoimmune disorder, it is no surprise that the interstitium has a significant population of lymphocytes. T cells predominant, but B cells and plasma cells are also present.

Cells with the potential to differentiate into adipocytes, preadipocyte fibroblasts, occupy the retro-orbital space. The cells, like the follicular cells of the thyroid gland, express the receptor for TSH. The precipitating event is invasion of mononuclear cells (predominately T cells and some B cells) into the retro-orbital space. The presence of the TSH receptors on the preadipocyte fibroblasts causes the mono-nuclear cells to mount an autoimmunologic attack against these receptors. This attack prompts the T cells to release various cytokines that stimulate proliferation and deposition of glycosaminoglycans (GAGs), specifically hyaluronic acid and chondroitin sulfate. The accumulation of hydrophilic GAGs expands the volume of the extracellular matrix within the confines of the retro-orbital space by hydration. Moreover, cytokines cause the preadipocyte fibroblasts to ramp up expression of TSH receptors on the surfaces of their plasma membranes. This process amplifies the autoimmune response. Other responses by the autoimmune attack are edema of the extraocular muscles and differentiation of preadipocyte fibroblasts into adipocytes. All these responses conspire to expand the volume of the retro-orbital space, thereby protruding the eye.

WHAT ARE THE EFFECTS OF GRAVES' DISEASE ON THE HEART?

Elevated thyroid hormones have several effects on the heart and cardiomyocytes. These effects include:

- Hypertrophy of the cardiac muscle cells
- Increase in mitochondrial volume density. This means that mitochondria comprise a greater percentage of the total volume of the cardiac myocyte. The research data also show that the increase in mitochondrial volume is greater than the enlargement of the cell.
- Myofibrillar volume remains unchanged from the euthyroid condition. This means that the myofibrils increase in proportion to the increase in cell size.
- Membrane growth (sarcolemma and sarcoplasmic reticulum) is proportional to the increase in cell volume
- Increase in capillary density (number of capillaries per mm^2). This enhances oxygen and nutrient delivery to more metabolically active cardiac myocytes.
- Alterations in the synthesis of myosin heavy chains and myosin isoenzymes in the ventricles but not the atria. Thyroid hormones and/or changes in myocardial workload cause myosin heavy chain synthesis to change from the beta to the alpha form. Switching to the alpha myosin heavy chain also changes the myosin isoenzyme to V_1, which is faster than the V_3 isoform (V_1 and V_3 isoforms are the ATPases associated with the heads of the myosin heavy chains) associated with the beta myosin heavy chain. Because of the increase in V_1, ATP is

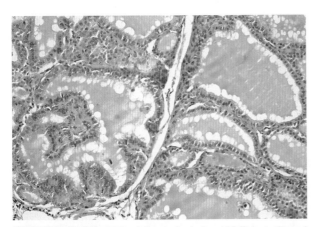

FIGURE 7-25 Diffusely hyperplastic thyroid follicles in Graves' disease. (Kumar V, Abbas A and Fausto N: *Robbins & Cotran Pathologic Basis of Disease*, 7e. WB Saunders, 2004. Fig. 24-12.)

enzymatically cleaved at a greater rate (this increases the energy consumption of the cardiac myocyte). This increase in energy cost, however, leads to a decrease in contractile efficiency.

- Thyroid hormones increase gene expression of Ca^{2+}-ATPase associated with the sarcoplasmic reticulum. This increases the calcium ion handling capacity of the sarcoplasmic reticulum.

- Thyroid hormones also increase gene expression of GLUT-4, an insulin-dependent glucose transporter.

GLUT-4 receptors are found on the target cells of insulin. Increased GLUT-4 enhances the rate of glucose influx by thyroid hormone-stimulated cardiac muscle cells.

- Lastly, gene expression of beta1-adrenergic receptors by thyroid hormones causes the myocardium to be more responsive to the action of the sympathetic nervous division.

A 66-year-old man presented to his physician with complaints of hand tremors and stiffness of movement. During the history, the patient revealed that he had difficulty walking, getting out of his chair, and swallowing. He also stated that he started drooling about a month ago. The physician noted that the patient answered his questions in a whispering, rapid speech pattern. The physical examination showed that the patient had pill-rolling bilateral hand tremor at rest that diminished with voluntary movement, muscle rigidity with a series of brief muscle relaxations (cogwheel rigidity), and bradykinesia. A minor degree of postural instability was observed as the patient slightly stumbled forward during ambulation and maintained a stooped-forward posture. The patient was diagnosed with Parkinson's disease and was treated with L-DOPA.

WHAT STRUCTURE OF THE BRAIN, WHEN DAMAGED, PRODUCES THE SYMPTOMS OF PARKINSON'S DISEASE?

Parkinson's disease is a lesion of the basal ganglia characterized by a loss of dopaminergic neurons in the substantia nigra, a bilateral nucleus that extends through the length of the midbrain (Fig. 7-26A). The neurons, which project to the corpus striatum (composed of the caudate nucleus, putamen, and globus pallidus), are responsible for inhibiting movements. Loss of this inhibition through the degeneration of the neurons in the substantia nigra permits movements that the patient does not want to perform but cannot prevent.

WHAT BRAIN NUCLEI CONSTITUTE THE BASAL GANGLIA?

There are five brain nuclei that are typically considered to be members of the basal ganglia. The family members are:

- Substantia nigra (Fig. 7-26A)
- Caudate nucleus (Fig. 7-27)
- Putamen (Fig. 7-27)
- Globus pallidus (Fig. 7-27)
- Subthalamic nucleus (not shown)

Collectively, the putamen and globus pallidus resemble a lentil and are aptly referred to as the *lentiform (lenticular) nucleus*. The corpus striatum is composed of the lentiform and caudate nuclei, and the caudate nucleus and putamen are collectively called the striatum.

WHAT ARE THE PATHOLOGIC FEATURES OF PARKINSON'S DISEASE?

Gross inspection of sections from the midbrain of a parkinsonian brain reveals overt depigmentation (melanin is the pigment that is lost) in the substantia nigra owing to the loss of dopaminergic neurons (Fig. 7-26B). Microscopic observation confirms neuronal loss that is accompanied by an excess number of astrocytes (gliosis). Surviving neurons may contain one or more eosinophilic inclusions known as Lewy bodies (Fig. 7-26C). Lewy bodies are elongated or round in appearance and often contain a dense eosinophilic core surrounded by a light halo. Lewy bodies contain filaments of α-synuclein, as well as neurofilaments, parkin, and ubiquitin.

WHY WAS THE PATIENT TREATED WITH L-DOPA RATHER THAN DOPAMINE?

Dopamine is unable to cross the blood-brain barrier in the central nervous system, whereas L-DOPA, being a smaller precursor molecule for the dopamine synthetic pathway, is capable of crossing the barrier into the neural interstitium. Once in the interstitium, it enters dopaminergic neurons to enter the synthetic pathway for dopamine.

The blood-brain barrier is established by the following structural features:

- Continuous capillaries, which are the least porous of the three types of capillaries

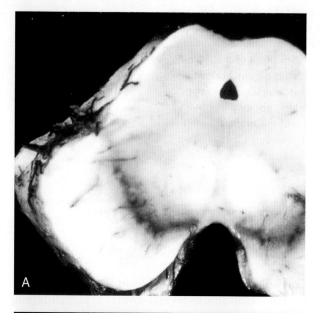

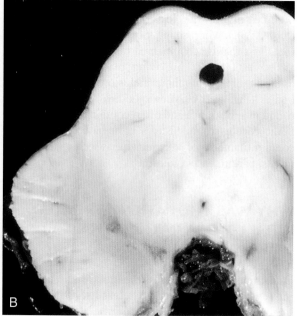

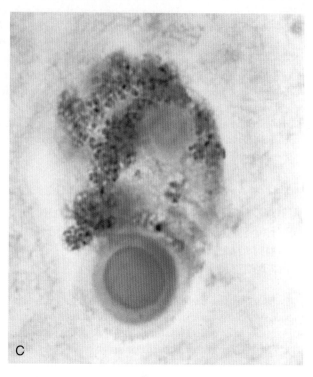

FIGURE 7-26 Parkinson's disease. **A,** Normal black-staining substantia nigra. **B,** Substantia nigra is depigmented. **C,** Bright eosinophilic Lewy bodies in a neuron of the substantia nigra. (Kumar V, Abbas A and Fausto N: *Robbins & Cotran Pathologic Basis of Disease, 7e.* WB Saunders, 2004. Fig. 28-37. Part C Courtesy of Dr. R. Kim, V.A. Medical Center, Long Beach, CA.)

- Fasciae occludentes tightly join endothelial cells to one another, reducing the intercellular space. This structural attribute restricts the passage of molecules through the intercellular space.
- Pinocytotic vesicles are relatively few in number. This feature limits vesicular transport of substances across the endothelium.

The basal lamina and astrocytes also play roles in selectively allowing chemicals into and out of the neural interstitium. These structures, however, are not structural elements of the blood-brain barrier.

WHAT IS THE BLOOD SUPPLY TO THE MIDBRAIN?

The major blood supply to the midbrain is from three arteries:

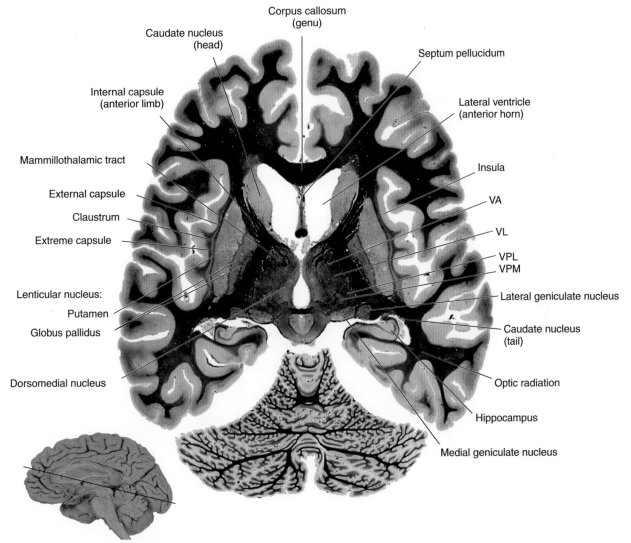

FIGURE 7-27 Basal ganglia in a horizontal section of the brain. (Nolte J: *The Human Brain*, 5e. Mosby, 2002. Fig. 19-1. Modified from Nolte J, Angevine JB Jr: *The Human Brain in Photographs and Diagrams*, ed 2, St. Louis, 2000; Mosby.)

- Basilar, which is formed by the union of the vertebral arteries
- Superior cerebellar arteries, which spring from the basilar artery prior to its terminal bifurcation

- Posterior cerebral arteries, which are the terminal branches of the bifurcation of the basilar artery

A 52-year-old woman presented to her physician with complaints of fatigue, weakness, constipation, and that she passed a small kidney stone 4 days ago. Her physical examination was unremarkable. The lab results showed elevations in the patient's blood calcium and parathyroid hormone levels. Radiologic findings revealed increased bone resorption. A technetium-99m-sestamibi radionuclide scan demonstrated increased uptake in the superior right parathyroid gland. The patient was diagnosed with primary hyperparathyroidism caused by an adenoma. A parathyroidectomy was performed.

WHAT ARE THE GROSS ANATOMICAL CHARACTERISTICS OF THE PARATHYROID GLANDS?

The parathyroid glands have the following gross anatomical characteristics:

- Although the number of parathyroid glands is variable, there are normally four: a pair of superior and a pair of inferior glands (Fig. 7-28).
- The mass of each yellow-brown gland is approximately 35 to 40 mg.
- Superior parathyroid glands are embedded in fat posterior to the superior lobe of the thyroid gland.
- Inferior parathyroid glands are more variable in location. They may be located in the fascial thyroid sheath caudal to the inferior thyroid artery; external to the thyroid sheath cranial to the inferior thyroid artery; and in the inferior pole of the thyroid gland. These locations are of surgical significance. Tumors of the parathyroid glands located in the fascial thyroid sheath may migrate along the

inferior thyroid veins into the superior mediastinum by passing anterior to the trachea. If the inferior parathyroid glands are located outside the sheath, a tumor may extend into the posterior mediastinum by descending posteroinferiorly to the esophagus.

WHAT IS THE ARTERIAL SUPPLY TO THE PARATHYROID GLANDS?

The rich arterial supply to the parathyroid glands is from the inferior thyroid artery or the anastomosis between the superior and inferior thyroid arteries (Fig. 7-28).

WHAT IS THE VENOUS DRAINAGE OF THE PARATHYROID GLANDS?

A venous plexus located on the anterior surface of the thyroid gland and trachea receives the superior, middle, and inferior parathyroid veins.

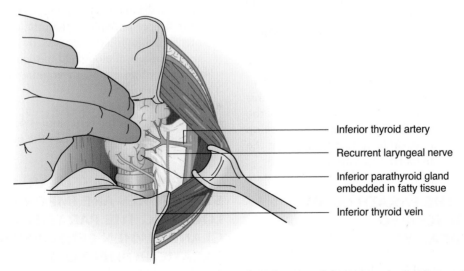

Inferior thyroid artery

Recurrent laryngeal nerve

Inferior parathyroid gland embedded in fatty tissue

Inferior thyroid vein

FIGURE 7-28 Relationship of parathyroid glands to the inferior thyroid artery and the recurrent laryngeal nerve. (Towsend C et al.: *Sabiston Textbook of Surgery, 17e.* WB Saunders, 2004. Fig. 35-9. From Yim JH, Doherty GM: Operative strategies in primary hyperparathyroidism. In doherty GM, Skogseld B (eds): *Surgical Endocrinology.* Philadelphia, Lippincott Williams & Wilkins, 2001, p. 167.)

WHAT IS THE LYMPHATIC DRAINAGE OF THE PARATHYROID GLANDS?

Lymphatic vessels drain into the deep cervical and paratracheal lymph nodes.

WHAT IS THE INNERVATION OF THE PARATHYROID GLANDS?

Sympathetic nerve fibers innervate the parathyroid. The fibers are vasomotor and the fibers are from the superior or middle cervical ganglia or from a plexus that follows the superior and inferior thyroid arteries.

HOW DO THE PARATHYROID GLANDS DEVELOP?

The parathyroid glands develop from the endoderm lining the third and fourth pharyngeal pouches. The inferior parathyroid glands derive from the third, and the superior parathyroid glands originate from the fourth. The parathyroid glands descend with the thymus gland. In the neck, the parathyroid glands separate from the thymus gland and assume their position on the dorsal surface of the thyroid gland. Because migration is variable, parathyroid glands do not always assume their normal positions. Ectopic inferior parathyroid glands may be found as high as the carotid artery bifurcation, or they may descend into the anterior mediastinum with the thymus gland.

The principal (chief) cells of the parathyroid gland develop during the embryonic period and assume an active functional role in regulating calcium homeostasis in the fetus. Oxyphil cells, on the other hand, do not differentiate until 5 to 7 years after birth. A third cell type found in the parenchyma of the thyroid gland is the parafollicular (also known as *clear or C*) cell. This cell type has a different embryonic origin than the principal and oxyphil cells. Parafollicular cells develop from the ultimopharyngeal body that forms from the ventral aspects of the fourth pharyngeal pouches.

HOW ARE THE PARATHYROID GLANDS DESCRIBED HISTOLOGICALLY?

Each parathyroid gland is enveloped by a thin capsule. Thin septa from the capsule penetrate the gland and serve to guide blood vessels, lymphatics, and nerves into and out of the gland. The septa also provide a network of reticular fibers to support the principal (chief) and oxyphil cells (Fig. 7-24). The parathyroid gland accumulates adipose tissue with increasing age. In some cases, adipose tissue may occupy 60% of the gland's total volume.

WHAT ARE THE CYTOLOGIC CHARACTERISTICS OF THE PRINCIPAL AND OXYPHIL CELLS?

The principal cell is actively involved in the synthesis and secretion of parathyroid hormone, a polypeptide. The active cell has the following constellation of features that are customarily observed in protein secretion:

- Small in diameter, 5 to 8 μm
- Lightly acidophilic cytoplasm
- Coarse granules in cytoplasm represent lipofuscin
- Juxtanuclear Golgi complex
- Abundant rough endoplasmic reticulum
- Elongated mitochondria
- Secretory granules
- Occasional desmosomes join neighboring principal cells.
- A cilium may be present.

Inactive principal cells possess a less elaborate array of organelles. These cells outnumber active ones by a ratio of 3–5 to 1.

The oxyphil cell, whose function remains to be elucidated, has the following characteristics:

- Larger in diameter, 6 to 10 μm, than the principal cell
- More deeply acidophilic than the principal cell
- Intense acidophilia is caused by the presence of large numbers of elongated mitochondria. The significance of an abundant volume of mitochondria remains an enigma.
- Golgi is poorly developed
- Rough endoplasmic reticulum is scanty.
- Glycogen is present between the mitochondria.

WHAT NEUROVASCULAR STRUCTURES ARE IMPORTANT IN LOCATING THE PARATHYROID GLANDS WHEN PERFORMING A PARATHYROIDECTOMY?

The inferior thyroid artery and the recurrent laryngeal nerve are important anatomical landmarks in locating the parathyroid glands (Fig. 7-28). The superior parathyroid glands are located within a 2-cm area cranial to the intersection of the inferior thyroid artery and the recurrent laryngeal nerve, whereas the inferior parathyroid glands are found proximate to the intersection.

WHAT IS THE MORPHOLOGY OF A PARATHYROID ADENOMA?

A parathyroid adenoma demonstrates the following morphology (Fig. 7-29):

- Predominately composed of well-differentiated chief cells. Well-differentiated tumor cells resemble normal cells.
- Adenoma is well circumscribed.
- Principal (chief) cells may arrange themselves in follicles.
- Few nests of oxyphil cells are visible.

- Mitotic figures are rarely seen.
- Some cells may contain oddly shaped nuclei.
- Normal principal cells outside of the adenoma appear normal in size or smaller than normal. The cells become smaller as a result of the negative feedback of elevated calcium (i.e., low calcium stimulates the cells and elevated calcium inhibits the cells).

WHAT ARE THE RADIOLOGIC FINDINGS THAT ACCOMPANY HYPERPARATHYROIDISM?

Hyperparathyroidism can result in increased subperiosteal bone resorption. This is best observed in the following osteologic sites:

- Lateral (radial) sides of the phalanges
- Tips of the distal phalanges
- Acromial ends of the clavicles

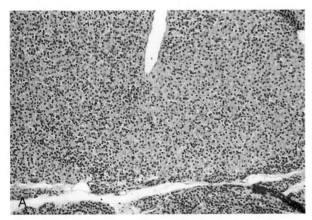 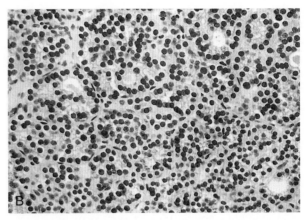

FIGURE 7-29 Parathyroid adenoma. **A,** Low power micrograph of a chief cell parathyroid adenoma. **B,** High power micrograph of a chief cell parathyroid adenoma. Nuclear size is fairly uniform. (Kumar V, Abbas A and Fausto N: *Robbins & Cotran Pathologic Basis of Disease,* 7e. WB Saunders, 2004. Fig. 24-25.)

A 3-month-old boy, delivered by caesarian section, was brought to the pediatrician. The mother was concerned about the peculiar tilt of her son's head. The pediatrician, after a brief examination, told the mother that her son had congenital torticollis and that it needed to be surgically corrected.

WHAT IS THE CAUSE OF CONGENITAL TORTICOLLIS?

As there was no birth trauma, the suspected cause of congenital torticollis is a deficient arterial blood supply to the sternocleidomastoid muscle during development. The resulting ischemia causes the underdeveloped muscle to be shorter than its fellow.

In cases of birth trauma, fibers of the sternocleidomastoid muscle may be torn. As a normal response to injury, the damaged muscle fibers are replaced by fibrous tissue, which causes the muscle to be shorter than normal.

THE AFFECTED MUSCLE CAN BE LENGTHENED BY SURGICAL DIVISION. WHERE SHOULD THE MUSCLE BE DIVIDED?

The sternocleidomastoid muscle should be divided inferior to its innervation by the accessory nerve (CN XI), which is accomplished at its inferior attachment. Dividing the muscle superior to its innervation will denervate the muscle by also dividing its nerve supply.

WHAT ARE THE ATTACHMENTS OF THE STERNOCLEIDOMASTOID MUSCLE?

The muscle originates as two heads. The sternal head is attached to the manubrium, and the clavicular head is attached to the medial one-third of the clavicle. The muscle inserts on the mastoid process and the lateral portion of the superior nuchal line of the occipital bone.

THE SHORTENED STERNOCLEIDOMASTOID MUSCLE MIMICS THE NORMAL ACTIONS OF THIS MUSCLE DURING CONTRACTION. WHAT POSITION WOULD THE HEAD BE IN IF THE RIGHT MUSCLE WAS AFFECTED?

Shortening of the right sternocleidomastoid muscle causes lateral flexion of the head to the same side and contralateral rotation of the head. The net result is that the chin points upward on the opposite side (Fig. 7-30).

WHAT IS THE BLOOD SUPPLY TO THE STERNOCLEIDOMASTOID MUSCLE?

The blood supply to the sternocleidomastoid muscle is from the:

● Sternocleidomastoid artery of the superior thyroid artery, a branch of the external carotid artery
● Sternocleidomastoid branches (usually two) of the occipital artery, a branch of the external carotid artery

WHAT IS THE INNERVATION TO THE STERNOCLEIDOMASTOID MUSCLE?

Motor innervation to the sternocleidomastoid muscle is provided by the accessory nerve (CN XI), and its proprioceptive (sensory) innervation is from the ventral primary rami of the second, third, and occasionally the fourth cervical nerves. It is now believed that some motor fibers are transmitted to the muscle via the cervical nerves.

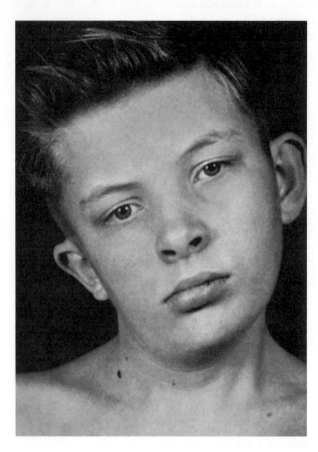

FIGURE 7-30 12-year-old boy with torticollis. (Moore K and Persaud TVN: *The Developing Human*, 7e. WB Saunders, 2003. Fig. 16-7. From Behman RE, Vaughan III VC: *Nelson Textbook of Pediatrics, 13th ed*. Philadelphia, WB Saunders, 1987.)

A 56-year-old woman presented to her physician with the chief complaint of excruciating facial pain that comes and goes. Triggered by eating, drinking, and face washing, the pain occurs on her nose, upper cheek, upper lip, and upper teeth. The patient has lost weight since her last visit 10 months ago and is dehydrated. The physical examination was unremarkable and a magnetic resonance imaging (MRI) study of the head revealed demyelination of a cranial nerve. Based on these findings, the patient was diagnosed with cranial nerve neuralgia and was initially treated with carbamazepine, an oral anticonvulsant. When the patient developed tolerance to this medication, microvascular decompression surgery was performed.

WHICH CRANIAL NERVE IS INVOLVED IN PRODUCING THE PATIENT'S SYMPTOMS?

The patient was diagnosed with neuralgia of the trigeminal nerve, which is also known as tic douloureux. The trigeminal nerve is composed of three divisions:

- Ophthalmic (V_1)
- Maxillary (V_2)
- Mandibular (V_3)

The specific division producing the symptoms in this scenario is the maxillary nerve, which conveys general sensory fibers. Trigeminal neuralgia frequently involves the maxillary or mandibular divisions, or both, but rarely affects the ophthalmic nerve.

WHAT ARE THE SENSORY AND MOTOR DISTRIBUTIONS OF THE TRIGEMINAL NERVE?

The motor and sensory distribution (Figs. 7-31 and 7-32) of the trigeminal nerve and its branches are described in Table 7-2.

THE MANDIBULAR DIVISION OF THE TRIGEMINAL NERVE SUPPLIES THE MUSCLES OF MASTICATION. WHAT ARE THE ATTACHMENTS AND ACTIONS OF THE MUSCLES OF MASTICATION?

The four muscles of mastication and their attachments and actions are described in Table 7-3.

WHICH CELL TYPE IS RESPONSIBLE FOR THE MYELINATION OF THE CRANIAL NERVE AND WHAT ARE ITS CYTOLOGIC CHARACTERISTICS?

Schwann cells are responsible for the myelination of peripheral nerves. Peripheral nerves are the 12 pairs of cranial nerves and the 31 pairs of spinal nerves. A myelinated axon consists of many individual Schwann cells, each forming myelin around a short segment of the axon. The minute gaps between the cells are the nodes of Ranvier. Schwann cells that myelinate axons possess the following characteristics (Fig. 7-33):

- Flattened cells with flattened nuclei
- Golgi apparatus is poorly developed.
- Mitochondria are few in number.
- Myelin is the plasmalemma of the cell.

Unmyelinated axons in the peripheral nervous system are also enveloped by Schwann cells. In contrast to myelinated axons, one Schwann can envelop several unmyelinated axons (Fig. 7-34).

WHAT IS THE PURPOSE OF MICROVASCULAR DECOMPRESSION SURGERY?

Trigeminal neuralgia is most likely caused by compression of the trigeminal nerve by a branch from the superior cerebellar artery. Compression of the root of the trigeminal nerve where it attaches to the pons causes it to lose its insulation of myelin. The loss of this insulation allows the bare axons to cross-communicate with one another. Access to the site of compression is made by performing a craniectomy posterior to the mastoid process. This point of access is at the junction of the sigmoid and transverse sinuses.

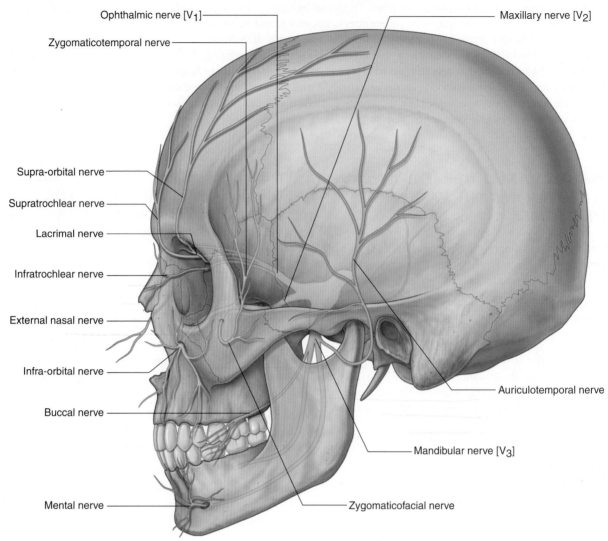

FIGURE 7-31 Trigeminal nerve (CN V). (Drake R, Vogl W and Mitchell A: *Gray's Anatomy for Students*. Churchill Livingstone, 2004. Fig. 8-58)

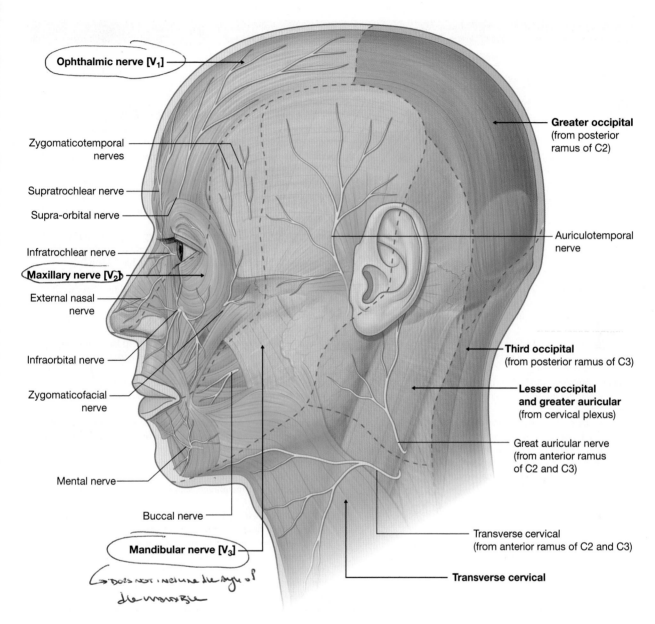

Ophthalmic nerve [V₁]

Zygomaticotemporal nerves

Supratrochlear nerve

Supra-orbital nerve

Infratrochlear nerve

Maxillary nerve [V₂]

External nasal nerve

Infraorbital nerve

Zygomaticofacial nerve

Mental nerve

Buccal nerve

Mandibular nerve [V₃]

→ Does not include the angle of the mandible

Greater occipital (from posterior ramus of C2)

Auriculotemporal nerve

Third occipital (from posterior ramus of C3)

Lesser occipital and greater auricular (from cervical plexus)

Great auricular nerve (from anterior ramus of C2 and C3)

Transverse cervical (from anterior ramus of C2 and C3)

Transverse cervical

FIGURE 7-32 Cutaneous distribution of the trigeminal nerve (CN V). (Drake R, Vogl W and Mitchell A: *Gray's Anatomy for Students.* Churchill Livingstone, 2004. Fig. 8-59)

TABLE 7-2 Sensory and Motor Distribution of the Trigeminal Nerve

Division	Branch of Division	Distribution
Ophthalmic nerve	Lacrimal nerve (smallest of the main branches of the ophthalmic nerve)	Sensory to lacrimal gland, adjoining conjunctiva, and upper eyelid
Ophthalmic nerve	Frontal nerve (largest branch of the ophthalmic nerve)	Sensory via supratrochlear nerve to conjunctiva, skin of upper eyelid, and skin of inferior forehead near midline
		Sensory via supraorbital nerve to conjunctiva and upper eyelid, skin of scalp back to lambdoid suture, and mucosa of frontal sinus
Ophthalmic nerve	Nasociliary nerve	Sensory via anterior ethmoidal nerve to medial and lateral nasal walls and to skin of nose
		Sensory via infratrochlear nerve to skin of eyelids, conjunctiva, lacrimal sac, and lacrimal caruncle
		Sensory via posterior ethmoidal nerve to ethmoidal and sphenoidal sinuses
		Sensory via long ciliary nerves to the ciliary body, iris, and cornea. Long ciliary nerves also convey sympathetic postganglionic fibers from the superior cervical ganglion to the dilator pupillae
Maxillary nerve	Middle meningeal nerve	Sensory to dura mater
Maxillary nerve	Posterior, middle, and anterior superior alveolar nerves	Sensory to the maxillary sinus, nasal septum, and maxillary teeth
Maxillary nerve	Palpebral, nasal, and superior labial nerves	Sensory to skin of lower eyelid, nose, anterior cheek, and upper lip. Also supplies the oral mucosa and labial glands
Maxillary nerve	Ganglionic branches (connect maxillary nerve to the pterygopalatine ganglion)	Ganglionic fibers contain secretomotor fibers to lacrimal gland. Sensory to periosteum of orbit and mucosae from nose, palate, and pharynx
Mandibular nerve	Meningeal branch (nervus spinosus)	Sensory to dura mater in the middle cranial fossa
Mandibular nerve	Nerve to medial pterygoid	Motor to medial pterygoid, tensor tympani, and tensor veli palatini muscles
Mandibular nerve	Buccal nerve (long buccal nerve)	Sensory to skin over buccinator muscle, buccal mucosa, and gingiva
Mandibular nerve	Masseteric nerve	Motor to masseter muscle and sensory to temporomandibular joint
Mandibular nerve	Deep temporal nerves (usually two)	Motor to the temporalis muscle
Mandibular nerve	Lateral pterygoid nerve	Motor to the lateral pterygoid muscle
Mandibular nerve	Auriculotemporal nerve	Sensory to the temporomandibular joint, auricle, external acoustic meatus, tympanic membrane, skin of temporal region and skin of lateral scalp
		Parotid branches carry postganglionic parasympathetic fibers. These secretomotor fibers are transmitted by the communication of the auriculotemporal nerve with the otic ganglion
Mandibular nerve	Lingual nerve	Sensory to the submandibular gland, mucosa of anterior two-thirds of tongue, adjacent mouth and gingivae, and sublingual gland
Mandibular nerve	Inferior alveolar nerve	Supplies mandibular teeth and its termination, the mental nerve, supplies skin of chin and skin and mucosa of inferior lip

TABLE 7-3 Muscles of Mastication

Muscle	Origin	Insertion	Action
Temporalis	Along inferior temporal line, temporal fossa, and temporal fascia	Coronoid process and ramus of mandible	Elevates mandible and retracts mandible following its protrusion
Masseter	Zygomatic arch	Lateral surface of mandibular ramus and coronoid process	Elevates, protracts mandible. Deep fibers of muscle retract mandible
Lateral pterygoid	Superior head: Inferior temporal surface and greater wing of sphenoid bone Inferior head: Lateral surface of lateral pterygoid plate of sphenoid bone	Neck of mandible and articular disc, and capsule of temporomandibular joint	Protrudes mandible and depresses mandible when acting bilaterally. Contracting alternately, they produce side-to-side movements of the mandible
Medial pterygoid	Superficial head: Tuberosity of maxilla Deep head: Medial aspect of lateral pterygoid plate and pyramidal process of palatine bone	Medial surface of mandibular ramus just inferior to mandibular foramen	Bilaterally, protrudes and elevates mandible. Unilaterally, muscle protrudes jaw ipsilaterally and when alternately contracting they produce a grinding action.

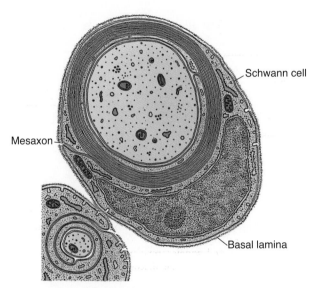

FIGURE 7-33 Myelinated nerve fiber. (Gartner L and Hiatt J: *Color Textbook of Histology, 2e*. WB Saunders, 2001. Fig. 9-7. From Lentz TL: *Cell Fine Structure: An Atlas of Drawings of Whole-Cell Structure*. Philadelphia, WB Saunders, 1971.)

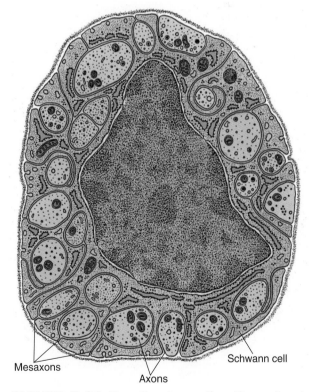

FIGURE 7-34 Unmyelinated nerve fiber. (Gartner L and Hiatt J: *Color Textbook of Histology, 2e*. WB Saunders, 2001. Fig. 9-8. From Lentz TL: *Cell Fine Structure: An Atlas of Drawings of Whole-Cell Structure*. Philadelphia, WB Saunders, 1971.)

A 55-year-old man was found in a closed garage with the car engine running. Police initially concluded it was a suicide attempt. He was treated for carbon monoxide poisoning. Upon questioning of his family, it was learned that everything had gone well over the holidays and everyone in the family was fine. He really had no reason to kill himself and had never discussed it. Further questioning of his family revealed certain behavioral changes to include forgetfulness and mild confusion, and complaints of headaches. A neurologic examination of cranial nerve function indicated extraocular muscle movements were limited. A magnetic resonance imaging (MRI) study was ordered. Results of the MRI showed bilateral watershed infarcts of the frontal lobes caused by a pituitary gland tumor (Fig. 7-35).

WHAT IS THE EMBRYOLOGIC ORIGIN OF THE PITUITARY GLAND?

The distinct histologic differences of the adenohypophysis and the neurohypophysis are explained by their dual embryologic origin (Fig. 7-36). The neurohypophysis, being composed of neural elements, is derived from the neuroectoderm of the diencephalon. The adenohypophysis, being glandular in nature, has an epithelial origin from the ectoderm lining the roof of the stomodeum (primitive mouth). A diverticulum, called the *hypophysial (Rathke's) pouch*, develops from the oral ectoderm, ultimately giving rise to the adenohypophysis.

SURGERY IS THE PREFERRED PROCEDURE FOR TREATING TUMORS OF THE PITUITARY GLAND. ONE METHOD OF ACCESSING THE GLAND IS BY ENTERING THE NOSTRIL. HOW IS THIS ANATOMICALLY POSSIBLE?

A transsphenoidal surgical approach is practical because of the anatomical relationships (remember, to know your anatomy is to know your anatomical neighbors!) of the pituitary gland, sphenoid sinus, and nasal cavity. Surgical instruments are inserted into the

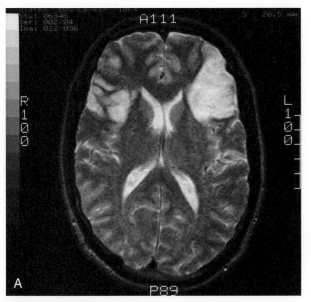

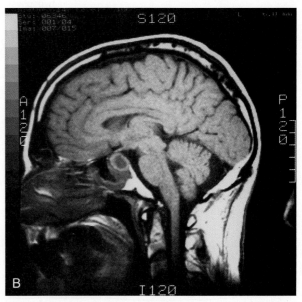

FIGURE 7-35 Watershed infarction secondary to a pituitary gland tumor. **A,** Watershed infarction of frontal lobes. **B,** Pituitary gland tumor is represented by a white halo.

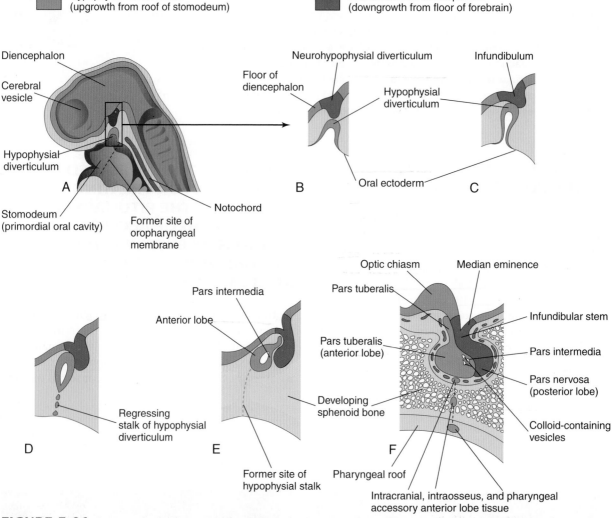

FIGURE 7-36 Stages in the development of the pituitary gland. **A,** Hypophysial diverticulum and neurohypophysial diverticulum is shown at 36 days. **B,** Enlarged view of **A. C to F,** Successive stages of pituitary gland development. (Moore K and Persaud TVN: *The Developing Human*, 7e. WB Saunders, 2003. Fig. 18-25.)

right nostril and passed along the superior margin of the nasal septum (Fig. 7-37). At the superior-posterior region of the right nasal cavity resides the sphenoid sinus. The mucosa of the anterior wall is incised, exposing the bone of the sinus. The bone is then surgically removed, permitting entry into the sinus. From here, the pituitary gland, sitting in the sella turcica, is accessed by cutting through the roof of the sphenoid sinus.

HOW DOES A PITUITARY GLAND TUMOR COMPROMISE ARTERIAL BLOOD FLOW TO THE FRONTAL LOBES AND LIMIT EXTRAOCULAR MUSCLE MOVEMENTS?

The anatomical relationships of the pituitary gland with the cavernous sinuses are shown in Figure 7-38. The structures traversing the cavernous sinuses are the:

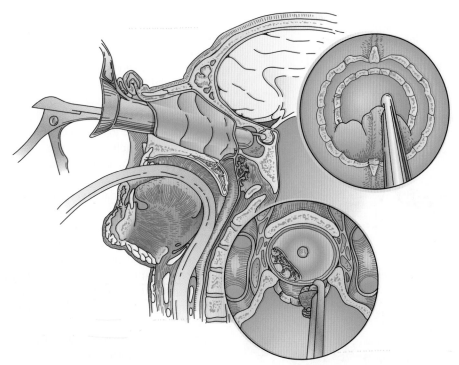

FIGURE 7-37 Transphenoidal approach to the pituitary gland. (Towsend C et al.: *Sabiston Textbook of Surgery, 17e.* WB Saunders, 2004. Fig. 37-9. Reported from Tindall GT, Barrow DL: *Disorders of the Pituitary.* St. Louis, CV Mosby, 1986.)

- Internal carotid artery
- Cranial nerve III (oculomotor)
- Cranial nerve IV (trochlear)
- Cranial nerve VI (abducent)
- Ophthalmic nerve (V_1)
- Maxillary nerve (V_2)

Expansion of the pituitary gland tumor into the cavernous sinuses compresses the internal carotid artery and cranial nerves III, IV, and VI. Compression of the internal carotid artery sufficiently reduced the perfusion pressure to the distal branches of the anterior and middle cerebral arteries to cause a watershed infarction of the frontal lobes.

Involvement of cranial nerves III, IV, and VI may limit extraocular movements, as these nerves supply the extraocular muscles. The extraocular muscles innervated by these cranial nerves, and their attachments and actions, are described in Table 7-4.

WHAT FUNCTIONS ARE ATTRIBUTED TO THE FRONTAL LOBES?

Many functions are attributed to the frontal lobes. These include behavior, emotion, motivation, planning, judgment, olfaction, problem solving, voluntary movements, and, in the left frontal lobe, language production. The lesions in this clinical scenario evoked behavioral changes, but the other functions remained intact.

HOW CAN THE FRONTAL CORTEX BE DESCRIBED HISTOLOGICALLY?

The neocortex, which includes the frontal cortex, is stratified into six layers. Residing in these cortical layers are neurons and the more numerous neuroglial cells. Comprising about 75% of the nerve population is the pyramidal cell, the principal projection nerve cell of the neocortex. The remaining neurons, which exhibit diverse morphology, are collectively referred to as *nonpyramidal cells.* The multipolar stellate (granule) cell, a type of interneuron, is the most common member of the nonpyramidal cell family. Other nerve cell members are identified on the basis of their shape and include basket cells, chandelier cells, bipolar cells, horizontal cells (of Cajal), double bouquet cells, Martinotti cells (triangular in shape), and other small, multipolar neurons.

From external to internal, the layers of the frontal cortex are:

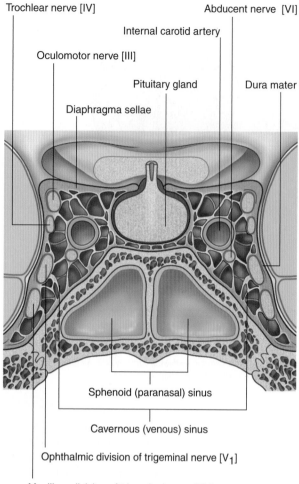

Trochlear nerve [IV]

Abducent nerve [VI]

Internal carotid artery

Oculomotor nerve [III]

Pituitary gland

Dura mater

Diaphragma sellae

Sphenoid (paranasal) sinus

Cavernous (venous) sinus

Ophthalmic division of trigeminal nerve [V₁]

Maxillary division of trigeminal nerve [V₂]

FIGURE 7-38 Relationship of pituitary gland to cavernous sinus. (Drake R, Vogl W and Mitchell A: *Gray's Anatomy for Students.* Churchill Livingstone, 2004. Fig. 8-44.)

- Molecular layer (I) — This layer is immediately deep to the pia mater and contains a few horizontal cells, neuroglia, and a dense plexus of axons and dendrites from the horizontal and other nonpyramidal cells.
- External granule layer (II) — Residing in this layer are granule (stellate) cells, small pyramidal cells, and neuroglia. The granule cells have apically directed dendrites, which end in the molecular layer, and axons that project into the deeper layers of the cortex.
- External pyramidal layer (III) — This layer is distinguished by the presence of the large pyramidal cells, which progressively get larger from the superficial to the deeper regions of this stratum. Nonpyramidal cells are also found in this lamina.
- Internal granule layer (IV) — Tightly packed granule cells, scattered pyramidal cells, and neuroglia occupy this cortical layer. This layer constitutes the chief input layer to the cortex and is thick in the primary sensory cortex and thin and indistinct in the primary motor cortex.
- Internal pyramidal layer (V) — Large pyramidal cells and neuroglia comprise this stratum. Layer V represents the principal projection (output) layer and is well developed in the primary motor cortex and thin in the primary sensory cortex.
- Multiform layer (VI) — This layer contains a few pyramidal cells, nonpyramidal cells, and neuroglia.

In the area of the watershed infarct, the neocortical layers are all well represented. This histologic architecture is called *homotypical.*

↳ All layers are well developed

Muscle	Origin	Insertion	Nerve Supply	Action
Superior oblique	Body of sphenoid bone	After passing through the trochlea, it attaches to the superior part of sclera deep to the attachment of the superior rectus muscle	Trochlear nerve (CN IV)	Abducts, depresses, and medially rotates eyeball
Inferior oblique	Anterior aspect of floor of orbit	Inferior part of sclera deep to inferior rectus muscle	Oculomotor nerve (CN III)	Abducts, elevates, and laterally rotates eyeball
Superior rectus	Common annular tendon	Superior part of sclera posterior to cornea	Oculomotor nerve (CN III)	Elevates, adducts, and medially rotates eyeball
Inferior rectus	Common annular tendon	Inferior part of sclera posterior to cornea	Oculomotor nerve (CN III)	Depresses, adducts, and medially rotates eyeball
Medial rectus	Common annular tendon	Medial part of sclera posterior to cornea	Oculomotor nerve (CN III)	Adducts eyeball
Lateral rectus	Common annular tendon	Lateral part of sclera posterior to cornea	Trochlear nerve (CN IV)	Abducts eyeball

TABLE 7-4 Extraocular Muscles

WHAT IS THE PATTERN OF NECROSIS THAT OFTEN OCCURS IN BRAIN TISSUE?

Hypoxic damage to brain tissue often causes liquefactive necrosis. Although the mechanism has not been elucidated for this pattern of cell death, it is characterized by the complete degradation of brain cells, forming a liquid mass.

SECTION 8

Multiple Choice Questions

1. The facial nerve is at risk of being compressed in the facial canal. Which bone contains the facial canal?

   A. Sphenoid bone

   B. Petrous portion of temporal bone

   C. Maxillary bone

   D. Occipital bone

   E. Ethmoid bone

2. What is the major constituent of Hirano bodies?

   A. Microtubules

   B. Neurofilaments

   C. Actin microfilaments

   D. Tau protein

   E. Cytokeratin

3. Which type of cell predominately morphs into foam cells in atherosclerosis?

   A. Smooth muscle cell   D. Fibroblast

   B. Neutrophil   E. Macrophage

   C. B lymphocyte

4. Which nerve is vulnerable to injury when the shoulder is dislocated?

   A. Axillary nerve

   B. Supra-scapular nerve

   C. Musculocutaneous nerve

   D. Thoracodorsal nerve

   E. Upper subscapular nerve

5. Which muscle separates the lateral collateral ligament from the lateral meniscus?

   A. Sartorius

   B. Plantaris

   C. Gracilis

   D. Lateral head of gastrocnemius

   E. Popliteus

6. What type of tissue is found in the organ of Zuckerkandl?

   A. Thyroid gland tissue

   B. Chromaffin tissue

   C. Adrenal cortical tissue

   D. Thymic tissue

   E. Pancreatic tissue

7. Winging of the scapula is a manifestation of Duchenne's muscular dystrophy. What muscle has atrophied so that winging of the scapula occurs?

   A. Rhomboid major   D. Subscapularis

   B. Serratus anterior   E. Teres major

   C. Levator scapulae

8. What ligament is damaged if a positive anterior drawer sign is observed?

   A. Posterior cruciate ligament

   B. Lateral collateral ligament

   C. Medial collateral ligament

   D. Anterior cruciate ligament

   E. Oblique popliteal ligament

9. What intracellular element does dystrophin anchor to the sarcolemma of a striated muscle fiber?

   A. Z line   D. Actin microfilaments

   B. a-Actinin   E. Vimentin

   C. Myosin filaments

10. Which nucleus is damaged in Alzheimer's disease that projects cholinergic fibers to the cerebral cortex?

    A. Putamen

    B. Nucleus of Meynert

    C. Substantia innominata

    D. Substantia nigra

    E. Caudate nucleus

11. Which artery is the main contributor to forming the anastomosis that supplies the femoral head?

A. Medial femoral circumflex artery
B. Lateral femoral circumflex artery
C. Artery to the head of the femur
D. Superior gluteal artery
E. Inferior gluteal artery

12. Clinically, glenohumeral dislocations occur in what direction?

A. Posterior
B. Superior
C. Inferior
D. Anterior
E. Posteroinferior

13. What joint is injured if the conoid and trapezoid ligaments are torn?

A. Hip
B. Glenohumeral
C. Acromioclavicular
D. Knee joint
E. Elbow

14. What is the weakest part of the fibrous capsule of the glenohumeral joint?

A. Anterior
B. Posterior
C. Inferior
D. Superior
E. Posteroinferior

15. Which one of the following cardiac defects is not one of the four cardinal features found in the tetralogy of Fallot?

A. Overriding aorta
B. Ventricular septal defect
C. Patent ductus arteriosus
D. Right ventricular hypertrophy
E. Pulmonary stenosis

16. Which segment of the intestines is most commonly aganglionic in Hirschsprung's disease?

A. Distal rectum
B. Ascending colon
C. Transverse colon
D. Sigmoid colon
E. Descending colon

17. Which regulatory molecule must be inhibited in order to form the joint cavity?

A. Gdf-5
B. Wnt-14
C. Noggin
D. Bone morphogenetic proteins
E. Wnt-7

18. Which layer of the skin is absent in thin skin?

A. Stratum basale
B. Stratum granulosum
C. Stratum corneum
D. Stratum spinosum
E. Stratum lucidum

19. When does the periderm form during development of the skin?

A. 2 weeks postfertilization
B. 3 weeks postfertilization
C. 4 weeks postfertilization
D. 5 weeks postfertilization
E. 6 weeks postfertilization

20. What is the layer that envelops an entire nerve?

A. Neurilemma
B. Endoneurium
C. Perineurium
D. Epineurium

21. What pharyngeal arch receives its innervation from the facial nerve?

A. First
B. Second
C. Third
D. Fourth
E. Sixth

22. Based on their staining characteristics, corticotrophs are:

A. Acidophils
B. Chromophobes
C. Basophils
D. Argyrophilic
E. PAS positive

23. Which of the following structures of the adrenal gland hypertrophy in response to elevated levels of ACTH?

A. Zona glomerulosa only
B. Zona reticularis only
C. Zona fasciculata only
D. Medulla only
E. Zona fasciculata and zona reticularis

24. What artery gives rise to the inferior suprarenal artery?

A. Inferior phrenic
B. Superior phrenic
C. Aorta
D. Superior mesenteric
E. Renal

25. Which structure is responsible for the production of aqueous humor?

    A. Ciliary processes   D. Trabecular meshwork

    B. Iris   E. Limbus

    C. Uvea

26. What structures form the outer nuclear layer of the retina?

    A. Ganglion cells   C. Rods and cones

    B. Bipolar cells   D. Müller cells

27. What is the predominant leukocyte in thyroid tissue from a patient with Graves' disease?

    A. Macrophage   D. Neutrophil

    B. B lymphocyte   E. T lymphocyte

    C. Plasma cell

28. What type of pathologic structure is found in the substantia nigra of Parkinson's disease patients?

    A. Mallory bodies   D. Herring bodies

    B. Lewy bodies   E. Howell-Jolly bodies

    C. Negri bodies

29. What type of capillary forms the blood-brain barrier?

    A. Fenestrated capillary with diaphragms

    B. Continuous capillary

    C. Sinusoidal capillary

    D. Fenestrated capillary without diaphragms

30. Which artery that supplies the midbrain is formed by the vertebral arteries?

    A. Basilar

    B. Superior cerebellar

    C. Anterior inferior cerebellar

    D. Posterior cerebral

    E. Posterior inferior cerebellar

31. Which malformed muscle results in congenital torticollis?

    A. Trapezius

    B. Splenius capitis

    C. Sternocleidomastoid

    D. Splenius cervicis

    E. Semispinalis capitis

32. A 56-year-old woman presented to her physician with the chief complaint of excruciating facial pain that comes and goes. Triggered by eating, drinking, and face washing, the pain occurs on her nose, upper cheek, upper lip, and upper teeth. What cranial nerve is involved in producing the patient's symptoms?

    A. Facial

    B. Ophthalmic division of trigeminal

    C. Maxillary division of trigeminal

    D. Mandibular division of trigeminal

    E. Glossopharyngeal

33. Which structure develops from Rathke's pouch?

    A. Thyroid gland   D. Adenohypophysis

    B. Parathyroid gland   E. Testicles

    C. Neurohypophysis

34. What type of nerve cell comprises 75% of the neocortex?

    A. Granule cell   D. Bipolar cells

    B. Pyramidal cell   E. Horizontal cells of Cajal

    C. Purkinje cell

35. What vertebral structure is represented by the eye of the Scottie dog in an oblique radiograph of the lumbar vertebrae?

    A. Pedicle

    B. Superior articular process

    C. Inferior articular process

    D. Spinous process

    E. Transverse process

36. Which embryonic vein gives rise to the prerenal segment of the inferior vena cava?

    A. Right supracardinal

    B. Right posteriorcardinal

    C. Right subcardinal

    D. Right vitelline

    E. Left vitelline

37. The _____ nerve conveys sensory information from the aortic bodies to the dorsal respiratory area of the _____.

    A. Vagus; pons

    B. Vagus; medulla oblongata

    C. Glossopharyngeal; pons

    D. Glossopharyngeal; medulla oblongata

    E. Glossopharyngeal; midbrain

38. What two arteries supply the sternocleidomastoid muscle?

    A. Inferior thyroid and occipital arteries

    B. Inferior thyroid and transverse cervical arteries

    C. S uperior thyroid and occipital arteries

    D. Superior thyroid and transverse cervical arteries

    E. Superior and inferior thyroid arteries

39. What are the structures that form the uterus?
    A. Paramesonephric ducts
    B. Mesonephric ducts
    C. Wolffian ducts
    D. Urogenital sinus
    E. Gartner ducts

40. Which ligament of the knee, when torn, is responsible for 80% of hemarthroses?
    A. Posterior cruciate ligament
    B. Medial collateral ligament
    C. Lateral collateral ligament
    D. Oblique popliteal ligament
    E. Anterior cruciate ligament

41. Which genicular artery pierces the fibrous capsule of the knee joint?
    A. Superior lateral genicular
    B. Superior medial genicular
    C. Middle genicular
    D. Inferior lateral genicular
    E. Inferior medial genicular

42. Damage to skeletal muscle fibers in Duchenne's muscular dystrophy results in release of creatine kinase into the blood. Which isoenzyme of creatine kinase would be elevated?
    A. CK_1
    B. CK_2
    C. CK_3
    D. CK_4

43. Which ligament of the hip is Y-shaped and checks hyperextension of the joint during standing?
    A. Iliofemoral
    B. Pubofemoral
    C. Ischiofemoral
    D. Ligamentum capitis femoris
    E. Annular

44. Which spinal cord tract is responsible for transmitting pain impulses?
    A. Corticospinal
    B. Fasciculus cuneatus
    C. Fasciculus gracilis
    D. Posterior columns
    E. Spinothalamic

45. What molecular moiety is predominately found in Mallory bodies?

    A. Neurofilaments
    B. Actin microfilaments
    C. Keratin filaments
    D. Microtubules
    E. Microtubule-associated proteins

46. Where are the cells of the macula densa located?
    A. Afferent arteriole
    B. Efferent arteriole
    C. Proximal convoluted tubule
    D. Distal convoluted tubule
    E. Loop of Henle

47. Which cell type is contractile and is responsible for clearing the particulate-clogged basal lamina in the renal corpuscle?
    A. Mesangial cell
    B. Podocyte
    C. Juxtaglomerular cell
    D. Cell of macula densa
    E. Principal cell

48. Which cell type is found in the intestinal glands of the ileum but is not found in the intestinal glands of the large intestine?
    A. Regenerative (stem) cell
    B. Paneth cell
    C. Absorptive cell
    D. Enteroendocrine cell
    E. Goblet cell

49. What is the origin of the primordial germ cells?
    A. Endoderm of dorsal part of yolk sac
    B. Endoderm of ventral part of the yolk sac
    C. Mesenchyme deep to the gonadal ridge
    D. Gonadal ridge
    E. Paramesonephric duct

50. Vestigial remnants of the cortex of the indifferent gonad in the male develop into the:
    A. Gubernaculum
    B. Seminiferous tubules
    C. Rete testis
    D. Efferent ductules
    E. Ductus epididymis

51. What is the most likely location of a cryptorchid testis?
    A. Inguinal canal
    B. Outside of the superficial inguinal ring
    C. Outside of the deep inguinal ring
    D. Immediately inferior to the kidney
    E. Between the kidney and the deep inguinal ring

52. Which structure forms the cremaster muscle and the cremasteric fascia of the spermatic cord?

    A. Aponeurosis of the internal abdominal oblique muscle

    B. Aponeurosis of the transversus abdominis muscle

    C. Aponeurosis of the external abdominal oblique muscle

    D. Transversalis fascia

    E. Processus vaginalis

53. Which structure principally forms the anterior wall of the inguinal canal?

    A. Fibers of the internal abdominal oblique muscle

    B. Conjoint tendon

    C. Transversalis fascia

    D. Aponeurosis of the external abdominal oblique muscle

    E. Fibers of the transversus abdominis muscle

54. What is the inferior limit of the parietal pleura in the midaxillary line?

    A. Rib 4   D. Rib 10

    B. Rib 6   E. Rib 12

    C. Rib 8

55. What type of epithelium is the mesothelium?

    A. Simple squamous

    B. Simple cuboidal

    C. Simple columnar

    D. Pseudostratified columnar

    E. Stratified cuboidal

56. What is the principal type of collagen found in ligaments?

    A. Type I   D. Type IV

    B. Type II   E. Type V

    C. Type III

57. What is the function of the macula densa in the distal convoluted tubule?

    A. Detect changes in the ionic composition of the ultrafiltrate

    B. Release renin

    C. Contract around the glomerular capillaries

    D. Remove basal lamina clogged with particulate matter via phagocytosis

    E. Reabsorb glucose from the ultrafiltrate

58. The secretions from mesothelial cells of the pleurae are rich in which type of glycosaminoglycan?

    A. Chondroitin sulfate

    B. Hyaluronic acid

    C. Keratan sulfate

    D. Heparan sulfate

    E. Dermatan sulfate

59. What coronary artery is most frequently involved in causing a myocardial infarction?

    A. Circumflex artery

    B. Right coronary artery

    C. Main trunk of the left coronary artery

    D. Anterior interventricular artery

    E. Posterior interventricular artery

60. Where would you expect to observe increased subperiosteal bone resorption in hyperparathyroidism?

    A. Medial sides of the phalanges

    B. Sternal ends of the clavicles

    C. Tips of the distal phalanges

    D. Acromion

    E. Sternum

61. The posterior longitudinal ligament extends from the sacrum to the:

    A. Vertebra prominens

    B. Occipital bone

    C. Axis

    D. Atlas

    E. Third cervical vertebra

62. A herniation of a cervical intervertebral disc is most likely to occur between:

    A. C1/C2   D. C4/C5

    B. C2/C3   E. C5/C6

    C. C3/C4

63. Which lymph nodes receive most of the lymph that drains from the deep surface of the breast?

    A. Apical group of axillary nodes

    B. Parasternal nodes

    C. Abdominal nodes

    D. Central group of axillary nodes

    E. Pectoral group of axillary nodes

64. Which one of the following structures does not form Guyon's canal?

    A. Lunate bone   D. Triquetral bone

    B. Hamate bone   E. Pisohamate ligament

    C. Pisiform bone

65. Which nerve is vulnerable to compression in Guyon's canal?

A. Radial nerve

B. Ulnar nerve

C. Median nerve

D. Anterior interosseous nerve

E. Posterior interosseous nerve

66. What is the pattern of necrosis in cardiac tissue following a myocardial infarction?

A. Fat necrosis

B. Liquefactive necrosis

C. Caseous necrosis

D. Coagulative necrosis

E. Suppurative necrosis

67. What is the pattern of necrosis in brain tissue following a cerebral infarction?

A. Fat necrosis

B. Liquefactive necrosis

C. Caseous necrosis

D. Coagulative necrosis

E. Suppurative necrosis

68. Which one of the following muscles would be paralyzed with avulsion of ventral roots C8 and T1 of the brachial plexus?

A. Abductor pollicis brevis

B. Deltoid

C. Extensor carpi radialis longus

D. Teres major

E. Extensor digitorum

69. Which root is infrequently injured in a brachial plexus injury?

A. C5

B. T1

C. C6

D. C8

E. C7

70. Which embryonic structure gives rise to most of the dermis?

A. Dermatome of somite

B. Intermediate mesoderm

C. Paraxial mesoderm

D. Endoderm

E. Lateral somatic mesoderm

71. If a patient had a lesion of her ventral primary ramus of C7, where would the sensory deficit be located?

A. Digit 1

B. Superior surface of deltoid

C. Cubital fossa

D. Digits 2, 3, and 4

E. Medial side of arm

72. If a patient had a lesion of his ventral primary ramus of T1, what motor deficit would you observe?

A. Extension of wrist

B. Supination of forearm

C. Abduction of shoulder

D. Movements of intrinsic hand muscles

E. Flexion of elbow

73. Which digit of the hand is most likely to suffer from a serious flexion deformity in Dupuytren's contracture?

A. First

B. Second

C. Third

D. Fourth

74. What causes the flexion contracture in Dupuytren's disease?

A. Shortening of the flexor digitorum superficialis tendons

B. Shortening of the flexor digitorum profundus tendons

C. Shortening of the interossei muscle tendons

D. Lengthening of the extensor digitorum longus tendons

E. Thickening of the palmar aponeurosis

75. What structure is most likely to fracture in posterior dislocation of the elbow joint?

A. Capitulum

B. Coronoid process

C. Trochlea

D. Olecranon

E. Head of radius

76. Which one of the following arteries that supplies the elbow joint is a branch of the profunda brachii artery?

A. Superior ulnar collateral

B. Inferior ulnar collateral

C. Radial collateral

D. Posterior ulnar recurrent

E. Radial recurrent

77. Which nerve has a lesion if the patient has clawhand?

A. Ulnar nerve

B. Median nerve

C. Radial nerve

D. Anterior interosseous nerve

E. Posterior interosseous nerve

78. Which cell type in the synovial layer is phagocytic?

    A. Type A cell
    B. Type B cell
    C. Type C cell
    D. Type D cell
    E. Type E cell

79. Which nerve may be injured during a reduction of a dislocation of the elbow?

    A. Ulnar nerve
    B. Median nerve
    C. Lateral cutaneous nerve of the forearm
    D. Radial nerve
    E. Superficial branch of the radial nerve

80. What two nerves principally supply the elbow joint?

    A. Anterior interosseous and ulnar nerves
    B. Radial and ulnar nerves
    C. Anterior interosseous and radial nerves
    D. Radial and musculocutaneous nerves
    E. Median and ulnar nerves

81. What is the first ossification center to appear in the elbow joint?

    A. Trochlea
    B. Capitulum
    C. Lateral epicondyle
    D. Medial epicondyle
    E. Olecranon

82. Where does the enzymatic cleavage of procollagen to tropocollagen occur?

    A. Rough endoplasmic reticulum
    B. Extracellular milieu
    C. Smooth endoplasmic reticulum
    D. Golgi complex
    E. Secretory vesicle

83. In insulitis of type I diabetes mellitus, what is the principal leukocyte that infiltrates the islet?

    A. Monocyte
    B. T lymphocyte
    C. B lymphocyte
    D. Neutrophil
    E. Plasma cell

84. What are the spinal cord levels that provide sympathetic output to the adrenal medulla?

    A. T8-L1
    B. T6-T10
    C. T7-T12
    D. T9-L2
    E. T10-L2

85. Which muscle of the rotator cuff group can medially rotate the humerus?

    A. Teres minor
    B. Supraspinatus
    C. Infraspinatus
    D. Subscapularis
    E. Teres major

86. What is the time band of reversible injury during a myocardial infarction?

    A. 0 to 15 minutes
    B. 0 to 30 minutes
    C. 0 to 1 hour
    D. 0 to 90 minutes
    E. 0 to 2 hours

87. Which zone of the active epiphyseal plate is characterized by death of the chondrocytes?

    A. Zone of rest
    B. Zone of hypertrophy
    C. Zone of ossification
    D. Zone of proliferation
    E. Zone of calcification

88. A lesion of the right medial lemniscus would result in a deficit of:

    A. Proprioception from the contralateral side
    B. Proprioception from the ipsilateral side
    C. Pain and temperature from the contralateral side
    D. Pain and temperature from the ipsilateral side
    E. Discriminative touch from the contralateral side

89. What is the deepest structure of the popliteal fossa?

    A. Popliteal vein
    B. Tibial nerve
    C. Popliteal artery
    D. Common fibular nerve
    E. Small saphenous vein

90. What produces the dimpling of peau d'orange that is characteristic of large invasive breast carcinomas?

    A. Lactiferous sinuses
    B. Areolar glands
    C. Increased lymphatic drainage of the breast
    D. Suspensory ligaments of the breast
    E. Mastitis

91. The breast is innervated by the:

    A. Long thoracic nerve
    B. 2nd to 6th intercostal nerves
    C. 1st to 4th intercostal nerves
    D. 3rd to 7th intercostal nerves
    E. Long thoracic and medial and lateral pectoral nerves

92. What is the most common type of emphysema resulting in clinically significant airflow obstruction?

    A. Paraseptal emphysema
    B. Centriacinar emphysema
    C. Panacinar emphysema
    D. Irregular emphysema

93. What structure forms the lateral border of the triangle of Calot?

    A. Cystic duct

    B. Common bile duct

    C. Common hepatic duct

    D. Right hepatic artery

    E. Liver

94. What spinal cord levels give rise to the preganglionic sympathetic neurons that innervate the gallbladder?

    A. T6-T8   D. T7-T11

    B. T5-T9   E. T7-T9

    C. T5-T7

95. Which one of the following structures does not pass through the carpal tunnel?

    A. Median nerve

    B. Tendon of the flexor carpi radialis muscle

    C. Tendon of the flexor pollicis longus muscle

    D. Tendons of the flexor digitorum superficialis muscles

    E. Tendons of the flexor digitorum profundus muscles

96. In addition to Meckel's diverticulum, where else does heterotopic gastric mucosa commonly occur?

    A. Appendix   D. Biliary tract

    B. Rectum   E. Duodenum

    C. Sigmoid colon

97. A patient with a brachial plexus lesion is a suitable candidate for a nerve transfer procedure. Which nerve is commonly transferred to restore some function to the rotator cuff?

    A. Phrenic nerve

    B. Third intercostal nerve

    C. Fourth intercostal nerve

    D. Accessory nerve

    E. Axillary nerve

98. Which segment of the small and large intestines is most commonly involved in the formation of diverticula?

    A. Descending colon

    B. Sigmoid colon

    C. Rectum

    D. Second part of duodenum

    E. Third part of duodenum

99. What type of emphysema is associated with alpha$_1$-antitrypsin deficiency?

    A. Paraseptal emphysema

    B. Centriacinar emphysema

    C. Panacinar emphysema

    D. Irregular emphysema

100. What is a fibroid or leiomyoma of the uterus?

    A. Benign growth of fibroblasts

    B. Cancerous growth of fibroblasts

    C. Benign growth of smooth muscle cells

    D. Cancerous growth of smooth muscle cells

    E. Cancerous growth of chondrocytes

101. What structure is damaged if a patient has a Bankart's lesion?

    A. Acetabular labrum

    B. Iliofemoral ligament

    C. Medial lemniscus

    D. Glenoid labrum

    E. Radial collateral ligament

102. What artery gives rise to the appendicular artery?

    A. Right colic   D. Superior mesenteric artery

    B. Middle colic   E. Inferior mesenteric artery

    C. Ileocolic

103. What is the most common location of the vermiform appendix?

    A. Subcecal

    B. Retrocecal and retrocolic

    C. Preileal

    D. Postileal

    E. Pelvic

104. What is the function of M cells?

    A. Transport of antigens across the intestinal epithelium

    B. Secrete mucus

    C. These are mitotic cells that regenerate cells that are shed

    D. Secrete various hormones

    E. Secrete lysozyme

105. Paresthesias are observed in Tinel's sign. Where are the observed paresthesias?

    A. Lateral three and one-half digits of the hand

    B. Medial one and one-half digit of the hand

    C. Lateral one and one-half digit of the foot

    D. Medial three and one-half digits of the foot

106. Where does the supraspinous ligament end superiorly?

A. External occipital protuberance

B. Posterior tubercle of atlas

C. Spinous process of axis

D. Spinous process of vertebra prominens

E. Spinous process of first thoracic vertebra

107. Which nerve is vulnerable to injury during harvesting of the great saphenous vein for a coronary bypass graft?

A. Genicular nerve

B. Superficial peroneal nerve

C. Sural nerve

D. Saphenous nerve

E. Medial femoral cutaneous nerve

108. Which zone of the prostate gland has the most frequent incidence of adenocarcinoma?

A. Peripheral zone   D. Periurethral zone

B. Central zone   E. Intermediate zone

C. Transition zone

109. Which muscle reflex is preferred for testing involvement of the root of the sixth cervical spinal nerve with a herniation of the intervertebral disc at C5-C6?

A. Biceps brachii   D. Brachialis

B. Brachioradialis   E. Flexor carpi radialis

C. Triceps brachii

110. A mutation in calcitonin gene-related peptide might cause the testis to:

A. Not develop properly

B. Arrest its transabdominal descent

C. Arrest its inguinoscrotal descent

D. Develop a seminoma

E. Undergo torsion

111. Which nerve releases calcitonin gene-related peptide?

A. Pudendal nerve

B. Genitofemoral nerve

C. Ilioinguinal nerve

D. Parasympathetic fibers from S2-S4

E. Sympathetic fibers

112. Which spinal root mediates the Achilles tendon reflex?

A. L3   D. S1

B. L4   E. S2

C. L5

113. Which spinal root mediates the patellar tendon reflex?

A. L3   D. S1

B. L4   E. S2

C. L5

114. Which spinal root supplies sensation to the dorsum of the foot and digits 2–4?

A. L3   D. S1

B. L4   E. S2

C. L5

115. Which reflex would be diminished with a lesion at the level of the fifth cervical spinal root?

A. Brachioradialis   D. Deltoid

B. Biceps brachii   E. Supraspinatus

C. Triceps brachii

116. What membrane proteins embedded in the plasmalemma of the clear zone of an osteoclast form a seal against the surface of neighboring bone?

A. Catenins   D. Desmoglein

B. Integrins   E. Vinculin

C. Desmoplakin

117. Which extraocular muscle would be affected with a lesion involving the trochlear nerve?

A. Superior rectus   D. Superior oblique

B. Lateral rectus   E. Inferior oblique

C. Medial rectus

118. What role does selectin play in the metastasis of cancer cells?

A. Underexpression allows cancer cells to dissociate from one another

B. Snags cancer cells as they travel through blood vessels

C. Underexpression allows cancer cells to dissociate from the basal lamina

D. Activation of proteases

E. Causes disorganization of the cytoskeleton in cancer cells

119. The valves of Houston are features of the:

A. Esophagus

B. Jejunum

C. Rectum

D. Stomach

E. Sigmoid colon

120. What is the clinical stage of breast cancer if it is invasive with a diameter of 4 cm with four axillary nodes involved?

 A. Stage 0   D. Stage 3
 B. Stage 1   E. Stage 4
 C. Stage 2

121. Where does breast carcinoma most commonly occur?

 A. Upper lateral quadrant
 B. Upper medial quadrant
 C. Lower lateral quadrant
 D. Lower medial quadrant
 E. Subareolar

122. Which mutated integral membrane protein has been implicated in increasing the activity of glycogen synthase kinase 3ß activity?

 A. Tau
 B. Amyloid precursor protein
 C. Presenilin I
 D. P-glycoprotein
 E. Synaptophysin

123. What is a gold standard characteristic of mesothelioma?

 A. Abundant staining keratin at the periphery of tumor cells
 B. Presence of CEA
 C. Long, slender microvilli are observed on the tumor cells
 D. Cells are columnar in appearance
 E. Pleomorphic nuclei are observed

124. Peroxiredoxins protect cells against _____ _____; however, some cancer cells overexpress peroxiredoxins thus desensitizing the cells to the effects of _____:

 A. Reactive oxygen species; radiation therapy
 B. Reactive oxygen species; chemotherapy
 C. Ribonucleases; radiation therapy
 D. Ribonucleases; chemotherapy

125. The pancreas lies across vertebral bodies:

 A. T10-T12   D. L1-L2
 B. T11-L1   E. L1-L3
 C. T12-L2

126. Most of the lymph from the pancreas drains first into the _____ nodes.

 A. Pyloric   D. Superior mesenteric
 B. Pancreaticosplenic   E. Hepatic
 C. Celiac

127. Which one of the following is a structural characteristic of a pancreatic acinar cell?

 A. Poorly developed Golgi complex
 B. Apical region is acidophilic
 C. Mitochondria are more abundant in the apical region
 D. Secretory vesicles accumulate in the basal region of the cell
 E. The nucleus is located in the apical region of the cell

128. Which segment(s) is (are) most frequently involved in Crohn's disease?

 A. Small intestine alone
 B. Small intestine and colon
 C. Colon alone
 D. Esophagus and stomach
 E. Descending colon and rectum

129. Which segment of the duodenum is most commonly involved in the formation of diverticula?

 A. First   C. Third
 B. Second   D. Fourth

130. Which muscle is necessary to initiate abduction of the humerus from the anatomical position?

 A. Teres minor   D. Supraspinatus
 B. Deltoid   E. Subscapularis
 C. Teres major

131. Which lobe of the cerebrum contains the hippocampal formation?

 A. Occipital   C. Parietal
 B. Frontal   D. Temporal

132. What anatomical landmark differentiates an anterior cleft palate from a posterior cleft palate?

 A. Lesser palatine foramen
 B. Incisive fossa
 C. Greater palatine foramen
 D. Uvula
 E. Median part of lip

133. What are the vertebral relationships of the thyroid gland?

 A. C3-C6   D. C6-T2
 B. C4-C7   E. C7-T3
 C. C5-T1

134. Which division of the trigeminal nerve is infrequently involved in tic douloureux?

A. Ophthalmic

B. Maxillary

C. Mandibular

135. What vertebral level corresponds to the beginning of the esophagus?

A. C4

B. C5

C. C6

D. C7

E. T1

136. A histologic section demonstrates an admixture of smooth and skeletal muscle in the muscularis externa. Which region of the esophagus is represented by this section?

A. Superior one-third

B. Middle one-third

C. Inferior one-third

137. The second esophageal constriction is caused by the:

A. Esophageal hiatus of the diaphragm

B. Aorta

C. Cricopharyngeus muscle

D. Left primary bronchus

E. Carina of the trachea

138. What is the most frequent location of an abdominal aortic aneurysm?

A. Just inferior to the diaphragm

B. Level of the celiac trunk

C. Level of the superior mesenteric artery

D. Level of the renal arteries

E. Inferior to the renal arteries

139. When performing microvascular decompression surgery to relieve trigeminal neuralgia, where is the craniectomy performed?

A. Adjacent to foramen rotundum

B. Adjacent to foramen ovale

C. Posterior to mastoid process

D. Posterior to styloid process

E. Posterior to external acoustic meatus

140. A newborn presented with a cystlike sac in the lumbar region of the vertebral column. The cyst contained meninges and the spinal cord. What is the most likely diagnosis?

A. Spina bifida occulta

B. Spina bifida with meningomyelocele

C. Spina bifida with meningocele

D. Rachischisis

E. Spina bifida with myeloschisis

141. What two vertebral levels are most frequently involved in spina bifida occulta?

A. L1 and L2

B. L2 and L3

C. L3 and L4

D. L4 and L5

E. L5 and S1

142. Which glucose transporter is found on target cells for insulin?

A. GLUT-1

B. GLUT-2

C. GLUT-3

D. GLUT-4

E. GLUT-5

143. Which one of the following structures forms the medial boundary of Hesselbach's triangle?

A. Rectus abdominis muscle

B. Inferior epigastric artery

C. Inguinal ligament

D. Conjoint tendon

E. Lacunar ligament

144. Which arteries must be divided when performing a fundoplication procedure to treat gastroesophageal reflux disease?

A. Left gastric

B. Right gastric

C. Short gastric

D. Right gastro-omental

E. Left gastro-omental

145. What gland is involved in a patient with a Bartholin's cyst?

A. Greater vestibular gland

B. Periurethral gland

C. Seminal vesicle

D. Glands of Littre

E. Bulbourethral gland

146. Prostate cancer has a tendency to metastasize to the axial skeleton. Which element of the axial skeleton is most frequently involved?

A. Ribs

B. Lumbar vertebrae

C. Os coxa

D. Thoracic vertebrae

E. Proximal extremity of femur

147. What molecular signal drives the metaplasia observed in Barrett's esophagus?

A. Human epidermal growth factor

B. Barx-1

C. Hoxa-2

D. Wnt

E. Pax-1

148. Most of the lymph from the stomach drains into the _____ nodes.
    - A. Celiac
    - B. Left gastric
    - C. Gastro-omental
    - D. Pyloric
    - E. Pancreaticosplenic

149. An endoscopy is performed on a patient with a suspected gastric ulcer. Where would you most likely observe a peptic ulcer in the stomach?
    - A. Fundus
    - B. Body along the greater curvature
    - C. Lesser curvature at or near the incisura angularis
    - D. Cardia
    - E. Pyloric antrum along the greater curvature

150. The acromioclavicular joint is innervated by the suprascapular and lateral pectoral nerves. What spinal cord segments contribute to the formation of the suprascapular nerve?
    - A. C2-C3
    - B. C3-C4
    - C. C4-C5
    - D. C5-C6
    - E. C7-C8

151. What is the signature feature of a type II pneumocyte?
    - A. Occluding junctions
    - B. Abundant mitochondria
    - C. Lamellar bodies
    - D. Apical microvilli
    - E. Abundant rough endoplasmic reticulum

152. During lung development, the single lung bud divides into _____ bronchial buds which are derived from _____.
    - A. Two; mesoderm
    - B. Two; endoderm
    - C. Four; mesoderm
    - D. Four; endoderm
    - E. Five; endoderm

153. Which phase of lung development is characterized by the initial presence of terminal sacs and respiratory bronchioles branching from terminal bronchioles?
    - A. Alveolar period
    - B. Terminal sac period
    - C. Canalicular period
    - D. Pseudoglandular period
    - E. Surfactant period

154. Which spinal cord root or roots may be involved in spondylolisthesis of the fifth lumbar vertebra?
    - A. L4
    - B. L5
    - C. S1
    - D. L4 and L5
    - E. L5 and S1

155. Spondylolisthesis of the fifth lumbar vertebra would result in a diminished _____ tendon reflex and diminished sensation of the _____.
    - A. Patellar; dorsal surface of foot
    - B. Patellar; lateral and dorsal surface of foot
    - C. Achilles; medial surface of leg
    - D. Achilles; dorsal surface of foot
    - E. Achilles; lateral and dorsal surface of foot

156. Which tendon of the rotator cuff muscle group is most likely to rupture?
    - A. Teres minor
    - B. Supraspinatus
    - C. Infraspinatus
    - D. Subscapularis
    - E. Teres major

157. What histologic structure is common to the small and large intestines?
    - A. Well-developed microvilli are associated with the columnar absorptive cells
    - B. Plicae circulares
    - C. Villi
    - D. Intestinal glands
    - E. Paneth cells

158. An incision is made at McBurney's point to perform an appendectomy. After penetrating through the skin, what is the next layer immediately deep to the dermis?
    - A. Scarpa's fascia
    - B. Camper's fascia
    - C. Transversalis fascia
    - D. Deep fascia
    - E. External abdominal oblique muscle

159. A patient with calculous cholecystitis has her gallbladder removed. Histologic examination revealed that the inflammation has penetrated into the third layer of the gallbladder's wall. What is the third layer of the gallbladder?
    - A. Serosa
    - B. Mucosa
    - C. Perimuscular connective tissue layer
    - D. Fibromuscular layer
    - E. Muscularis mucosae

160. The infrarenal segment of the abdominal aorta is missing structures that may contribute to the formation of an abdominal aortic aneurysm. What structure is missing?

A. Internal elastic lamina

B. Vasa vasorum in the tunica media

C. External elastic lamina

D. Elastic lamellae in the tunica media

E. Nerve fibers

161. A positive Rovsing's sign elicits pain in which abdominal quadrant?

A. Right upper quadrant

B. Right lower quadrant

C. Left upper quadrant

D. Left lower quadrant

162. What embryologic structure gives rise to the adrenal medulla?

A. Endoderm

B. Somatic mesoderm

C. Neural crest cells

D. Splanchnic mesoderm

E. Dermomyotome

163. Where do most abdominal aortic aneurysms rupture?

A. Peritoneal cavity

B. Right retroperitoneum

C. Left retroperitoneum

D. Omental bursa

E. Foramen of Winslow

164. What is the most common type of atrial septal defect?

A. Ostium primum defect

B. Ostium secundum defect

C. Sinus venosus defect

D. Coronary sinus defect

165. The valve of the foramen ovale is formed by the _____ and the foramen ovale forms in the _____.

A. Septum primum; septum primum

B. Septum primum; septum secundum

C. Septum secundum; septum secundum

D. Septum secundum; septum primum

166. What embryonic structure forms the smooth wall of the right atrium?

A. Left horn of the sinus venosus

B. Right horn of the sinus venosus

C. Right common cardinal vein

D. Left common cardinal vein

E. Primitive atrium

167. What is the embryologic basis of the tetralogy of Fallot?

A. Unequal division of the truncus arteriosus

B. Fusion of the pulmonic semilunar valve cusps

C. Perforated aorticopulmonary septum

D. Hypoplastic (underdeveloped) left ventricle

E. Stenotic bulbous cordis and truncus arteriosus

168. A positive Thompson test would most likely indicate a torn:

A. Ulnar collateral ligament

B. Patellar tendon

C. Medial meniscus

D. Coracoclavicular ligament

E. Calcaneal tendon

169. What is the mechanism of action of alendronate for the treatment of osteoporosis?

A. Activates osteoblasts

B. Inhibits recruitment of osteoclasts

C. Inhibits the hydrogen pump in osteoclasts

D. Prevents osteoclasts from forming lysosomes

E. Prevents osteoclasts from developing ruffled borders

170. Which lobe of the lung is the first to show cystic fibrosis–related changes?

A. Superior lobe of left lung

B. Inferior lobe of left lung

C. Superior lobe of right lung

D. Middle lobe of right lung

E. Inferior lobe of right lung

171. Cystic fibrosis is caused by a defective ion transport protein. What ion transport is directly affected by this defective transporter?

A. Calcium

B. Potassium

C. Sodium

D. Bicarbonate

E. Chloride

172. During portal hypertension, a patient may exhibit caput medusae. Which veins are distended causing this appearance?

A. Paraumbilical veins

B. Inferior rectal veins

C. Esophageal veins

D. Superior rectal veins

173. What structure fails to migrate causing a unilateral posterior cleft palate?

    A. Median palatine process
    B. Nasal septum
    C. Primary palate
    D. Lateral palatine process

174. What gene is expressed by inducible endothelial cells that line the atrioventricular tract where endocardial cushions form?

    A. Msx-1   D. Hoxa-2
    B. Wnt-7   E. Barx-1
    C. Pax-1

175. What muscle element is thickened in hypertrophic pyloric stenosis?

    A. Muscularis mucosae
    B. Oblique layer of muscularis externa
    C. Circular layer of muscularis externa
    D. Longitudinal layer of muscularis externa

176. Which one of the following muscles does not contribute to the formation of the calcaneal (Achilles) tendon?

    A. Soleus
    B. Plantaris
    C. Popliteus
    D. Gastrocnemius

177. What is the most common mechanism of popliteal artery entrapment syndrome?

    A. Fibrosis of the tunica intima of the popliteal artery due to repetitive flexion-extension movements of the hip joint.
    B. Popliteal artery develops within the substance of the medial head of the gastrocnemius muscle.
    C. Superior migration of the medial head of the gastrocnemius muscle during its development moves the popliteal artery medially.
    D. The primitive distal popliteal axial artery persists rather than regresses.

178. What artery or arteries would be involved with posterior compartment syndrome of the leg?

    A. Anterior tibial artery
    B. Posterior tibial artery
    C. Fibular artery
    D. Posterior tibial and fibular arteries
    E. Anterior and posterior tibial arteries

179. What isoform of creatine kinase would be elevated in posterior compartment syndrome of the leg?

    A. CK-MM (CK_3)
    B. CK-BB (CK_1)
    C. CK-MB (CK_2)

180. What cell type is responsible for the fibrotic remodeling of the cirrhotic liver?

    A. Kupffer cell
    B. Hepatocyte
    C. Endothelial cell
    D. Perisinusoidal cell (hepatic stellate cell)

181. A radiologist observes a coeur en sabot image on a radiograph. What is the most likely diagnosis?

    A. Achalasia
    B. Sinus venosus type of atrial septal defect
    C. Emphysema
    D. Hirschsprung's disease
    E. Tetralogy of Fallot

182. The ovarian and testicular arteries branch from the abdominal aorta at what vertebral level?

    A. T12   D. L3
    B. L1   E. L4
    C. L2

183. What cell type is responsible for secreting human chorionic gonadotropin that is detected in the blood of a patient with choriocarcinoma of the testis?

    A. Syncytiotrophoblast
    B. Cytotrophoblast
    C. Sertoli cell
    D. Interstitial cell of Leydig

184. What is the most likely location of a leiomyoma of the uterus?

    A. Cervix
    B. Fundus
    C. Body

185. What are the most important ligaments supporting the uterus?

    A. Uterosacral
    B. Mesometrium
    C. Pubocervical
    D. Round
    E. Transverse cervical (cardinal)

ANSWERS TO MULTIPLE CHOICE QUESTIONS

Question #	Answer	Reference page #	Question #	Answer	Reference page #
1	B	243	42	C	178
2	C	234	43	A	171–172
3	E	61	44	E	186
4	A	224	45	C	85
5	E	181	46	D	108
6	B	129	47	A	106
7	B	178	48	B	90
8	D	184	49	A	137
9	D	177	50	C	138
10	B	233	51	A	137
11	A	173	52	A	165
12	D	224	53	D	111
13	C	225	54	D	51
14	C	222	55	A	51
15	C	67	56	A	222–223
16	A	144	57	A	108
17	A	188	58	B	51
18	E	239	59	D	57
19	C	237	60	C	273
20	D	243	61	C	5
21	B	244	62	E	4
22	C	252	63	A	31
23	E	255	64	A	227
24	E	255	65	B	227
25	A	258	66	D	62
26	C	260	67	B	287
27	E	265	68	A	201–202
28	B	267	69	E	199
29	B	267	70	E	238
30	A	269	71	D	201
31	C	275	72	D	201–202
32	C	277	73	D	209
33	D	283	74	E	209
34	B	285	75	B	214
35	A	11	76	C	213
36	C	132	77	A	227
37	B	41	78	A	212
38	C	275	79	B	213
39	A	149–150	80	D	214
40	E	186	81	B	214
41	C	186	82	B	223

ANSWERS TO MULTIPLE CHOICE QUESTIONS

Question #	Answer	Reference page #	Question #	Answer	Reference page #
83	B	93	124	A	35
84	A	130	125	E	119
85	D	219	126	B	120
86	B	62	127	B	121
87	E	214	128	A	91
88	A	184–185	129	B	117
89	C	190	130	D	219
90	D	31	131	D	233
91	B	31	132	B	247
92	B	44	133	C	263
93	A	97	134	A	277
94	E	99	135	C	19
95	B	205	136	B	22
96	E	116	137	B	21
97	D	201–202	138	E	71
98	B	116	139	C	277
99	C	46	140	B	8
100	C	150	141	E	8
101	D	224	142	D	94
102	C	77	143	A	111
103	B	76	144	C	101
104	A	79	145	A	135
105	A	205	146	B	160–161
106	D	4	147	D	101
107	D	58	148	B	124
108	A	158	149	C	125
109	B	6	150	D	225
110	C	141	151	C	50
111	B	141	152	B	47
112	D	6	153	C	49
113	B	6	154	E	11
114	C	6	155	E	6
115	B	6	156	B	219
116	B	14	157	D	90
117	D	286	158	B	75
118	B	240	159	C	99
119	C	144	160	B	74
120	E	34	161	B	75
121	A	31	162	C	129
122	C	236	163	C	71
123	C	53	164	B	27

ANSWERS TO MULTIPLE CHOICE QUESTIONS

Question #	Answer	Reference page #	Question #	Answer	Reference page #
165	B	27	176	C	169
166	B	27	177	C	189
167	A	67	178	D	194
168	E	169	179	A	194
169	E	15	180	D	86
170	C	37	181	E	67
171	E	37	182	C	153
172	A	83	183	A	165
173	D	247	184	C	150
174	A	23	185	E	147
175	C	87			

BIBLIOGRAPHY

Adams JC, Hamblen DL. *Outline of Orthopaedics.* 13th ed. Edinburgh: Churchill Livingstone; 2001.

Alberts B, et al. *Molecular Biology of the Cell.* 4th ed. New York: Garland Science; 2002.

Alder MN, et al. Gene silencing in Caenorhabditis elegans by transitive RNA interference. *RNA* 9:25–32, 2003.

Bannister LH, et al. *Gray's Anatomy. The Anatomical Basis of Medicine and Surgery.* 38th ed. New York: Churchill Livingstone; 1995.

Bell A, et al. Functional TSH receptor in human abdominal preadipocytes and orbital fibroblasts. *Am J Physiol Cell Physiol* 279:C335–C340, 2000.

Bergman RA, et al. Illustrated Encyclopedia of Human Anatomic Variation. www.vh.org/adult/provider/anatomy/AnatomicVariants/AnatomyHP.html

Bezold LI. Atrial Septal Defect, Coronary Sinus. *www.emedicine.com/ped/topic2493.htm,* 2004.

Braunwald E, ed. *Heart Disease. A Textbook of Cardiovascular Medicine.* 5th ed. Philadelphia: Saunders; 1997.

Canby CA, et al. Incidence of a duplicated inferior vena cava. Abstract submitted to Experimental Biology 2005 meeting in San Diego, Calif.

Carlson BM. *Human Embryology and Developmental Biology.* 3rd ed. Philadelphia: Mosby; 2004.

Clemente CD. *Gray's Anatomy. 30th American edition.* Philadelphia: Lea and Febiger; 1985

Dandy DJ, Edwards DJ. *Essential Orthopaedics and Trauma.* 4th ed. Edinburgh: Churchill Livingstone; 2003.

Clayton J. Wnt signaling and the developmental fate of lung cells. *J Biol* 3:9, 2004.

Drake RL, et al. *Gray's Anatomy for Students.* Philadelphia: Elsevier Churchill Livingstone; 2005.

Fabry HFJ, et al. Clinical relevance of parasternal uptake in sentinel node procedure for breast cancer. *J Surg Oncol* 87:13–18, 2004.

Fawcett D. *Bloom and Fawcett Textbook of Histology.* 12th ed. New York: Chapman and Hall; 1994.

Foresta C, Ferlin A. Role of INSL3 and LGR8 in cryptorchidism and testicular functions. *Reproductive BioMedicine Online* 2004 Volume 9, No. 3, 294–298.

Gartner LP, Hiatt JL. *Color Textbook of Histology.* 2nd ed. Philadelphia: W.B. Saunders; 2001.

Gilman AG, et al. *Goodman and Gilman's The Pharmacological Basis of Therapeutics.* 8th ed. New York: Pergamon Press; 1990.

Goldman L, Ausiello D. *Cecil Textbook of Medicine.* 22nd ed. Philadelphia: Saunders; 2004.

Greenfield LJ, et al. *Surgery Scientific Principles and Practice.* 2nd ed. Philadelphia: Lippincott-Raven; 1997.

Halstead ME, Bernhardt DT. Elbow dislocation. www.emedicine.com/sports/topic31.htm, 2004.

Hoppenfeld S. *Orthopaedic Neurology. A Diagnostic Guide to Neurologic Levels.* Philadelphia: Lippincott Williams and Wilkins; 1997.

Illenberger S, et al. The endogenous and cell cycle-dependent phosphorylation of tau protein in living cells: implications for Alzheimer's disease. *Mol Biol Cell* 9:1495–1512, 1998.

Junqueira LC, Carneiro J. *Basic Histology.* Text and Atlas. 10th ed. New York: Lange; 2003.

Halstead ME. Elbow Dislocation. www.emedicine.com/sports/topic31.htm.

Kierszenbaum AL. *Histology and Cell Biology. An Introduction to Pathology.* St. Louis: Mosby; 2002.

Kim ED, Grayhack JT. Clinical signs and symptoms of prostate cancer. In: *Comprehensive Therapy of Genitourinary Oncology.* Vogelzang NJ, Scardino PT, Shipley WU, et al, eds. Baltimore: Williams and Wilkins; 1995.

Kim H-S, et al. Rat lung peroxiredoxins I and II are differentially regulated during development and by hyperoxia. *Am J Physiol Lung Cell Mol Physiol* 280:L1212–L1217, 2001.

Kimberly WT, et al. The intracellular domain of the ß-amyloid precursor protein is stabilized by Fe65 and translocates to the nucleus in a notch-like manner. *J Biol Chem* 276:40288–40292, 2001.

Kumar V, et al. Robbins Basic Pathology. 7th ed. Philadelphia: Saunders; 2003.

Kumar V, et al. *Robbins and Cotran Pathologic Basis of Disease.* 7th ed. Philadelphia: Elsevier Saunders; 2005.

Kuwahara F, et al. Hypoxia-inducible factor-1a/vascular endothelial growth factor pathway for adventitial vasa vasorum formation in hypertensive rat aorta. *Hypertension* 39:46–50, 2002.

Lachman E. *Case Studies in Anatomy.* 3rd ed. New York: Oxford University Press, Inc.; 1981.

Lawless MW. Midshaft humeral fractures. www.emedicine.com/orthoped/topic199.htm, 2004.

Legato MJ, ed. *The Stressed Heart.* Boston: Martinus Nijhoff Publishing; 1987.

Lerwill MF. Current practical applications of diagnostic immunohistochemistry in breast pathology. *Am J Surg Pathol* 28:1076–1091, 2004

Lin DY, et al. Achilles Tendon Rupture. www.emedicine.com/sports/topic1.htm, 2004.

Lucentini J. Silencing cancer. *The Scientist* 18(17):14–15, 2004.

Mani NBS, et al. Case report: duplication of IVC and associated renal anomalies. *Ind J Radiol Imag* 10:Case 3, 2000.

McMilan S, et al. Porcine small intestine submucosa for modeling elbow ulnar collateral ligament regeneration. *JAOA* 104:348 (C19), 2004.

Marcus ML. *The Coronary Circulation in Health and Disease.* New York: McGraw-Hill; 1983.

Moore KL, Dalley AF. *Clinically Oriented Anatomy.* 4th ed. Philadelphia: Lippincott Williams and Wilkins; 1999.

Moore KL, Persaud TVN. *The Developing Human. Clinically Oriented Embryology.* 7th ed. Philadelphia: Saunders; 2003.

Noh DY, et al. Overexpression of peroxiredoxin in human breast cancer. *Anticancer Res* 21(3B):2085–2090, 2001.

Nolte J. *The Human Brain. An Introduction to Its Functional Anatomy.* 5th ed. St. Louis: Mosby; 2002.

Park SH, et al. Effects of thyroid state on AMP-activated protein kinase and acetyl-CoA carboxylase expression in muscle. *J Appl Physiol* 93:2081–2088, 2002.

Physicians' Desk Reference. Montvale: Thomson PDR; 2004.

Pigino G, et al. Alzheimer's presenilin 1 mutations impair kinesin-based axonal transport. *J Neurosci* 23:4499–4508, 2003.

Pillai A. Popliteal artery entrapment syndrome: diagnosis by MRI. *Ind J Radiol Imag* 12(1):91–93, 2002.

Plasschaert SLA, et al. Influence of functional polymorphisms of the MDR1 gene on vincristine pharmacokinetics in childhood acute lymphoblastic leukemia. *Clin Pharmacol Ther* 76:220–229, 2004.

Podnos YD, Tessier DJ. Popliteal artery thrombosis. www.emedicine.com/med/topic2769.htm, 2004.

Provost P, et al. Ribonuclease activity and RNA binding of recombinant human Dicer. *EMBO J* 21:5864–5874, 2002.

Rosse C, Gaddum-Rosse P. *Hollinshead's Textbook of Anatomy.* 5th ed. Lippincott-Raven, Philadelphia, 1997.

Shen C, Nathan C. Nonredundant antioxidant defense by multiple two-cysteine peroxiredoxins in human prostate cancer cells. *Molecular Med* 8(2):95–102, 2002.

Stadelmann C, et al. Activation of caspase-3 in single neurons and autophagic granules of granulovacuolar degeneration in Alzheimer's disease. Evidence for apoptotic cell death. *Am J Pathol* 155:1459–1466, 1999.

Thompson JC. *Netter's Concise Atlas of Orthopaedic Anatomy.* ICON Learning Systems, 2002.

Sabiston DC. Textbook of Surgery: *The Biological Basis of Modern Surgical Practice.* 14th ed. Saunders, Philadelphia, 1991.

Standring S, et al. *Gray's Anatomy. The Anatomical Basis of Clinical Practice*. 39th ed. Edinburgh: Churchill Livingstone, 2005.

Stefanadis C, et al. Effect of vasa vasorum flow on structure and function of the aorta in experimental animals. *Circulation* 91:2669–2678, 1995.

Stein JH (editor-in-chief). *Internal Medicine*. 4th ed. St. Louis: Mosby; 1994.

Thompson, JC. *Netter's Concise Atlas of Orthopaedic Anatomy*. Teterboro: Icon Learning Systems; 2002.

Townsend CM, et al, eds. *Sabiston Textbook of Surgery*. 17th ed. Philadelphia: Elsevier Saunders; 2004.

Van Noorden CJF, et al. *Metastasis. American Scientist* 86(2):130–141, 1998.

Wallace S, et al. Compartment Syndrome, Lower Extremity. www.emedicine.com/orthoped/topic596.htm, 2004.

Weiss L. *Cell and Tissue Biology. A Textbook of Histology*. 6th ed. Baltimore: Urban and Schwarzenberg; 1988.

Williams PL, et al. *Gray's Anatomy*. 37th ed. Edinburgh: Churchill Livingstone; 1989.

Young PA, Young PH. *Basic Clinical Anatomy*. Baltimore: William and Wilkins; 1997.

Zipes DP, et al. *Braunwald's Heart Disease. A Textbook of Cardiovascular Medicine*. 7th ed. Philadelphia: Elsevier Saunders; 2005.

I N D E X

Note: Page numbers followed by *f* indicate illustrations; those followed by *t* indicate tables.

A

Abdomen, 69–132. *See also under* Abdominal; Stomach
Abdominal aorta
  branches of, 71
  infrarenal, histologic characteristics of, 71–73, 73f
Abdominal aortic aneurysm, 71–74, 72f–74f
  rupture of, sites of, 71
  sites of, 71, 72f, 73f
    causes of, 74
  vertebral levels of, 71
Aberrant obturator artery, 111
AC joint. *See* Acromioclavicular (AC) joint
Acetabulum
  deepening of, structure in, 171f, 172
  fracture of, 173
Achalasia, 19–22, 19f
  "bird beak" appearance in, 19f, 21
  dyspnea in, 21
  morphologic changes in esophagus and, 22
Achilles tendon. *See* Calcaneal tendon
Acinar cells, cellular features of, 121
Acinus, structure of, 45f
Acromioclavicular (AC) joint
  anatomical description of, 225, 226f
  arterial supply to, 225
  nerve supply to, 225
  radiographs of, 225f
  separation of, ligaments torn in, 225, 225f
ACTH
  excessive level of, adrenal gland response to, 255, 255f
  target cells for, sites of, 254–255, 254f
ACTH-secreting cells, in pituitary gland
  histologic description of, 251–252
  sites of, 251–252
ACTH-secreting pituitary gland tumor, 251–256, 251f,
    253f–256f. *See also* Cushing's disease
Acute calculous cholecystitis, 97–99, 97f, 98f, 100f
  perforation of gallbladder due to, 99
Adaptin(s), 59
Adenocarcinoma, prostate, morphology of, 159
Adenohypophysis, 251
Adenoma(s), parathyroid, morphology of, 273, 273f
Adheron(s), 23
Adrenal gland, response to excessive level of ACTH, 255, 255f
Adrenal medulla, sympathetic outflow to, spinal cord segments
    in, 130

AFP. *See* Alpha-fetoprotein (AFP)
Alcoholic cirrhosis, 81–86, 82f, 83t, 84f, 85f
Alcoholic hyalin, 85, 85f
Alendronate, osteoclasts affected by, 15
Alpha-fetoprotein (AFP), synthesis of, structures involved in, 7
Alzheimer's disease, 233–236, 233f, 234f, 236f
  axonal transport in neurons disruption in, 236–237
  cholinergic neurons in, degeneration of, 233–234, 234f
  described, 233
  neuronal death in, apoptosis in, 235
  pathogenesis of, amyloid precursor protein in, 235, 236f
Amyloid precursor protein, in Alzheimer's disease, 235, 236f
Anal canal
  hindgut-derived, *vs.* anal canal derived from proctodeum,
      145–146
  rectum and, 145, 145f
Anal pecten, 145, 145f
Anastomosis(es), portosystemic
  distention of, 81, 82f, 83t
  sites of, 81, 82f, 83t
Aneurysm(s), aortic, abdominal, 71–74, 72f–74f. *See also*
    Abdominal aortic aneurysm
Angle closure glaucoma, causes of, 260–261
Anterograde transport, 235
Aorta, abdominal
  branches of, 71
  infrarenal, histologic characteristics of, 71–73, 73f
Aortic aneurysm, abdominal, 71–74, 72f–74f. *See also*
    Abdominal aortic aneurysm
Aortic bodies, 41
Aortic sinus, function of, 55
Apoptosis, in neuronal death in Alzheimer's disease, 235
Appendicitis, 75–79, 75t, 76f–78f
  referred pain in, 78, 78f
Appendix
  layers of, 78–79
  vermiform. *See* Vermiform appendix
Aqueous humor
  draining of, 257–258, 257f
  production of, structure in, 257–258, 257f
  return to right atrium, 258
Arterial blood flow, pituitary gland tumor effects on, 284–285,
    286f, 286t
Arterial chemoreceptors, sites of, 41
Arterial supply
  to AC joint, 225
  to breast, 29, 30f
  to colon, 89

Arterial supply (*contd.*)
    to elbow joint, 213
    to gallbladder, 97
    to heart, 55, 56f
    to hip joint, 171f, 173, 173f
    to ileum, 89
    to kidney, 105
    to knee joint, 186, 188f
    to lungs, 42
    to ovary, 153, 154f
    to parathyroid glands, 271, 271f
    of parietal pleura, 51
    to pituitary gland, 251, 251f
    to prostate gland, 157
    to rectum, 143
    to shoulder joint, 224
    to stomach, 123
    to testicle, 163
    to thyroid gland, 263, 263f
    of visceral pleura, 51
Arteriole(s), histologic characteristics of, 60t
Artery(ies)
    coronary, 55, 56f, 57
    dorsalis pedis, palpability of, 190, 191f
    elastic, histologic characteristics of, 60t
    genicular, 186, 188f
    muscular, histologic characteristics of, 60t
    obturator, aberrant, 111
    popliteal. *See* Popliteal artery
    suprarenal, parent vessels of, sites of, 255
    thoracic, internal, 58
        as conduit for coronary bypass, arterial flow to intercostal
            spaces maintained when, 58
Atherosclerosis, development of, cytologic events in, 61, 63f
Atrial septal defects, embryological basis of, 27, 28f
Atrium(a)
    formation of, structures in, 27
    primitive, septation of, normal events in, 23–27, 23f–26f
Axillary lymph nodes, dissection of, lymphedema of upper
    extremity due to, 31

B

Back, 1–15
Bankart's lesion, described, 224
Barrett's esophagus, metaplasia in, 101
Bartholin gland(s), 135, 135f, 136f
    described, 135, 135f, 136f
    development of, 135, 136f
Basal cell carcinoma, 237–241, 237f–239f, 241f, 242f
    pathologic characteristics of, 237f–238f, 240
    removal of, cutaneous wound healing after, 241, 242f
Basal ganglia, brain nuclei and, 267, 268f, 269f
Bell's palsy, 243–245, 243f–245f, 245t
    cranial nerve in, 243, 243f, 244f, 245t
    eye care related to, 245
"Bird's beak" appearance, in achalasia, 19f, 21
Bladder, urinary, innervation of, 160f, 161
Blood supply
    to esophagus, 19
    to liver, 81
    to midbrain, 268–269
    to pancreas, 120
    to retina, 258–259
    to sternocleidomastoid muscle, 275
    to vermiform appendix, 77
Blood—air barrier, structural elements of, 44, 44f
Bochdalek hernia, lung hypoplasia due to, 47–50, 49f
Bone fractures, healing of, events accompanying, 216–217

Bone resorption, osteoclasts in, 14–15
Bowman's capsule, 105–106, 105f
Brachial plexus
    anatomical levels of, sensory and motor function of, 199,
        201t
    components of, damage to, 199
    formation of, muscles innervated by ventral primary rami
        contributing to, 199, 202t
    organization of, 199, 200f
Brachial plexus injury, 199–202, 200f, 201t, 202t, 203f
    surgical nerve transfers for, 201–202
Brain, nuclei of, basal ganglia and, 267, 268f, 269f
Brain tissue, necrosis of, pattern of, 287
Breast(s), female
    arterial supply to, 29, 30f
    histologic characteristics of, 32–33, 32f
    internal structure of, 32f
    invasive carcinoma of no special type, 33, 33f
    invasive ductal carcinoma of, 29, 29f
    lymphatic drainage of, 30–31, 30f
    nerve supply of, 31
    venous drainage of, 30
Breast cancer
    chemotherapeutic agent resistance in, MDR-1 and, 35
    clinical staging of, 34, 34t, 35t
    invasive carcinoma of no special type, 33, 33f
    peau d'orange appearance in, 31, 32f
    radiation for, resistance to, 35
    sites of, 31
Bundle(s), 243, 245f

C

CABG. *See* Coronary artery bypass graft (CABG)
Calcaneal (Achilles) tendon
    formation of, muscles in, 169, 169t
    rupture of
        causes of, 169, 170f
        immobilization of lower limb with foot in equinus after,
           169
        site of, 169, 170f
Calf muscles, enlargement of, 178
Canal of Schlemm, 257f, 258
Cancer
    breast. *See* Breast cancer
    prostate. *See* Prostate cancer
Capillary(ies), cardiac, 58–59, 60t, 61t
Cardiac. *See also* Heart
Cardiac tissue, infarcted, morphologic characteristics of, 62t,
    64, 65f
Cardiomyocyte(s), contractile, histologic characteristics of, 64
Carpal tunnel
    boundaries of, structures forming, 205, 206f
    structures transmitted through, 205, 206f
    tendons transmitted through, attachments, innervation, and
        actions of muscles with, 205, 207t
Carpal tunnel syndrome, 205, 206f, 207t, 208f
    neurologic deficits with, 205, 207t
CDH. *See* Congenital diaphragmatic hernia (CDH)
Celiac trunk, occlusion of, stomach effects of, 123
Cell(s). *See specific types*, e.g. Sustentacular cells
    clear of C, 272
    foam, 61
    follicular, characteristics of, 264–265
    nonpyramidal, 285
    oxyphil, cytologic characteristics of, 272
    parafollicular, 272
    principal, cytologic characteristics of, 272
    renin secreted by, 108, 109f

Cell cycle, checkpoints in, 36
Cerebral amyloid angiopathy, 234
CFTR. *See* Cystic fibrosis transmembrane conductance regulator (CFTR)
Chemoreceptor(s)
  arterial, sites of, 41
  peripheral, histologic characteristics of, 41–42
Chemotherapy, for breast cancer, resistance to, 35
Chloride, in sweat, 39, 40f
Chloride ion secretion, in cystic fibrosis, 39, 40f
Cholecystectomy, considerations prior to, arterial variations, 97–98
Cholecystitis, acute calculous, 97–99, 97f, 98f, 100f
Cholinergic neurons, in Alzheimer's disease, degeneration of, 233–234, 234f
Choriocarcinoma, testicular, morphology of, 165, 165f
Chromaffin cells
  cortisol for epinephrine synthesis in, 129–130
  germ layer giving rise to, 129
  sites of, 129, 129f
Chromogranin A, elevation of, pheochromocytoma and, 129
Ciliary body, 257, 257f
Circulatory system, arterial and venous segments of, histologic characteristics of, 58, 60t
Cirrhosis, alcoholic, 81–86, 82f, 83t, 84f, 85f
Cirrhotic liver, healing of, 85f, 86
Clawhand, 227
Clear of C cell, 272
Cleft palate, 247, 248f, 249f
  development of, 247
  posterior, embryologic basis of, 247, 249f
Colitis, ulcerative
  characteristics of, 91t
  Crohn's disease and, morphologic comparison between, 91f
Collagen, type I, synthesis of, steps in, 223
Collateral ligaments, functions of, 181, 183, 183f, 184f
Colon
  arterial supply to, 89
  histologic characteristics of, 89, 90t
  radiologic features of, 89, 90f
Conduction system, cardiac, structural elements of, 62–63
Congenital diaphragmatic hernia (CDH), lung hypoplasia due to, 47–50, 49f
Congenital hypertrophic pyloric stenosis, 87, 87f, 88f
Congenital torticollis, causes of, 275
Connective tissue investments, of nerve, 243, 245f
Contractile cardiomyocytes, histologic characteristics of, 64
Contracture(s), Dupuytren's, 209, 210f
Coronary artery(ies), 55, 56f
  narrowing of, 57
  thrombosing of, 57
  variations in, 55
Coronary artery bypass graft (CABG), blood vessels used in, 57–58
Coronary bypass, internal thoracic artery as conduit for, arterial flow to intercostal spaces maintained when, 58
Coronoid process, fracture of, 211f, 214
Corpuscle(s), renal, histology of, 105–106, 105f
Cortex
  frontal, histologic description of, 285–286
  of lymph node, 34
Corticotroph(s), 251
Cortisol, for epinephrine synthesis, in chromaffin cells, 129–130
Cranial nerve
  in Bell's palsy, 243, 243f, 244f, 245t
  myelination of, 277, 281f
  in neuralgia of congenital torticollis, 277
Creatine kinase, elevation of, causes of, 178

Cricopharyngeus muscle, thyropharyngeous muscle and, transition in fiber orientation between, clinical relevance of, 21
CRITOE, 214, 214t
Crohn's disease, 89, 90f, 90t, 91f, 91t
  characteristics of, 91t
  ulcerative colitis and, morphologic comparison between, 91f
Cruciate ligaments, functions of, 181, 183, 183f, 184f
Cryptochid testis, 137–141, 137f–140f
  morphologic characteristics of, 137
  orchiopexy for, timing of, 137
  site of, 137, 137f
Cubitus valgus, ulnar nerve compression due to, 227, 228f
Cushing's disease, 251–256, 251f, 253f–256f
  pituitary gland in, pathologic characteristics of, 252
  vs. Cushing's syndrome, 252
Cushing's syndrome, *vs.* Cushing's disease, 252
Cutaneous wound healing, after basal cell carcinoma removal, 241, 242f
Cystadenocarcinoma, serous
  of ovary, morphologic characteristics of, 153f, 154
  papillary, of ovary, 153, 153f
Cystic duct, lymphatic drainage of, 99
Cystic fibrosis, 37–40, 38f–40f
  causes of, 37, 40f
  CFTR and, 37, 40f
    chloride ion secretion decrease in, 39, 40f
    lung lobes effects of, 37, 39f
    pancreatic insufficiency and, 37, 40f
Cystic fibrosis transmembrane conductance regulator (CFTR), 37, 40f

D

Death receptor—initiated pathway, 235
Deep plexus, 42
Dentate line, defined, 145, 145f
Desmosome(s), structural elements of, 239
Diabetes mellitus
  type I, pancreatic islets in, morphological characteristics of, 93–94, 93f
  type II, 93–95, 93f, 94f
    development of
      GLUT-2 in, 95
      GLUT-4 in, 95
      insulin receptors in, 95
    pancreatic islets in, morphological characteristics of, 93–94, 93f
Diarthrosis, 221
Digital rectal examination, structures palpated during, 157, 157t
Dihydrotestosterone, in prostate gland development, 158–159
Disc(s)
  herniated, MRI of, 3, 3f
  intervertebral. *See* Intervertebral discs
Dislocation(s)
  of elbow joint. *See* Elbow joint, dislocations of
  of glenohumeral joint, direction of, 224
  hip, sciatic nerve injury due to, 174
  of shoulder joint, nerves vulnerable to injury with, 224
Diverticulum(a)
  in large intestine
    reasons for, 116f, 117
    sites of, 116–117
  Meckel's. *See* Meckel's diverticulum
  in small intestine, sites of, 116–117
  true *vs.* false, 115–116
DOPA decarboxylase, 130
Dopamine
  to norepinephrine, enzymes for conversion of, sites of, 130
  tyrosine to, enzymes for conversion of, sites of, 130

Dopamine beta-hydroxylase, 130
Dorsalis pedis artery, palpability of, 190, 191f
Dorsiflexor muscles, of foot, 174–175, 176t
Double inferior vena cava, development of, 130–132, 131f
Duchenne's muscular dystrophy
    skeletal muscle in, histologic characteristics of, 178, 178f
    winging of scapulae in, causes of, 178–179
Dupuytren's contracture, 209, 210f
Dupuytren's disease, 209, 210f
    digits contracted in, 209
Dyspnea, in achalasia, 21
Dystrophin
    described, 177
    function of, 177, 177f

E

Elastic artery, histologic characteristics of, 60t
Elbow(s)
    posterior dislocation of, 211, 211f
    ulnar nerve relationship to, 228f
Elbow joint, 211–216, 211f–213f, 214t
    arterial supply to, 213
    dislocations of
        classification of, 213
        complications of, 213
        nerves involved in, 213
        radiographs of, assessment of, 214, 214t
    formation of, 211–212, 212f
    ligaments associated with, 211–212, 212f
    nerve supply to, 214
Emphysema, 41–46, 41t, 42t, 43f–45f, 46t
    centriacinar, 45f
        characteristics of, 46t
    distal acinar, characteristics of, 46t
    irregular, characteristics of, 46t
    morphologic changes of lung with, 44, 45f, 46t
    paracinar, characteristics of, 46t
    types of, characteristics of, 46t
Endocardial cushions, development of, 23–27, 23f–26f
Endochondral ossification, stages of, 214
Endoneurium, 243, 245f
Endothelium, monocytes' adherence to, cellular mechanisms in, 62
Epigastrium, referred pain to, anatomical basis of, 126–127
Epinephrine
    norepinephrine to, enzymes for conversion of, sites of, 130
    synthesis of, cortisol for, in chromaffin cells, 129–130
Epineurium, 243, 245f
Epithelium(a)
    of esophagus, 101, 102f, 103f
    gastric, embryonic germ layer and, 127
    germinal, 153, 155f
Esophagus
    Barrett's, metaplasia in, 101
    blood supply to, 19
    characteristics of, histologic, 21–22
    constriction points of, 21, 21f
    innervation of, 20
    layers of, 21–22
    lining of, 101, 102f, 103f
    lymphatic drainage of, 20–21
    morphologic changes in, achalasia due to, 22
    segments of, 21, 21f
    venous drainage of, 20
    vertebral relationships of, 19
Eversion muscles, of foot, 174–175, 176t
Expiration, inferior limits of parietal pleura, visceral pleura, and lungs after, 51, 52f, 53f

Extraocular muscle movements, pituitary gland tumor effects on, 284–285, 286f, 286t
Extremity(ies)
    lower, 167–195. See Lower extremities
    upper, 197–230
Eye(s), Bell's palsy and, 245

F

Facial nerve
    branches of, muscular distribution of, 243, 245t
    structures innervated by, embryologic basis of, 244
Fascicle(s), 243, 245f
Femoral vein, site of, 252–253, 253f
Fiber(s), muscle, skeletal, type 1 vs. type 2, histologic differences, 178, 179t
Fibroblast(s), active, cytologic features of, 223
Fibroid(s), microscopic morphology of, 151, 151f
Fibrosis(es), cystic, 37–40, 38f–40f. See also Cystic fibrosis
Foam cells, 61
Follicular cells, characteristics of, 264–265
Foot
    dorsiflexor muscles of, 174–175, 176t
    eversion muscles of, 174–175, 176t
Foramen cecum, 264
Foramen ovale, 24, 26f
    valve of, 26f, 27
Foramen primum, 24, 25f
Foramen secundum, 24, 26f
Forearm, anterior compartment of, muscles of, 228t
Fosamax, for osteoporosis, 14
Fracture(s)
    acetabulum, 173
    of coronoid process, 211f, 214
    healing of, events accompanying, 216–217
Frontal cortex, histologic description of, 285–286
Frontal lobes, functions of, 285
Fundoplication, described, 101, 103f

G

Gallbladder
    arterial supply to, 97
    cross morphologic characteristics of, 97
    developmemt of, 99, 100f
    innervation of, 99
        referred pain and, 99
    lymphatic drainage of, 99
    perforation of, acute calculous cholecystitis and, 99
    venous drainage of, 98
    wall of, layers of, 99
Gallstone(s), pancreatitis due to, 99
Ganglion(a), basal, brain nuclei and, 267, 268f, 269f
Gastric epithelium, embryonic germ layer and, 127
Gastric glands, 126
Gastric pits, occurrence of, 127
Gastric ulcers, sites of, 125
Gastroesophageal reflux disease (GERD), 101–102, 102f, 103f
Gene mutation, in primary open angle glaucoma, 261
Genicular arteries, 186, 188f
Genitofemoral nerves
    genital branch of
        distribution of, 113t
        injury to, assessment of, 113
    iliohypogastric branch of, distribution of, 113t
    ilioinguinal branch of, distribution of, 113t
GERD. See Gastroesophageal reflux disease (GERD)
Germinal epithelium, 153, 155f

Gland(s)
adrenal, response to excessive level of ACTH, 255, 255f
gastric, 126
parathyroid, 271–273, 271f, 273f. *See also* Parathyroid glands
pituitary, tumor of, ACTH-secreting, 251–256, 251f, 253f–256f. *See also* Cushing's disease
prostate. *See* Prostate gland
suprarenal, on CT imaging, appearance of, 256, 256f
thyroid. *See* Thyroid gland
Glaucoma
angle closure, causes of, 260–261
morphologic changes with, 261, 261f
open angle
causes of, 260–261
primary, 257–261, 257f, 259f, 261f
Glenohumeral joint
dislocations of, direction of, 224
functional and anatomical classifications of, 221–222, 222f
nerves innervating, 223
Glenoid labrum, 221
Glomerular capsule
parietal layer of, 105–106, 105f
visceral layer of, 105–106
Glomerulonephritis, histologic alterations in, 107, 107f, 108f
Glomus cells, 41
Glucose transporters. *See also under* GLUT-2; GLUT-4
GLUT-2, in type II diabetes mellitus development, 95
GLUT-4, in type II diabetes mellitus development, 95
Granulation tissue, described, 240–241, 241f
Grave's disease, 263–266, 263f–265f
cardiac effects of, 265–266
pathologic changes of thyroid gland associated with, 265, 265f
Great saphenous vein, harvesting of, sensory deficits in lower extremity after, 58, 59f
Gubernaculum, 140f, 141
Guyon's canal, 227

H

Hand(s)
median nerve in, distribution of, 208f
ulnar nerve damage effects on, 227
HCl, secretion of, cell type in, 126
Head and neck, 231–287
Heart. *See also under* Cardiac
arterial supply to, 55, 56f
capillaries in, 58–59, 60t, 61t
conduction system of, structural elements of, 62–63
Grave's disease effects on, 265–266
histologic characteristics of, 63–64
innervation of, 57
muscle cells of, histologic characteristics of, 64
tissue of, infarcted, morphologic characteristics of, 62t, 64, 65f
venous drainage of, 57
Hemidesmosome(s), structural elements of, 239
Hepatocystic triangle of Calot, borders of, 97, 98f
Hepatocyte(s)
attributes of, 84
characteristics of, 84
Hernia(s)
Bochdalek, lung hypoplasia due to, 47–50, 49f
congenital diaphragmatic, lung hypoplasia due to, 47–50, 49f
inguinal
direct *vs.* indirect, inguinal triangle landmarks in differentiation of, 111
surgical repair of, nerves vulnerable to injury during, 111, 113, 113f

surgical repair of, anterior approach to, blood vessels to be retracted or ligated during, 113
Herniated disc, MRI of, (s)3, 3f
Herniation(s), of intervertebral discs
direction of, 5
sites of, 3, 4f
Herniation, of stomach through diaphragm, vertebral level of, 50
Hip(s), dislocation of, sciatic nerve injury due to, 174
Hip joint, 171–175, 171f–173f, 174t–176t
arterial supply to, 171f, 173, 173f
ligaments comprising, 171–172, 171f, 172f
muscles across, 173, 174t–176t
nerve supply to, 172
Hirano bodies, 234
Hirschsprung's disease
barium contrast radiograph of, 143, 143f, 144
intestinal segments exhibiting aganglionosis in, 144
pathogenesis of, 144
Homotypical, 286
Hormone(s), thyroid, transport to right atrium, 264
Humerus, midshaft fracture of, neurovascular structures vulnerable to injury in, 215, 215f
Hyalin, 107
alcoholic, 85, 85f
Hydrochloric acid, parietal cell secretion of, timing of, 127
Hyperparathyroidism, radiologic findings with, 273
Hypertension, portal, surgical relief of, 81
Hypophyseal pouch, 283
Hypoplasia, lung, 47–50, 47f–49f, 50t. *See also* Lung hypoplasia

I

Ileum
arterial supply to, 89
histologic characteristics of, 89, 90t
radiologic features of, 89, 90f
Impotence, prostate surgery and, 160f, 161
Incontinence, urinary, prostate surgery and, 160f, 161
Infant(s), premature, survival of, surfactant production and, 50
Infarction(s), watershed, secondary to pituitary gland tumor, 283, 283f
Inferior vena cava, derivative of, 132, 132t
Infrarenal abdominal aorta, histologic characteristics of, 71–73, 73f
Inguinal canal
anterior and posterior walls of, structures forming, 111
development of, 140f, 141
roof and floor of, structures forming, 111
Inguinal hernia
direct *vs.* indirect, inguinal triangle landmarks in differentiation of, 111
surgical repair of, nerves vulnerable to injury during, 111, 113, 113f
Inguinal triangle
boundaries of, structures defining, 111, 112f
landmarks of, in differentiation of direct *vs.* indirect inguinal hernia, 111
Insulin action, regulation on target cells, transporter proteins in, 94, 94f
Insulin receptors, in type II diabetes mellitus development, 95
Insulin secretion, regulation on target cells, transporter proteins in, 94, 94f
Insulinsecreting cells, cellular characteristics of, 93
Internal thoracic artery, as conduit for coronary bypass, arterial flow to intercostal spaces maintained when, 58
Interspinous ligaments, 4
Intertransverse ligaments, 4
Intervertebral discs
formation of, embryological, 7, 8f, 9f

Intervertebral discs (*contd.*)
  herniation of
    direction of, 5
      neurologic examination results of, 5, 6t
      sites of, 4
  histology of, 3–4
  location of, 3, 4f
  secure positioning of, structures involved in, 5, 5f
Intervertebral joints, 3, 4f
Invasive ductal carcinoma, of female breast, 29, 29f

J

Jejunum, radiologic features of, 89, 90f
Joint(s)
  AC. *See* Acromioclavicular (AC) joint
  glenohumeral. *See* Glenohumeral joint
  hip, 171–175, 171f–173f, 174t–176t. *See also* Hip joint
  intervertebral, 3, 4f
  knee. *See* Knee joint
  shoulder. *See* Shoulder joint
  synovial, embryologic formation of, 186, 188

K

Keratinocyte(s), 239
Kidney(s)
  arterial supply to, 105
  filtration apparatus of, structures in, 106–107, 106f
Knee joint
  arterial supply to, 186, 188f
  embryologic formation of, 186, 188
  functional and anatomical classification of, 181
  nerves innervating, 184

L

Lamellar bodies, 50
Large intestine, diverticula in
  reasons for, 116f, 117
  sites of, 116–117
Law of Hilton, 223
LDL. *See* Low-density lipoprotein (LDL)
L-DOPA, for Parkinson's disease, 267–268
Leg(s), compartments of, 193, 193f, 194t
  posterior, muscles of deep division of, 193, 194t
  structures contained in, 193, 193f, 194t
Leiomyoma(s)
  microscopic morphology of, 151, 151f
  uterine, sites of, 150
Lentiform nucleus, 267
LES. *See* Lower esophageal sphincter (LES)
Ligament(s)
  collateral, functions of, 181, 183, 183f, 184f
  cruciate, functions of, 181, 183, 183f, 184f
  of hip joint, 171–172, 171f, 172f
  histologic description of, 222–223, 223f
  interspinous, 4
  intertransverse, 4
  of ovaries, 147–149, 147f–149f
  supraspinous, 4
  of uterine tubes, 147–149, 147f–149f
  of uterus, 147–149, 147f–149f
  in vertebral column, 4
Ligamentum flava, 4
Ligamentum nuchae, 4
Limb(s), lower, 167–195

Liver
  biopsy of, obtaining of, 83
  blood supply to, 81
  cirrhotic, healing of, 85f, 86
  development of, 83
  histologic architectures of, 83–84, 84f
  innervation of, 81–82
  lymphatic drainage of, 82–83
  venous drainage of, 81
Low-density lipoprotein (LDL), in cell, process of uptake, 59–60
Lower esophageal sphincter (LES), 101–102
Lower extremities, 167–195
  muscles of, segmental innervation of, 194, 195t
  sensory deficits in, after harvesting of great saphenous vein, 58, 59f
Lung(s)
  arterial supply to, 42
  development of, 47, 47f, 48f, 49t
  fluid in, reduction of, lung hypoplasia due to, 48–49
  inferior limits of, surface markings after expiration, 51, 52f, 53f
  left, gross anatomical characteristics of, 42, 42t
  lobes of, cystic fibrosis effects on, 37, 39f
  lymphatic drainage of, 42, 43f
  maturation of, periods of, 49t
  morphologic changes of, emphysema and, 44, 45f, 46t
  right, gross anatomical characteristics of, 42, 42t
  venous drainage of, 42
Lung hypoplasia, 47–50, 47f–49f, 50t
  causes of, 47–50, 49f
  conditions associated with, 49–50
  embryonic basis of, 47–50, 49f
  lung fluid reduction and, 48–49
Lymph nodes, of female breast, morphology of, 33–34
Lymphatic drainage
  of cystic duct, 99
  of esophagus, 20–21
  of female breast, 30–31, 30f
  of gallbladder, 99
  of liver, 82–83
  of lungs, 42, 43f
  of ovary, 153
  of pancreas, 120
  of parathyroid glands, 272
  of parietal pleura, 51–52
  of prostate gland, 157
  of rectum, 143
  of stomach, 124, 125f
  of testicle, 163
  of vermiform appendix, 77
  of visceral pleura, 51–52
Lymphedema, of upper extremity, dissection of axillary lymph nodes and, 31

M

M cells, 79
Magnetic resonance imaging (MRI), of herniated disc, 3, 3f
Malignant mesothelioma, 51–53, 52f, 53f
  morphologic characteristics of, 52–53, 53f
Mallory bodies, 85, 85f
Malpighian layer, 239
Mastectomy, nerves vulnerable to injury during, 32
Mastication, muscles of, attachments and actions of, 277, 281t
McBurney's point
  described, 75
  incision of abdominal wall over, to gain access to abdominal cavity, layers involved in, 75, 77f
  site of, 75

MDR-1 (P-glycoprotein), in breast cancer resistance to chemotherapeutic agents, 35
Meckel's diverticulum
  embryologic basis of, 115, 115f
  ulceration of, reasons for, 116, 116f
Median nerve, in hand, distribution of, 208f
Medulla
  adrenal, sympathetic outflow to, spinal cord segments in, 130
  of lymph node, 34
Meningocele, spina bifida with, 8, 10f
Meniscus(i)
  functions of, 181, 183, 183f, 184f
  histological description of, 186
  secured to tibia, means of, 186
Mesothelioma, malignant, 51–53, 52f, 53f
  morphologic characteristics of, 52–53, 53f
Metastasis, mechanisms of, 239–240
Microfold cells, 79
Microvascular decompression surgery, purpose of, 277
Midbrain, blood supply to, 268–269
Mitochondrial pathway, 235
Mitosis, prevention of mutated cell from entering, 36
Monocyte(s), adherence to endothelium, cellular mechanisms in, 62
MRI. *See* Magnetic resonance imaging (MRI)
Muscle(s)
  across hip joint, 173, 174t–176t
  acting across shoulder joint, 221, 222t
  of anterior compartment of forearm, 228t
  calf, enlargement of, 178
  cricopharyngeous, thyropharyngeous muscle and, transition in fiber orientation between, clinical relevance of, 21
  dorsiflexor, of foot, 174–175, 176t
  eversion, of foot, 174–175, 176t
  extraocular, movements of, pituitary gland tumor effects on, 284–285, 286f, 286t
  of lower extremity, segmental innervation of, 194, 195t
  of mastication, attachments and actions of, 277, 281t
  plantaris, 169, 169t
  radial nerve innervation of, 215–216, 216t, 217t
  in rotator cuff muscle group, 219, 219t, 220f
  of scapular region, 219, 220t
  skeletal, in Duchenne's muscular dystrophy, histologic characteristics of, 178, 178f
  sternocleidomastoid. *See* Sternocleidomastoid muscle
  tensor, 258
  tissue investments of, 177
  triceps surae, 169, 169t
Muscle fibers, skeletal, type 1 *vs.* type 2, histologic differences, 178, 179t
Muscle of Brücke, 258
Muscular artery, histologic characteristics of, 60t
Mutation, gene, in primary open angle glaucoma, 261
Myocardial infarction, ventricular fibrillation after, 62–63
Myofibroblast(s), 260

N

Neck, head and, 231–287
Nerve(s)
  connective tissue investments of, 243, 245f
  cranial, in Bell's palsy, 243, 243f, 244f, 245t
  facial
    branches of, muscular distribution of, 243, 245t
    structures innervated by, embryologic basis of, 244
  genitofemoral. *See* Genitofemoral nerves
  in glenohumeral joint innervation, 223
  mastectomy effects on, 32

  median, in hand, distribution of, 208f
  radial, muscles innervated by, 215–216, 216t, 217t
  sciatic, injury of, dislocation of hip and, 174
  trigeminal. *See* Trigeminal nerve
  ulnar. *See* Ulnar nerve
  vagus, in vagal trunk formation, 20
Nerve root compression, with spondylolisthesis of fifth lumbar vertebra, nerve root compression with, 12
Nerve supply
  to AC joint, 225
  to elbow joint, 214
  of female breast, 31
  to hip joint, 172
  to ovary, 153
  to pancreas, 121
  of vermiform appendix, 77–78
Nerve transfers, surgical, for brachial plexus injury, 201–202
Neuron(s)
  axonal transport in, disruption of, in Alzheimer's disease, 236–237
  cholinergic, in Alzheimer's disease, degeneration of, 233–234, 234f
Nonpyramidal cells, 285
Norepinephrine
  dopamine to, enzymes for conversion of, sites of, 130
  to epinephrine, enzymes for conversion of, sites of, 130
Nose, skin on, histologic description of, 238–239, 239f
Nucleus(i)
  brain, basal ganglia and, 267, 268f, 269f
  lentiform, 267

O

Obturator artery, aberrant, 111
Obturator sign, described, 75t
Omeprazole, mechanism of action of, 126
Open angle glaucoma
  causes of, 260–261
  primary, 257–261, 257f, 259f, 261f
Orchiopexy, for cryptochid testis, timing of, 137
Ossification, zones of, 214
Osteoclast(s)
  in bone resorption, 14–15
  characteristics of, 14
Osteoporosis
  alendronate effects on, 15
  kyphosis of vertebral column in, 13–15, 13f
  skeletal elements most severely damaged by, 13
Ovary(ies)
  arterial supply to, 153, 154f
  ligaments attached to, 147–149, 147f–149f
  lymphatic drainage of, 153
  morphology of, 153, 155f
  nerve supply to, 153
  papillary serous cystadenocarcinoma of, 153, 153f
  serous cystadenocarcinoma of, morphologic characteristics of, 153f, 154
  structure of, 155f
  venous drainage of, 153
Oxyphil cell, cytologic characteristics of, 272

P

Pain
  perception of, pathway for, 186, 187f
  referred
    in appendicitis, 78, 78f

Pain (*contd.*)
　　to epigastrium, anatomical basis of, 126–127
　　innervation of gallbladder and, 99
Palate(s), cleft, 247, 248f, 249f
Palmar aponeurosis, thickening of, in Dupuytren's disease, 209, 210f
Pancreas, 119–121, 119f, 120f, 122f
　　anatomical relationships of, 119–120, 120f
　　blood supply to, 120
　　exocrine, histologic appearance of, 121
　　lymphatic drainage of, 120
　　nerve supply to, 121
　　parts of, 119, 119f
　　protection against self digestion by, 121
　　venous drainage of, 120
Pancreatic ducts, sites of, 39–40
Pancreatic insufficiency, cystic fibrosis due to, 37, 40f
Pancreatic islets, in types I and II diabetes mellitus, morphological characteristics of, 93–94, 93f
Pancreatitis
　　chronic, morphologic alterations of, 121, 122f
　　gallstone and, 99
Papillary serous cystadenocarcinoma, of ovary, 153, 153f
Paracortex, of lymph node, 34
Parafollicular cell, 272
Paranasal sinuses
　　described, 37
　　drainage from, 37, 38f, 39f
Parathyroid adenoma, morphology of, 273, 273f
Parathyroid glands, 271–273, 271f, 273f
　　arterial supply to, 271, 271f
　　development of, 272
　　gross anatomical characteristics of, 271, 271f
　　histologic description of, 272
　　innervation of, 272
　　location of, during parathyroidectomy, neurovascular structures in, 271f, 272–273
　　lymphatic drainage of, 272
　　venous drainage of, 271
Parathyroidectomy, parathyroid gland location during, neurovascular structures in, 271f, 272–273
Parietal cells, hydrochloric acid secretion from, timing of, 127
Parietal layer of glomerular capsule, 105–106, 105f
Parietal pleura
　　arterial supply of, 51
　　histologic characteristics of, 51
　　inferior limits of, surface markings after expiration, 51, 52f, 53f
　　innervation of, 52
　　lymphatic drainage of, 51–52
Parkinson's disease, 267–269, 268f, 269f
　　brain damage associated with, 267, 267f
　　L-DOPA for, 267–268
　　pathologic features of, 267, 268f
Pars ciliaris, 258
Pars interarticularis, 11
Peau d'orange, in breast cancer, 31, 32f
Pectinate line, in rectal biopsy, 145
Pelvis, 133–165
Penis, innervation of, 160f, 161
Peptic ulcers, defined, 125
Perception of pain, pathway for, 186, 187f
Perineum, 133–165
Perineurium, 243, 245f
Peripheral chemoreceptors, histologic characteristics of, 41–42
P-glycoprotein (MDR-1), in breast cancer resistance to chemotherapeutic agents, 35

Pheochromocytoma, chromogranin A elevation with, 129
Pituitary gland
　　ACTH-secreting cells in
　　　　histologic description of, 251–252
　　　　sites of, 251–252
　　arterial supply to, 251, 251f
　　in Cushing's disease, pathologic characteristics of, 252
　　embryologic origin of, 283, 284f
　　tumors of
　　　　ACTH-secreting, 251–256, 251f, 253f–256f. *See also* Cushing's disease
　　　　arterial blood flow effects of, 284–285, 286f, 286t
　　　　extraocular muscle movements effects of, 284–285, 286f, 286t
　　　　surgery for, procedure for, 283–284, 285f
　　　　watershed infarction secondary to, 283, 283f
Plantaris muscles, 169, 169t
Pleura
　　parietal. *See* Parietal pleura
　　visceral. *See* Visceral pleura
Pneumocyte(s), type II, cytologic characteristics of, 50
Podocyte(s), 106
Popliteal artery
　　described, 190
　　development of, 189
　　stenosis of, collateral circulation available in, 189–190
Popliteal artery entrapment syndrome, 189–191, 190f, 191f
　　anatomical basis of, 193–194, 193f
　　causes of, 189
　　dorsalis pedis arterial pulse and blood flow velocity effects of, 191
Popliteal fossa
　　boundaries of, 190
　　structures in, 190, 190f
Portal hypertension, surgical relief of, 81
Portosystemic anastomoses
　　distention of, 81, 82f, 83t
　　sites of, 81, 82f, 83t
Positive anterior drawer sign, described, 184
　　clinical significance of, 184
Positive Thompson test, 169
Posterior cleft palate, embryologic basis of, 247, 249f
Posterior compartment syndrome, 193–194, 193f, 194t, 195t
Premature infants, survival of, surfactant production and, 50
Primary open angle glaucoma, 257–261, 257f, 259f, 261f
　　gene mutation in, 261
Principal cell, cytologic characteristics of, 272
Proctodeum, anal canal derived from, *vs.* hindgut-derived anal canal, 145–146
Proenzyme(s), 121
Proprioception, pathway for, 184–186, 185f
Prostate adenocarcinoma, morphology of, 159
Prostate cancer
　　lymphatic spread of, 161
　　metastases of, sites of, 159, 159f, 161
　　rectal invasion of, 161
　　spread of, 159
　　surgery for, complications of, 160f, 161
Prostate gland
　　arterial supply to, 157
　　development of, hormone in, 158–159
　　embryonic derivation of, 158, 158f
　　histologic description of, 157–158, 157f
　　innervation of, 160f, 161
　　lymphatic drainage of, 157
　　venous drainage of, 157
　　zones of, 157, 157f
Prostate serum acid phosphatase (PSAP), 159

Prostate-specific antigen (PSA)
  cytologic origin of, 159
  function of, 159
Protein(s)
  amyloid precursor, in Alzheimer's disease, 235, 236f
  transporter, in regulation of insulin secretion and insulin
    action on target cells, 94, 94f
PSA. *See* Prostate-specific antigen (PSA)
PSAP. *See* Prostate serum acid phosphatase (PSAP)
Pseudocyst(s), defined, 121
Pseudohypertrophy, 178
Psoas sign, described, 75t
Pulmonic sinus, function of, 55
Pyloric antrum, mucosa of, histologic characteristics of, 126
Pyloromyotomy, performance of, 87, 87f, 88f
Pylorus, constriction of, gastric wall layer responsible for, 87

R

Radial nerve, muscles innervated by, 215–216, 216t, 217t
Radiation, for breast cancer, resistance to, 35
Rathke's pouch, 283
Receptor(s), Wnt, 101
Rectum
  anal canal and, 145, 145f
  anterior and posterior relationships of, 145, 145t
  arterial supply to, 143
  biopsy of, site of, 145
  gross and light microscopic characteristics of, 144
  innervation of, 144
  lymphatic drainage of, 143
  venous drainage of, 143
Referred pain
  in appendicitis, 78, 78f
  to epigastrium, anatomical basis of, 126–127
  innervation of gallbladder and, 99
Renal corpuscle, histology of, 105–106, 105f
Renin, cells secreting, 108, 109f
Respiration, accessory muscles of, 41, 41t
Retina
  blood supply to, 258–259
  development of, 260
  layers of, 259–260, 259f
Retrograde transport, 235
RNA(s), small interfering, 35
RNA-induced silencer complex, 35
Rotator cuff muscle group
  muscles in, 219, 219t, 220f
  tendon rupturing in, 219
Rovsings' sign, described, 75t

S

Saphenous vein, great, harvesting of, sensory deficits in lower
    extremity after, 58, 59f
Scapular region, muscles of, 219, 220t
Sciatic nerve, injury of, dislocation of hip and, 174
"Scottie dog," 11, 12f
  collar of, 11
Scrotum, testes descending into, 140f, 141
Seminiferous cords, 138, 139f
Sentinel node biopsy, 31
Septum secundum, 24, 26f
Serous cystadenocarcinoma
  of ovary, morphologic characteristics of, 153f, 154
  papillary, of ovary, 153, 153f
Shoulder joint
  arterial supply to, 224
  capsule of, 222f

dislocation of, nerves vulnerable to injury with, 224
  muscles acting across, 221, 222t
  normal, 221f
Sinus(es)
  aortic, function of, 55
  paranasal
    described, 37
    drainage from, 37, 38f, 39f
  pulmonic, function of, 55
Skeletal muscle, in Duchenne's muscular dystrophy, histologic
    characteristics of, 178, 178f
Skeletal muscle fibers, type 1 *vs.* type 2, histologic differences,
    178, 179t
Skin
  embryologic formation of, 237–238, 238f
  on nose, histologic description of, 238–239, 239f
Small interfering RNAs, 35
Small intestine, diverticula in, sites of, 116–117
Spermatic cord
  coverings of, 164f, 165
  layers of, 164f, 165
Spina bifida
  embryological basis of, 7–8
  types of, 8, 10f
Spina bifida cystica, defined, 8, 10f
Spina bifida occulta, defined, 8
Spina bifida with meningocele, 8, 10f
Spondylolisthesis
  example of, 11
  of fifth lumbar vertebra, nerve root compression with,
    neurological symptoms of, 12
  spondylolysis *vs.*, 11
Spondylolysis, spondylolisthesis *vs.*, 11
Spongiocyte(s), 255
Sternocleidomastoid muscle
  attachments of, 275
  blood supply to, 275
  in congenital torticollis, 275
  innervation to, 275
  lengthening of, 275
  shortening of, 275, 276f
Stomach, 123–127, 123f–125f
  arterial supply to, 123
  celiac trunk occlusion effects on, 123
  development of, 124–125
  herniation of, through diaphragm, vertebral level of, 50
  innervation of, 124, 124f
  lymphatic drainage of, 124, 125f
  venous drainage of, 123–124
  wall of, ulcers perforating through, stomach layers involved
    in, 125–126
Stratum germinativum, 237
Stratum lucidum, 239
Subepicardium, 63
Superficial plexus, 42
Suprarenal arteries, parent vessels of, sites of, 255
Suprarenal gland, on CT imaging, appearance of, 256, 256f
Supraspinous ligament, 4
Surfactant, production of, premature infants survival and, 50
Surgical nerve transfers, for brachial plexus injury, 201–202
Sustentacular cells, 41
Sweat, chloride in, 39, 40f
Synovial joint, embryologic formation of, 186, 188
Synovial membrane, histologic description of, 212–213, 213f

T

Target cells, transporter proteins in regulation of insulin
    secretion and insulin action on, 94, 94f

Tc 99m-pertechnetate scan, purpose of, 115, 115f
TDF. *See* Testis-determining factor (TDF)
Telangiectasis, 240
Tendon(s)
    Achilles. *See* Calcaneal tendon
    calcaneal. *See* Calcaneal tendon
    in rotator cuff muscle group, rupture of, 219
Tensor muscle, 258
Terminal hepatic vein, 84
Testicle(s), 163–165, 164f, 165f
    arterial supply to, 163
    lymphatic drainage of, 163
    venous drainage of, 163
Testicular choriocarcinoma, morphology of, 165, 165f
Testis(es)
    cryptochid, 137–141, 137f–140f. *See also* Cryptochid testis
    descending of, 140f, 141
    development of, 137–138, 138f–140f
    histologic characteristics of, 165
    innervation of, 163, 165
Testis-determining factor (TDF), 137
Tetralogy of Fallot, 67–68, 67f
    cardinal cardiac defects of, 67, 67f
        embryologic basis for, 67
    pulmonary outflow tract obstruction in, site of, 68
    radiographic findings in, 68
Thompson test, positive, 169
Thoracic artery, internal, as conduit for coronary bypass,
    arterial flow to intercostal spaces maintained when, 58
Thorax, 17–63
Thyroglobulin, 264
Thyroid gland
    anatomical characteristics of, 263
    anatomical relationships of, 263
    arterial supply to, 263, 263f
    embryologic formation of, 264
    histologic characteristics of, 264, 264f
    pathologic changes of, Grave's disease and, 265, 265f
Thyroid hormones, transport to right atrium, 264
Thyropharyngeous muscle, cricopharyngeus muscle and,
    transition in fiber orientation between, clinical relevance of, 21
Tinel's sign, 205
Tissue(s)
    brain, necrosis of, pattern of, 287
    cardiac, infarcted, morphologic characteristics of, 62t, 64,
        65f
    granulation, described, 240–241, 241f
Tissue investments, of muscle, 177
Tonofibril(s), 239
Torticollis, congenital, causes of, 275
Trachea, anatomical relationships of, 44, 44f
Tracheobronchial nodes, 42, 43f
Transporter proteins, in regulation of insulin secretion and
    insulin action on target cells, 94, 94f
Transverse rectal folds, 144
Triceps surae muscles, 169, 169t
Trigeminal nerve
    cutaneous distribution of, 279f
    neuralgia of, cranial nerve in, 277
    sensory and motor distributions of, 280t
Tumor(s), pituitary gland. *See* Pituitary gland, tumors of
Tunica adventitia, 72–73, 73f
Tunica albuginea, 138
Tunica intima, 71–72
    smooth muscle cells in subendothelial layer of, significance
        of, 73, 74f
Tunica media, 72, 73f
Tyrosine, to dopamine, enzymes for conversion of, sites of, 130
Tyrosine hydroxylase, 130

U

Ulcer(s)
    gastric, sites of, 125
    peptic, defined, 125
Ulcerative colitis
    characteristics of, 91t
    Crohn's disease and, morphologic comparison between, 91f
Ulnar nerve
    motor distribution of, 227, 228t, 229t
    relationship to elbow, 228f
    sensory distribution of, 227, 230f
    severe damage to, effects on hand, 227
Ulnar nerve compression
    cubitus valgus and, 227, 228f
    sites of, 227
"Unhappy triad," 181, 182f
Upper extremities, 197–230
    dermatomes of, 203f
    lymphedema of, dissection of axillary lymph nodes and, 31
Urinary bladder, innervation of, 160f, 161
Urinary incontinence, prostate surgery and, 160f, 161
Uterine leiomyomas, sites of, 150
Uterine tubes, ligaments attached to, 147–149, 147f–149f
Uterus
    development of, 150, 150f
    innervation of, 150
    ligaments attached to, 147–149, 147f–149f
    removal of, blood vessels divided in, 150

V

Vagal trunk, formation of, 20
Vagus nerves, in vagal trunk formation, 20
Valgus, defined, 227
Valve of the foramen ovale, 26f, 27
Varicocele(s), 163
Vasa vasorum, 73
Vein(s)
    femoral, site of, 252–253, 253f
    great saphenous, harvesting of, sensory deficits in lower
        extremity after, 58, 59f
    histologic characteristics of, 60t
    terminal hepatic, 84
Vena cava
    double inferior, development of, 130–132, 131f
    inferior, derivative of, 132, 132t
Venous drainage
    of esophagus, 20
    of female breast, 30
    of gallbladder, 98
    of heart, 57
    of liver, 81
    of lungs, 42
    of ovary, 153
    of pancreas, 120
    of parathyroid glands, 271
    of prostate gland, 157
    of rectum, 143
    of stomach, 123–124
    of testicle, 163
    of vermiform appendix, 77
Ventral primary rami, muscles innervated by, contributing to
    brachial plexus formation, 199, 202t
Ventricular fibrillation, myocardial infarction and, 62–63
Venule(s), histologic characteristics of, 60t
Vermiform appendix
    blood supply to, 77
    gross morphologic characteristics of, 76, 78f

histologic architecture of, 78–79
lymphatic drainage of, 77
nerve supply of, 77–78
venous drainage of, 77
Vertebra(ae)
classification of, 9f
formation of, embryological, 7, 8f, 9f
ossification of, 9f
Vertebral column
curvatures of, development of, 13
kyphosis of, in osteoporosis, 13–15, 13f
ligaments in, 4
Visceral layer of glomerular capsule, 105–106
Visceral pleura
arterial supply of, 51
histologic characteristics of, 51
inferior limits of, surface markings after expiration, 51, 52f, 53f
innervation of, 52
lymphatic drainage of, 51–52

W

Watershed infarction, secondary to pituitary gland tumor, 283, 283f
Wnt receptors, 101
Wound healing, cutaneous, after basal cell carcinoma removal, 241, 242f